Oh! 505 Homemade Cupcake Recipes

(Oh! 505 Homemade Cupcake Recipes - Volume 1)

Angela Lopez

Copyright: Published in the United States by Angela Lopez/ © ANGELA LOPEZ

Published on October, 12 2020

All rights reserved. No part of this publication may be reproduced, stored in retrieval system, copied in any form or by any means, electronic, mechanical, photocopying, recording or otherwise transmitted without written permission from the publisher. Please do not participate in or encourage piracy of this material in any way. You must not circulate this book in any format. ANGELA LOPEZ does not control or direct users' actions and is not responsible for the information or content shared, harm and/or actions of the book readers.

In accordance with the U.S. Copyright Act of 1976, the scanning, uploading and electronic sharing of any part of this book without the permission of the publisher constitute unlawful piracy and theft of the author's intellectual property. If you would like to use material from the book (other than just simply for reviewing the book), prior permission must be obtained by contacting the author at author@ashkenazirecipes.com

Thank you for your support of the author's rights.

Content

CHAPTER 1: CHOCOLATE CUPCAKE RECIPES 10

1. "Zuccotto" Cupcakes 10
2. 4th Of July Star Cupcakes 11
3. Banana Chocolate Chip Cupcakes With Cream Cheese Frosting 11
4. Bat Cupcakes 12
5. Black Bottom Cupcakes I 12
6. Black Bottom Cupcakes II 13
7. Black Forest Cupcakes 13
8. Brownie Cupcakes 14
9. CINfully Delicious Chocolate Cupcakes ... 15
10. Carlee's Celebrate Spring Cupcakes 15
11. Carrot Cupcakes With White Chocolate Cream Cheese Icing 16
12. Chef John's Red Velvet Cupcakes 17
13. Choco Coco Cupcakes 17
14. Chocolate Beer Cupcakes With Whiskey Filling And Irish Cream Icing 18
15. Chocolate Brownie Cupcake 19
16. Chocolate Chip Cookie Dough + Cupcake = The BEST Cupcake. Ever. 20
17. Chocolate Cornflake Cupcakes 20
18. Chocolate Cupcakes 21
19. Chocolate Cupcakes With Caramel Frosting 21
20. Chocolate Fudge Cupcakes 22
21. Chocolate Hazelnut Cupcakes 22
22. Chocolate Muck Muck Cake 23
23. Chocolate Raspberry Cupcakes 23
24. Chocolate Dipped Strawberry Cupcakes ... 24
25. Chocolate Orange Cupcakes With Pistachio Buttercream 25
26. Chocolate Zucchini Cupcakes 25
27. Christmas Santa Cupcakes 26
28. Christmas Tree Mini Cupcakes 26
29. Cinco De Chili Chocolate Cupcakes With Chili Cream Cheese Frosting 27
30. Coconut Chocolate Chip Cupcakes 28
31. Cream Filled Chocolate Cupcakes 28
32. Cream Filled Cupcakes 29
33. Creamy Chocolate Cupcakes 30
34. Cupcake Graveyard 30
35. Cupcake Surprise 31
36. Dark Chocolate Bacon Cupcakes 31
37. Easter Bird Nest Cupcakes 32
38. Easter Lamb Cupcakes 32
39. Easy Black Bottom Cupcakes 33
40. Easy Chocolate Cupcakes 33
41. Everything Cupcakes 34
42. Flourless Chocolate Cupcakes 34
43. German Chocolate Cupcakes 35
44. Gingerbread Cupcakes With Cream Cheese Frosting 36
45. Gluten Free Chocolate Cupcakes 36
46. Gluten Free Chocolate Chickpea Cupcakes 37
47. Gluten Free Chocolate Whiskey Bacon Cupcakes 37
48. Gluten Free Cocoa Coconut Cupcakes ... 38
49. Gluten Free Dark Chocolate Cupcakes ... 39
50. Gluten Free, Sugar Free Red Velvet Cupcakes With Sugar Free Cream Cheese Frosting 39
51. Grandma Gudgel's Black Bottom Cupcakes 40
52. Halloween Cyclops Cupcakes 41
53. Jama's Fancy Cakes 42
54. Joey's Mini Cupcakes 42
55. Keto Friendly Brownie Cakes 43
56. Lemon Daisy Cupcakes 43
57. Little French Fudge Cakes 44
58. Mexican Chocolate Cupcakes 44
59. Mexican Hot Chocolate Cupcakes (Vegan) 45
60. Mini Egg Cupcakes 46
61. Mini OREO Surprise Cupcakes 47
62. Mini Panda Cupcakes 47
63. Mint Chocolate Cupcakes 48
64. Mint Devil's Food Cupcakes 49
65. Molten Chocolate Cakes With Sugar Coated Raspberries 50
66. Monster Mini Cupcakes 50
67. Peanut Butter Cup Chocolate Cupcakes With Toasted Peanut Butter Meringue Frosting 51
68. Peanut Butter And Chocolate Chip Cupcakes 52
69. Peppermint Cupcakes With Marshmallow Fluff White Chocolate Frosting 53
70. Raspberry White Chocolate Buttercream

Cupcakes 53
71. Red Velvet Cupcakes 54
72. Rice Flour Mexican Chocolate Cupcakes (Gluten Free) 55
73. Salad Dressing Cupcakes 55
74. Self Filled Cupcakes I 56
75. Simple 'N' Delicious Chocolate Cake 56
76. Spider Cupcakes 57
77. Strawberry Chocolate Cream Cheese Cupcakes 57
78. Super Easy Chocolate Cupcakes 58
79. Toasted Marshmallow Cupcakes 58
80. White Chococonut Cupcakes 59
81. White Chocolate Cranberry Poke Cupcakes 59
82. Zucchini Chocolate Chip Cupcakes 60
83. Zucchini Raspberry Cupcakes 60

CHAPTER 2: CHEESECAKE CUPCAKE RECIPES 61

84. Bite Sized Cheesecake Cupcakes 61
85. Brownie Cheesecake Cupcakes 62
86. Cheesecake Cupcakes 62
87. Cheesecake Cups 63
88. Cherry Cheesecake Cupcakes 63
89. Chocolate Chip Cheesecake Cupcakes 64
90. Chocolate Cupcakes With Pumpkin Cheesecake Filling 64
91. Chocolate Peppermint Cheesecake Bites .. 65
92. Decadent Cheesecake Cups 66
93. Maille® Mini Cheesecakes 66
94. Mini Cheesecake Cups With Sour Cream Topping 67
95. Mini Cheesecakes 67
96. Mini Cheesecakes II 68
97. Mini Cheesecakes III 68
98. Mini Cherry Cheesecakes 69
99. Mini Chocolate Hazelnut Cheesecakes 69
100. Mini Pumpkin Cheesecake 70
101. Mini Pumpkin Cheesecakes From Reddi Wip® 70
102. Miniature Cheesecakes 71
103. Morgan's Reduced Fat Cheesecake Cups ..72
104. OREO Mini PHILLY Cheesecakes 72
105. Oreo® Mini Cheesecakes 72
106. Pumpkin Cheesecake Cupcakes 73
107. RITZ New York Style Mini Crumb Cheesecakes 74
108. S'mores Cheesecake Cupcakes 75
109. Samoa® Cheesecake Cupcakes 75
110. Triple Strawberry Cheesecake Cupcakes ...76

CHAPTER 3: LEMON CUPCAKE RECIPES 77

111. Frosted Pink Lemonade Cupcakes 77
112. Gluten Free Lemon Cupcakes 77
113. Lemon Cream Cupcakes 78
114. Lemon Cupcake With Blackberry Buttercream 79
115. Lemon Cupcakes With Lemon Frosting ... 79
116. Lemon PHILLY Cupcakes 80
117. Lemon Pineapple Daisy Bites 80
118. Lemon Cream Cheese Cupcakes 81
119. Lemon Lime Cupcakes 81
120. Mattie's Strawberry Lemonade Cupcakes ..82
121. One Bowl Lemon Cupcakes 82
122. Pink Lemonade Cupcakes 83
123. Raspberry Lemonade Cupcakes 83
124. Too Much Lemon Lemon Meringue Cupcakes 84

CHAPTER 4: BROWNIE CUPCAKE RECIPES 85

125. Brownie Cups 85
126. Brownie Ice Cream Cones 85
127. Brownie Kiss Cupcakes 86
128. Brownie Tarts 86
129. Brownie Turtles 87
130. Brownies In A Cone 87
131. Caramel Blondie Cups 88
132. Cherry Brownie Cups 88
133. Chocolate Cherry Brownie Cups 89
134. Chocolate Hazelnut Brownie Bites 90
135. Coconut Almond Fudge Cups 90
136. Cupcake Brownies 91
137. Frosted Walnut Brownie Cups 91
138. Mint Brownie Cheesecake Cups 92
139. Peanut Butter Brownie 92
140. Peanut Butter Brownie Bites 93
141. Peanut Butter Brownie Cups 94
142. Peppermint Brownie Cups 94

CHAPTER 5: CAKE MIX CUPCAKE RECIPES 95

143. Apple Upside Down Cakes 95
144. Autumn Harvest Cupcakes 95
145. Brownie Batter + Cupcake = The SECOND BEST Cupcake. Ever 96
146. Cake In A Mug 97
147. Classic Red Velvet Cupcakes 97
148. Filled Cupcakes With Cherry Flavored Filled DelightFulls™ 98
149. Frog Cupcakes 98
150. Grad Cupcakes 99
151. Ice Cream Cone Treats 100
152. Maharani Cupcakes 100
153. Margarita Cupcakes 101
154. PHILLY Blackforest Stuffed Cupcakes .. 101
155. Pineapple Upside Down Cupcakes 102
156. Rainbow Cupcake Cones 103
157. SPAM® A Licious Cupcakes With Salted Caramel Frosting 103
158. Sopapilla Cupcakes 104
159. Sushi Cupcakes 105

CHAPTER 6: HOLIDAY CUPCAKE RECIPES 105

160. 4th Of July Cupcakes 105
161. Almond Cupcake With Salted Caramel Buttercream Frosting 106
162. Aloha Cupcakes 107
163. Ann's Chocolate Chip Carrot Cake Pumpkins 107
164. Arnold Palmer Cupcakes 108
165. Autumn Pumpkin Cupcakes 109
166. Black Cat Cupcakes 110
167. Boston Creme Mini Cupcakes 110
168. Candied Holly Cupcakes 111
169. Candied Yam Cupcakes 111
170. Candy Corn Cupcakes 112
171. Candy'D Sweet Potato Cupcakes With Brown Sugar Icing 113
172. Cannoli Cupcakes 114
173. Carrot Cake Cupcakes With Cream Cheese Icing 114
174. Carrot Cake Cupcakes With Lemon Cream Cheese Frosting 115
175. Carrot Pineapple Cupcakes 115
176. Carrot Topped Cupcakes 116
177. Champagne Cupcakes 117
178. Cherry Amish Friendship Bread Cupcakes With Buttercream Frosting 117
179. Cherry Cheese Cupcakes 118
180. Chesscakes 118
181. Chocolate Chai Cupcakes 119
182. Chocolate Gingerbread Cupcakes 119
183. Chocolate And Red Wine Cupcakes 120
184. Christmas Reindeer Cupcakes 121
185. Christmas Tree Cupcakes 122
186. Cinnabon® Cupcakes 122
187. Creepy Halloween Skull Cupcakes 123
188. Cupcake Princess' Vanilla Cupcakes 124
189. Cute Bunny Cupcakes 124
190. Easter Bunny Cupcakes 125
191. Easter Nests 126
192. Easter Surprise Cupcakes 126
193. Easy Eggnog Cupcakes 127
194. Easy Halloween Mummy Cupcakes 128
195. Eggnog Cupcakes 128
196. Eggnog Chai Cupcakes 129
197. Firecracker Cupcakes 129
198. Flower Garden Cupcakes 130
199. Fluffy Pumpkin Spiced Cupcakes 130
200. Fruity Mini Cupcakes 131
201. Gingerbread Cupcakes 131
202. Gluten Free Lovely Lemon Cupcakes 132
203. Grownup Chai Chocolate Cupcakes 133
204. Halloween Chocolate Cupcakes With Monster Peanut Butter Eyes 133
205. Halloween Fondant Ghost Cupcakes 134
206. Halloween Gingerbread Cupcakes 135
207. Harvest Pumpkin Cupcakes 136
208. Hummingbird Cupcakes 136
209. Independence Day Cupcakes 137
210. Jelly Doughnut Cupcakes 138
211. Key Lime Cupcakes 138
212. Lemon Frosted Carrot Cake Cupcakes ... 139
213. Lemon Filled Cupcakes 140
214. Lemon Yogurt Tea Cakes 141
215. Light And Airy Strawberry Cupcakes 141
216. Mascarpone Strawberry Cupcakes 142
217. Mini Christmas Cakes 142
218. Monster Chocolate Cupcakes For Halloween 143
219. Moon Rocks 144
220. Nana's Chocolate Cupcakes With Mint Frosting 144
221. Neapolitan Cupcakes 145

222. Pecan Pie Cupcakes 146
223. Pineapple Upside Down Cupcakes 146
224. Pink Lemonade Cupcakes With Pink Buttercream Frosting 147
225. Pink Peppermint Cupcake 148
226. Pull Apart Spider Web Cupcakes 148
227. Pumpkin Cupcakes With Cream Cheese Frosting 149
228. Pumpkin Ginger Cupcakes 150
229. Pumpkin Pie Cupcakes 150
230. Pumpkin Spice Cupcakes With Cream Cheese Frosting 151
231. Pumpkin Streusel Cupcakes 151
232. REALLY Real Strawberry Cupcakes 152
233. Raspberry Iced Tea Cupcakes 153
234. Real Strawberry Cupcakes 154
235. Santa Hat Cupcakes 154
236. Spiced Spider Cupcakes 155
237. Strawberry Cupcakes 156
238. Strawberry Cupcakes With Lemon Zest Cream Cheese Icing 157
239. Strawberry Chocolate Mini Cupcakes With White Chocolate Ganache 157
240. Sweet Potato Cupcakes With Toasted Marshmallow Frosting 158
241. Sweet Pumpkin Cupcakes With Cream Cheese Frosting 159
242. Sweetheart Cupcakes 160
243. White Chocolate Chip Pumpkin Cupcakes 160
244. Zucchini Cupcakes 161

CHAPTER 7: CUPCAKE RECIPES FOR KIDS 161

245. Baby Rattles 161
246. Banana Chip Mini Cupcakes 162
247. Berry Surprise Cupcakes 163
248. Bunny Carrot Cakes & Cookies 163
249. Bunny Cupcakes 164
250. Buried Surprise Cupcakes 165
251. Butterfly Cupcakes 165
252. Candy Corn Flower Cupcakes 166
253. Caramel Apple Cupcakes 166
254. Chocolate Candy Corn Cupcakes 167
255. Chocolate Caramel Cupcakes 168
256. Chocolate Chip Cupcakes 168
257. Chocolate Cookie Cupcakes 169

258. Chocolate Cupcakes With Marshmallow Cream Filling 169
259. Chocolate Ganache Peanut Butter Cupcakes 170
260. Chocolate Dipped Ice Cream Cone Cupcakes 171
261. Chunky Monkey Cupcakes 172
262. Classic Yellow Cupcakes 172
263. Clown Cupcakes 173
264. Cocoa Banana Cupcakes 173
265. Coconut Orange Cupcakes 174
266. Cookie Cupcakes 175
267. Cream Filled Chocolate Cupcakes 175
268. Cream Filled Cupcakes 176
269. Creepy Crawly Cupcakes 176
270. Cupcake Christmas Tree 177
271. Cupcake Cones 178
272. Cupcakes With Peanut Butter Frosting ... 178
273. Cupcakes With Whipped Cream Frosting 179
274. Curveball Cupcakes 179
275. Devil's Food Cupcakes With Chocolaty Frosting 180
276. Dreamy Orange Cupcakes 180
277. Easter Basket Cupcakes 181
278. Elf Cupcakes 182
279. Fancy Cream Cupcakes 183
280. Frosted Banana Cupcakes 184
281. Fruit Filled Cupcakes 184
282. Fun Party Cupcakes 185
283. Gluten Free Chocolate Cupcakes 185
284. Golden Orange Cupcakes 186
285. Hidden Treasure Cupcakes 186
286. Holiday Gingerbread Cupcakes 187
287. Lady Bug Chocolate Cupcakes 187
288. Lemon Butterfly Cupcakes 188
289. Lemon Cupcakes With Strawberry Frosting 189
290. Lemon Tea Cakes 189
291. Little Holiday Cakes 190
292. Marshmallow Filled Banana Cupcakes 190
293. Mice Cupcakes 191
294. Mini Choco Cupcakes 192
295. Mint Brownie Cupcakes 192
296. Monkey Cupcakes 193
297. Mortarboard Cupcakes 193
298. Out Of This World Cupcakes 194

299. Owl Tree..194
300. Patriotic Cupcake Cones.........................195
301. Patriotic Cupcakes 196
302. Patriotic Ice Cream Cupcakes 197
303. Peanut & Banana Cupcakes 197
304. Peanut Butter & Jelly Cupcakes...............198
305. Peanut Butter Cup Cupcakes 199
306. Peanut Butter Filled Brownie Cupcakes..199
307. Picnic Cupcakes......................................200
308. Pumpkin Caramel Cupcakes 200
309. Pumpkin Cupcakes 201
310. Rainbow Cupcakes..................................201
311. Root Beer Cupcakes 202
312. Rudolph Cupcakes 202
313. Santa Cupcakes.......................................203
314. Slime Filled Cupcakes.............................203
315. St. Patrick's Day Cupcakes 204
316. St. Patrick's Day Pistachio Cupcakes 205
317. Strawberry Muffin Cones........................205
318. Strawberry Surprise Cupcakes.................206
319. Sunshine Cupcakes.................................206
320. Surprise Cupcakes 207
321. Truffle Filled Cupcakes...........................208
322. Wicked Witch Cupcakes 208
323. Wide Eyed Owl Cupcakes 209
324. Witch Cupcakes......................................209
325. Yellow Cupcakes.....................................210

CHAPTER 8: CUPCAKE FROSTING RECIPES 211

326. Apple Spice Cupcakes 211
327. Banana Cupcakes 211
328. Bananas Foster Surprise Cupcakes...........212
329. Baseball Cupcakes...................................213
330. Berry Topped White Cupcakes................213
331. Box Of Chocolates Cupcakes 214
332. Carrot & Raisin Spice Cupcakes...............215
333. Carrot Cake Cupcakes 216
334. Carrot Cupcakes With Cream Cheese Frosting..216
335. Chai Cupcakes 217
336. Cherry Chocolate Coconut Cupcakes......218
337. Cherry Gingerbread Cupcakes.................219
338. Chip Lover's Cupcakes............................219
339. Chocolate Angel Cupcakes With Coconut Cream Frosting..220
340. Chocolate Banana Split Cupcakes 220
341. Chocolate Cream Cheese Cupcakes.........221
342. Chocolate Cream Cupcakes.....................222
343. Chocolate Cupcake Cones.......................222
344. Chocolate Frosted Peanut Butter Cupcakes 223
345. Chocolate Peanut Butter Cupcakes..........223
346. Chocolate Toffee Cupcakes 224
347. Chocolate Glazed Cupcakes.....................225
348. Chocolate Mint Shamrock Cupcakes.......225
349. Cinnamon Cupcakes...............................226
350. Coconut Cupcakes 227
351. Coconut Pecan Cupcakes 227
352. Coconut Filled Chocolate Cupcakes........228
353. Coconut Frosted Chocolate Cupcakes 229
354. Conversation Cupcakes...........................229
355. Cookie Dough Cupcakes With Ganache Frosting..230
356. Cream Filled Banana Cupcakes 231
357. Creepy Cupcakes....................................231
358. Cupcake Easter Baskets 232
359. Elvis Cupcakes 233
360. Famous Chocolate Cupcakes 233
361. Gin & Tonic Cupcakes 234
362. Heavenly Surprise Cupcakes 235
363. Heavenly Surprise Mini Cupcakes...........235
364. Jalapeno Popper Corn Cupcakes..............236
365. Key Lime Pie Cupcakes 237
366. Kitty Cat Cupcakes 237
367. Lemon Coconut Cupcakes 238
368. Lemon Cupcakes....................................239
369. Lemon Curd Cupcakes............................240
370. Maple Carrot Cupcakes...........................241
371. Mocha Cupcakes....................................241
372. Moist Carrot Cupcakes............................242
373. Orange Applesauce Cupcakes..................242
374. Orange Cream Filled Cupcakes 243
375. Orange Date Cupcakes 244
376. Orange Dream Mini Cupcakes................244
377. Pad Thai Cupcakes 245
378. Peanut Butter Chocolate Cupcakes..........246
379. Peanut Butter Cup Chocolate Cupcakes .246
380. Peanut Butter Cupcakes..........................247
381. Peanut Butter Cupcakes With Creamy Chocolate Frosting...................................247
382. Peanut Butter Truffle Cupcakes 248
383. Peanut Filled Devil's Food Cupcakes 249
384. Peppermint Red Velvet Cupcakes............250

385. Pink Velvet Cupcakes.................................250
386. Pumpkin Pecan Bites................................251
387. Pumpkin Spice Cupcakes.........................251
388. Pumpkin Spice Cupcakes With Cream Cheese Frosting..252
389. Raisin Zucchini Spice Cupcakes 253
390. Raspberry Peach Cupcakes......................253
391. Raspberry Swirl Cupcakes 254
392. Red Velvet Cupcakes With Coconut Frosting..255
393. Red Wine And Chocolate Cupcakes........255
394. Rich Chocolate Cupcakes 256
395. Simply Decorated Cupcakes....................257
396. Sour Cream Chocolate Cupcakes 257
397. Special Mocha Cupcakes.........................258
398. Spice Cupcakes..258
399. Spice Cupcakes With Mocha Frosting.....259
400. Spiced Apple Cupcakes...........................260
401. Spiced Carrot Cupcakes 260
402. Spooky Spider Cupcakes.........................261
403. Strawberry Cheesecake Cupcakes...........262
404. Sugar Ghost Cupcakes 262
405. Sugar Plum Fairy Cupcakes 263
406. Surprise Red Cupcakes............................264
407. Sweet Potato Cupcakes...........................265
408. Texas Chocolate Cupcakes......................265
409. Walnut Banana Cupcakes 266

CHAPTER 9: AWESOME CUPCAKE RECIPES 267

410. Apple Banana Cupcakes 267
411. Apple Pie Cupcakes.................................267
412. Apple And Coconut Milk Cupcakes 268
413. Banana Cupcakes With Ganache Frosting 268
414. Banana Nut Cupcakes 269
415. Banana And Vanilla Cupcakes With Buttercream Frosting...270
416. Black Bottom Cupcakes..........................270
417. Black Sesame Cupcakes 271
418. Blueberry Angel Cupcakes......................271
419. Boston Cream Cupcakes.........................272
420. Bride And Groom Cupcakes...................273
421. British Butterfly Cakes 273
422. Brownie Graduation Caps 274
423. Butter Free Peanut Butter Cupcakes........274
424. Butterfly Cakes 275

425. Buttermilk Chocolate Cupcakes 276
426. Cappuccino Cupcakes 276
427. Carrot Blueberry Cupcakes......................277
428. Carrot Cupcakes......................................277
429. Carrot Cupcakes Or Cake With Cream Cheese Frosting..278
430. Cherry Banana Cupcakes........................279
431. Chocolate Cherry Cupcakes 279
432. Chocolate Orange Cupcakes 280
433. Chocolate Raspberry Tea Cakes 280
434. Chocolate Zucchini Cupcakes 281
435. Chocolate Bottom Mini Cupcakes...........281
436. Chocolate Coconut Angel Cupcakes 282
437. Cinnamon Mocha Cupcakes 282
438. Citrus Chocolate Cupcakes 283
439. Cone Cupcakes..284
440. Cookout Brownies 284
441. Cream Cheese Chocolate Cupcakes.........285
442. Cream Cheese Cupcakes 285
443. Cream Cheese Cupcakes With Sour Cream Topping 286
444. Cream Filled Pumpkin Cupcakes 286
445. Creme De Menthe Cupcakes 287
446. Double Chocolate Cupcakes....................288
447. Easy Chocolate Zucchini Cupcakes.........288
448. Easy Strawberry Cupcakes......................289
449. Fluffernutter Cupcakes 289
450. French Toast Cupcakes...........................290
451. Fresh Strawberry Shortcake Cupcakes 291
452. Frost Me Nots 291
453. Gluten Free Banana Cupcakes.................292
454. Gluten Free, Vegan, Banana Chocolate Cupcakes..292
455. Green Tea Cupcakes 293
456. Halfway Healthy Hanukkah Cupcakes 293
457. Hazelnut Truffle Cupcakes......................294
458. Honey Cupcakes With Strawberries........295
459. How To Decorate Soccer Cupcakes........295
460. Irish Cream Cupcakes 296
461. Key Lime Coconut Cupcakes 296
462. Lemon Sparkle Cupcakes........................297
463. Mardi Gras Cupcakes 298
464. Marissa's Gluten Free Strawberry Banana Coconut Cupcakes 298
465. Mini Coconut Cupcakes With Passion Fruit Icing 299
466. Moist Banana Cupcakes 299

467. Mountain Dew® Strawberry Cupcakes...300
468. One Bowl Vanilla Cupcakes For Two.....300
469. Orange Pudding Cakes With Marmalade Drizzle..................301
470. Paleo Jelly Donut Cupcakes 302
471. Perfect Cake Mix Cupcakes.......................302
472. Pineapple Marzipan Cupcakes 303
473. Posy Cupcakes...303
474. Pudding Filled Butterfly Cupcakes...........304
475. Pumpkin Chip Cupcakes 304
476. Raspberry Cup Cakes 305
477. Real Pistachio Cupcakes 305
478. Rosy Rhubarb Cupcakes 306
479. Salted Caramel Cupcakes 306
480. Shoofly Cupcakes.......................................307
481. Shortcake Cupcakes With Berries 308
482. Simple White Cake.....................................308
483. Sour Cream Cupcakes 309
484. Spice Cupcakes With Dates.......................309
485. Spiced Cocoa Cupcakes 310
486. Spiced Cupcakes With Cinnamon Cream Cheese Frosting.......................................310
487. Steamed Rainbow Cupcakes 311
488. Strawberry Champagne Cupcakes............312
489. Strawberry Cupcakes With Strawberry Icing 312
490. Strawberry Shortcake Cupcakes................313
491. Surprise Pumpkin Cupcakes......................313
492. Surprise Inside Cupcakes 314
493. Tres Leches Cupcakes 315
494. Truffle Chocolate Cupcakes......................315
495. Vanilla Cupcakes With Rhubarb Compote 316
496. Vanilla Cupcakes With Vanilla Whipped Cream Frosting.......................................317
497. Vegan Cupcakes 317
498. Vegan Red Velvet Cupcakes 318
499. Winter Fantasy Cupcakes..........................319
500. Winter Fantasy Poinsettia Cupcakes........319
501. Winter Fantasy Snowflake Cupcakes.......320
502. Winter Fantasy Star Cupcakes 320
503. Yazdi Cakes..321
504. Zucchini Chip Cupcakes...........................321
505. Zucchini Cupcakes With Cream Cheese Frosting...322

INDEX **324**

CONCLUSION..**328**

Chapter 1: Chocolate Cupcake Recipes

***

1. "Zuccotto" Cupcakes

Serving: 24 | Prep: 45mins | Cook: 15mins | Ready in:

Ingredients

- For Cupcakes:
- 1 (18.25 ounce) package white cake mix with pudding
- 1/3 cup vegetable oil
- 3 egg whites
- 1 1/4 cups water
- 6 ounces bittersweet chocolate, chopped fine
- For Filling:
- 1 cup cold heavy whipping cream
- 2 tablespoons confectioners' sugar
- 1/2 cup frozen unsweetened raspberries
- 1/4 cup chocolate-coated toffee bits
- 1/2 cup finely chopped toasted hazelnuts, skins removed
- For Ganache:
- 1/2 cup heavy cream
- 6 ounces semisweet chocolate, chopped
- For Frosting:
- 1 (12 ounce) package white chocolate chips
- 1 cup unsalted butter, at room temperature
- 2 (8 ounce) packages cream cheese, softened
- 2 teaspoons vanilla extract
- food coloring, if desired (optional)

Direction

- Heat the oven to 175°C or 350°F. Line 2-dozen cupcake liners on muffin tins.
- In mixing bowl, mix water, egg whites, oil and cake mix. Whip at low speed of an electric mixer for half a minute, then raise speed to moderate and whip, about 2 minutes, scrap down bowl sides. Mix in chopped bittersweet chocolate; spoon batter in cupcake liners, fill them 2/3 full.
- Bake for 15 to 20 minutes in prepped oven till golden in color and tops bounce back once slightly tapped. An inserted toothpick in the middle of one cupcake must exit clean. Take cupcakes out of pans and cool fully on the wire racks.
- Whip a cup of cold whipping cream for a minute on moderately-high speed till cream thickens. Put in confectioners' sugar; whip till firm peaks create. Mix in toffee bits, chopped toasted hazelnuts and frozen raspberries.
- Use paring knife or apple corer to remove the cupcakes' middles, grasp the knife at 45° angle to cut out centers in shape of a funnel. Pipe or spoon filling in cupcakes. Chill cupcakes while preparing ganache.
- In a heat-proof bowl, put pieces of semisweet chocolate. Boil half cup of heavy cream. Add hot cream on chocolate; put on bowl a cover and rest, about 5 minutes. Mix cream and chocolate till thoroughly incorporated; let ganache cool for an hour, till it attains spreading consistency. Smear 1 spoonful of ganache smoothly on every cupcake. Chill cupcakes while preparing the icing.
- Heat white chocolate chips about a minute in a microwavable bowl to melt, mixing after half a minute. Cool white chocolate till nearly at room temperature yet stay fluid. Beat cream cheese and butter together. Mix in vanilla extract, food coloring (optional) and liquified white chocolate. Smear frosting over cupcakes. Serve right away, or chill then serve.

Nutrition Information

- Calories: 487 calories;
- Total Fat: 36.2
- Sodium: 242
- Total Carbohydrate: 37.9

- Cholesterol: 66
- Protein: 5.3

2. 4th Of July Star Cupcakes

Serving: 12 | Prep: 45mins | Cook: 25mins | Ready in:

Ingredients

- 1 (18.25 ounce) package chocolate cake mix
- 1 1/3 cups water
- 1/2 cup vegetable oil
- 3 eggs
- 15 large fresh strawberries
- 2 cups white frosting
- 36 fresh blueberries, rinsed and dried

Direction

- Preheat the oven to 175 ° C or 350 ° F. Line paper liners on a dozen cupcake cups. Grease cupcake pan top to aid take baked cupcakes out.
- In a big mixing bowl, put in eggs, vegetable oil, water and cake mix, and combine on low speed using electric mixer for half a minute to incorporate the ingredients. Raise the speed to moderate, and whip for an additional of 1 minute, scraping down bowl sides from time to time. Fill lined cupcake cups to the brim with batter. Cupcakes will rise and bake above liners, creating round, wide surfaces on top.
- Bake for 25 minutes in prepped oven till an inserted toothpick in the middle of one cupcake gets out clean; monitor 20 minutes after. Cool cupcakes fully in pan. Slowly trace a knife beneath tops of cupcake to separate them from the pan so cupcakes may be taken, however retain them in pan.
- Slice green stem end from every berry, keeping a smooth platform on end. Halve berry, then rotate and cut in half once more crosswise to quarter each berry. To have 60 triangle-shaped pieces of berry in total.
- To decorate, use a sharp paring knife to cut out five shallow triangles in the wide rim of a cupcake top, equally spaced around top to make a star shape. Keep the center of cupcake uncut, and throw cut-out parts. Use white frosting to frost the cupcake, then the shape of a star of the top and keep the cut-out parts not frosted. Put 3 blueberries in the middle of cupcake, and put 5 slices of strawberry around the blueberries, points towards outward and cut sides facing down, into a big star of strawberry. Redo for the rest of the cupcakes.

Nutrition Information

- Calories: 449 calories;
- Total Fat: 23.2
- Sodium: 443
- Total Carbohydrate: 59.3
- Cholesterol: 46
- Protein: 4.3

3. Banana Chocolate Chip Cupcakes With Cream Cheese Frosting

Serving: 12 | Prep: 25mins | Cook: 20mins | Ready in:

Ingredients

- 1 1/4 cups all-purpose flour
- 1/2 teaspoon baking soda
- 1/4 teaspoon baking powder
- 1 pinch salt
- 1/2 cup white sugar
- 6 tablespoons lightly packed brown sugar
- 1/4 cup unsalted butter, softened
- 1 egg
- 2 ripe bananas, mashed
- 1/3 cup buttermilk
- 1/2 cup chocolate chips, or to taste (optional)
- Frosting:
- 1 (3 ounce) package cream cheese, softened

- 3 tablespoons butter, softened
- 1 teaspoon vanilla extract
- 2 cups confectioners' sugar, or more to taste

Direction

- Preheat oven to 175°C or 350°F and use paper liners to line a muffin tin.
- In a bowl, whisk together salt, baking powder, baking soda and flour.
- In another bowl, mix together 1/4 cup butter, brown sugar and white sugar, then use an electric mixer to beat until get a creamy mixture. Beat in egg then combine in mashed bananas. Put in flour mixture in 3 batches, alternating with buttermilk while stirring after each addition. Fold into the batter with chocolate chips.
- Transfer batter into the prepared muffin tin.
- In the preheated oven, bake for 20 minutes, until a toothpick tucked in the center comes out clean. Allow cupcakes to cool for a half hour on a wire rack.
- In a bowl, beat 3 tbsp. butter with cream cheese until smooth. Put in vanilla extract, then beat in confectioners' sugar with 1 cup at a time, until get a smooth frosting.
- Spread frosting over cupcakes.

Nutrition Information

- Calories: 332 calories;
- Total Fat: 12
- Sodium: 134
- Total Carbohydrate: 55.3
- Cholesterol: 41
- Protein: 3.2

4. Bat Cupcakes

Serving: 24 | Prep: 10mins | Cook: 20mins | Ready in:

Ingredients

- 1 (18.25 ounce) package chocolate cake mix
- 1 (16 ounce) container prepared chocolate frosting
- 1 (11.5 ounce) package fudge stripe cookies
- 1 (6 ounce) bag milk chocolate candy kisses, unwrapped
- 1 tablespoon red gel icing

Direction

- Prep cake mix following packaging instructions for cupcakes. Cool down. Use chocolate frosting to frost the cupcakes.
- Break cookies in 1/2, and push 2 halves in top of every cupcake to serve as wings, stripes towards the frosting. Put one chocolate kiss in front of cookies, point toward forward for body. Use red gel icing to create 2 beady little eyes facing to the point of kiss.

Nutrition Information

- Calories: 273 calories;
- Sodium: 272
- Total Carbohydrate: 41
- Cholesterol: 2
- Protein: 2.8
- Total Fat: 11.8

5. Black Bottom Cupcakes I

Serving: 24 | Prep: 30mins | Cook: 30mins | Ready in:

Ingredients

- 1 (8 ounce) package cream cheese, softened
- 1 egg
- 1/3 cup white sugar
- 1/8 teaspoon salt
- 1 cup miniature semisweet chocolate chips
- 1 1/2 cups all-purpose flour
- 1 cup white sugar
- 1/4 cup unsweetened cocoa powder
- 1 teaspoon baking soda

- 1/2 teaspoon salt
- 1 cup water
- 1/3 cup vegetable oil
- 1 tablespoon cider vinegar
- 1 teaspoon vanilla extract

Direction

- Set the oven to 175°C or 350°F to preheat. Use paper cups to line muffin tins or use nonstick cooking spray to spritz them lightly.
- Beat together 1/8 tsp. of salt, 1/3 cup of sugar, egg and cream cheese in a medium bowl until the mixture becomes fluffy and light. Stir in chocolate chips and put aside.
- Combine together 1/2 tsp. of salt, baking soda, cocoa, 1 cup of sugar and flour in a big bowl. Form a well in the center and put in vanilla, vinegar, oil and water. Stir together until well-combined. Fill the batter into muffin tins until 1/3 full and put a dollop of cream cheese mixture on top.
- In the preheated oven, bake about 25-30 minutes.

Nutrition Information

- Calories: 171 calories;
- Total Fat: 8.9
- Sodium: 145
- Total Carbohydrate: 22.4
- Cholesterol: 18
- Protein: 2.3

6. Black Bottom Cupcakes II

Serving: 24 | Prep: 10mins | Cook: 20mins | Ready in:

Ingredients

- 1 1/2 cups all-purpose flour
- 1 teaspoon baking soda
- 1/4 cup unsweetened cocoa powder
- 1/2 teaspoon salt
- 1 cup white sugar
- 1/3 cup vegetable oil
- 1 cup water
- 1 tablespoon vinegar
- 1 teaspoon vanilla extract
- 1 (8 ounce) package cream cheese, softened
- 1 egg
- 1/3 cup white sugar
- 1/8 teaspoon salt
- 1 cup miniature semisweet chocolate chips

Direction

- Set the oven to 350°F or 175°C for preheating. Use paper liners to line the two 12-cup muffin pans. Sift the salt, cocoa powder, flour, and baking soda. Put the mixture aside.
- Beat the oil, water, and a cup of sugar in a large bowl till combined. Mix in the vanilla and vinegar. Whisk in flour mixture until well-incorporated. Put the mixture aside.
- Whisk the cream cheese, salt, egg, and 1/3 cup of sugar in a medium bowl. Mix in the chocolate chips.
- Distribute the chocolate batter among the muffin cups, filling them 1/3 full. Top the batter with a heaping tablespoon of cream cheese mixture. Let them bake inside the preheated oven for 20-25 minutes until their tops spring back when they are pressed lightly.

Nutrition Information

- Calories: 171 calories;
- Cholesterol: 18
- Protein: 2.3
- Total Fat: 8.9
- Sodium: 145
- Total Carbohydrate: 22.4

7. Black Forest Cupcakes

Serving: 24 | Prep: 35mins | Cook: 12mins | Ready in:

Ingredients

- 1 cup butter, softened
- 1 cup white sugar
- 4 eggs
- 1/4 cup milk
- 1 1/4 cups all-purpose flour
- 6 tablespoons unsweetened cocoa powder
- 1 teaspoon baking soda
- Filling:
- 1 (12 ounce) jar black cherry jam
- Topping:
- 1 pint heavy whipping cream
- 2 tablespoons sucralose sweetener (such as Splenda®), or to taste
- 1 teaspoon vanilla extract
- 1 (6 ounce) jar maraschino cherries
- 1/2 cup grated milk chocolate, or to taste

Direction

- Set oven to 190° C (375° F) and start preheating. Line cupcake liners onto 2 muffin tins.
- In a big bowl, beat sugar and butter until fluffy and light. Whisk in eggs, an egg at a time; blend in milk. Add baking soda, cocoa powder, and flour; whisk till batter is smooth.
- Divide batter among prepared muffin tins to fill each liner half-full.
- Put into the preheated oven and bake for 12-15 minutes, or until you insert a toothpick into the center and it comes out clean. Remove to a wire rack, let rest for 25 minutes, or until completely cool.
- Cut off the tops of cooled cupcakes. Take out a little bit of the center of every cupcake and fill in a small dab of black cherry jam. Put back on the cut-off tops, covering the jam.
- In a big bowl, combine vanilla extract, sucralose sweetener and heavy cream; whisk until forming soft peaks. Keep in the fridge until chilled.
- Pour whipped cream into a piping bag fitted with a star or round tip. Frost every cupcake together with a swirl of the whipped cream.
- Put grated chocolate and a maraschino cherry on top of each.

Nutrition Information

- Calories: 275 calories;
- Total Fat: 17.3
- Sodium: 132
- Total Carbohydrate: 29
- Cholesterol: 80
- Protein: 2.9

8. Brownie Cupcakes

Serving: 18 | Prep: 15mins | Cook: 35mins | Ready in:

Ingredients

- 1 cup butter
- 1 cup chocolate chips
- 4 eggs
- 1 1/2 cups white sugar
- 1 cup all-purpose flour
- 1 teaspoon vanilla extract

Direction

- Start preheating the oven to 165°C (325°F). Prepare 18 paper liner-lined cupcake cups.
- In a saucepan, heat chocolate chips and butter over low heat, stirring until smooth; set aside to cool down.
- In a mixing bowl, whisk together sugar and eggs until well blended. Stir in vanilla extract and flour. Pour in chocolate mixture and fold until batter becomes smooth. Fill lined cupcake cups with the batter until about half full.
- In the prepared oven, bake for half an hour until there is no residue left or only moist crumbs when poke a toothpick inside the cupcakes.

Nutrition Information

- Calories: 241 calories;
- Total Carbohydrate: 28
- Cholesterol: 68
- Protein: 2.6
- Total Fat: 14.2
- Sodium: 89

9. CINfully Delicious Chocolate Cupcakes

Serving: 24 | Prep: 20mins | Cook: 15mins | Ready in:

Ingredients

- 1 (18.25 ounce) package chocolate cake mix
- 1 cup milk
- 3 eggs
- 1/2 cup butter, melted
- 1 teaspoon ground cinnamon
- 1 teaspoon vanilla extract
- 1 teaspoon cinnamon sugar, or as needed
- 1/2 cup butter
- 1/2 cup butter-flavored shortening
- 1 pinch sea salt
- 1 teaspoon vanilla extract
- 1 tablespoon ground cinnamon
- 1 tablespoon unsweetened cocoa powder
- 3 cups confectioners' sugar
- 1/4 cup milk
- 2 cups confectioners' sugar, or more as needed

Direction

- Set the oven to 175°C or 350°F to preheat.
- Use paper liners to line 24 muffin cups.
- Use an electric mixer to beat 1 tsp. of vanilla extract, 1 tsp. of cinnamon, 1/2 cup of melted butter, eggs, 1 cup of milk, and chocolate cake mix together in a bowl on low speed until moist. Beat on medium speed about 2 minutes longer.
- Pour batter into each muffin cup until 2/3 full.
- Sprinkle cinnamon sugar over cupcakes.
- In the preheated oven, bake for 15 minutes, until a toothpick exits clean after being inserted into the center.
- Allow to cool in pans about 10 minutes prior to transferring to a wire rack to cool through.
- In a bowl, cream together shortening and 1/2 cup of butter until smooth.
- Stir in 3 cups of confectioners' sugar, cocoa powder, 1 tbsp. of cinnamon, 1 tsp. of vanilla extract and sea salt.
- Stir in milk.
- Combine in 2 additional cups of confectioners' sugar or as necessary until preferred consistency is attained.
- Spread cooled cupcakes with frosting.

Nutrition Information

- Calories: 320 calories;
- Protein: 2.6
- Total Fat: 16.4
- Sodium: 260
- Total Carbohydrate: 43
- Cholesterol: 45

10. Carlee's Celebrate Spring Cupcakes

Serving: 24 | Prep: 30mins | Cook: 20mins | Ready in:

Ingredients

- 1 (18.25 ounce) package chocolate cake mix
- 1 1/4 cups water
- 1/3 cup vegetable oil
- 3 eggs
- 2 (3.9 ounce) packages instant chocolate pudding mix
- 2 cups milk
- 2 cups frozen whipped topping, thawed
- 1 tablespoon chocolate sprinkles
- 72 mini chocolate candy-coated Easter eggs

Direction

- Preheat an oven to 175°C/350°F.
- Grease/use paper liners to line 24 muffin cups.
- Beat eggs, vegetable oil, water and chocolate cake mix with electric mixer at medium speed for 2 minutes till combined thoroughly in a mixing bowl.
- Use batter to fill prepped muffin cups to 2/3 full.
- In preheated oven, bake for 19-23 minutes till inserted toothpick in middle of cupcake exits clean.
- Thoroughly cool cupcakes.
- Beat milk and 2 pudding mix packages using electric mixer for 2 minutes till thick in a bowl.
- To make creamy filling, beat thawed whipped topping into the pudding mixture.
- Put 1 1/2 cup of chocolate pudding filling in pastry bag with big piping tip.
- Press piping tip into middle of each cupcake; use 1 1/2 tbsp. pudding mixture to fill cupcake.
- Put heaping 1 tbsp. leftover pudding mixture 1 1/2-in. across into middle of every cupcake to create a nest. Into edges of nests, press chocolate sprinkles; into each nest, put 3 mini chocolate eggs.

Nutrition Information

- Calories: 211 calories;
- Total Carbohydrate: 28.7
- Cholesterol: 25
- Protein: 3.2
- Total Fat: 10
- Sodium: 329

11. Carrot Cupcakes With White Chocolate Cream Cheese Icing

Serving: 12 | Prep: 30mins | Cook: 25mins | Ready in:

Ingredients

- Cream Cheese Icing:
- 2 ounces white chocolate
- 1 (8 ounce) package cream cheese, softened
- 1/2 cup unsalted butter, softened
- 1 teaspoon vanilla extract
- 1/2 teaspoon orange extract
- 4 cups confectioners' sugar
- 2 tablespoons heavy cream
- Carrot Cake:
- 2 eggs, lightly beaten
- 1 1/8 cups white sugar
- 1/3 cup brown sugar
- 1/2 cup vegetable oil
- 1 teaspoon vanilla extract
- 2 cups shredded carrots
- 1/2 cup crushed pineapple
- 1 1/2 cups all-purpose flour
- 1 1/4 teaspoons baking soda
- 1/2 teaspoon salt
- 1 1/2 teaspoons ground cinnamon
- 1/2 teaspoon ground nutmeg
- 1/4 teaspoon ground ginger
- 1 cup chopped walnuts

Direction

- Preheat an oven to 175°C/350°F then grease 12 muffin cups lightly.
- Melt white chocolate in small saucepan on low heat; mix till smooth. Cool to room temperature.
- Beat butter and cream cheese till smooth in bowl; mix orange extract, 1 tsp. vanilla and white chocolate in. Beat confectioners' sugar in slowly till mixture is fluffy. Mix heavy cream in.
- Beat brown sugar, white sugar and eggs in bowl; mix vanilla and oil in. Fold pineapple and carrots in. Mix ginger, nutmeg, cinnamon, salt, baking soda and flour in another bowl; stir flour mixture into carrot mixture till evenly moist. Fold 1/2 cup walnuts in; put in prepped muffin cups.
- In preheated oven, bake for 25 minutes or till inserted toothpick in middle of muffin exits clean. On wire racks, completely cool; top with icing. Sprinkle leftover walnuts.

Nutrition Information

- Calories: 639 calories;
- Total Fat: 32.2
- Sodium: 317
- Total Carbohydrate: 84.7
- Cholesterol: 76
- Protein: 6

12. Chef John's Red Velvet Cupcakes

Serving: 12 | Prep: 20mins | Cook: 20mins | Ready in:

Ingredients

- Dry ingredients:
- 1 1/3 cups all-purpose flour
- 3 tablespoons unsweetened cocoa powder
- 1/4 teaspoon baking soda
- 1/2 teaspoon salt
- 1 teaspoon baking powder
- Wet ingredients:
- 1/4 cup butter, softened
- 1 cup white sugar
- 2 large eggs
- 3/4 cup buttermilk
- 2 teaspoons white vinegar
- 1 teaspoon vanilla extract
- 1 tablespoon red food coloring

Direction

- Set the oven to 350°F or 175°C for preheating. Use paper liners to line the 12 muffin cups.
- In a large mixing bowl, sift the cocoa, baking powder, salt, flour, and baking soda until blended.
- Combine sugar and butter into a work bowl of a large stand mixer with a whisk attachment fitted into it. Beat the sugar and butter until fluffy and light. Scrape the attachment and bowl down. Add the eggs to the mixture, one at a time and whisking well after each addition. Make sure to scrape the bowl's sides as you work.
- Whisk the vinegar and buttermilk into the moist ingredients. Add the red food coloring and vanilla extract. Whisk the mixture until the color is even.
- Whisk the dry ingredients into the wet ingredients gently using your hands until the batter turns smooth. Pour the batter into the prepared muffin cups, filling them up to 3/4 full.
- Bake them inside the preheated oven for 20-25 minutes until the inserted toothpick into the cupcake's center will come out clean. Allow them to rest in the pan for 10 minutes. Get the cupcakes from the pan and transfer them onto a cooling rack to cool completely prior to serving. Before frosting them, make sure to unwrap the cupcakes.

Nutrition Information

- Calories: 171 calories;
- Total Fat: 5.1
- Sodium: 219
- Total Carbohydrate: 29
- Cholesterol: 42
- Protein: 3.3

13. Choco Coco Cupcakes

Serving: 24 | Prep: 30mins | Cook: 30mins | Ready in:

Ingredients

- 2 1/3 cups all-purpose flour
- 1 1/2 tablespoons all-purpose flour
- 1 1/2 cups white sugar
- 1 1/2 tablespoons white sugar
- 1 teaspoon baking powder
- 1 teaspoon salt
- 1 cup vegetable oil
- 3 eggs, beaten

- 1/3 cup coconut milk
- 1 1/3 cups dried shredded coconut
- 1 teaspoon vanilla extract
- Chocolate Ganache:
- 6 1/4 ounces 85% dark chocolate, chopped
- 1 cup heavy whipping cream

Direction

- Set the oven for preheating to 350°F (175°C). Prepare a muffin tin and line it with paper liners.
- Mix together 1 1/2 cup plus 1 1/2 tablespoon white sugar, 2 1/3 cups plus 1 1/2 tablespoon flour, salt and baking powder in a big bowl.
- Combine eggs, vegetable oil, and coconut milk together in a separate bowl. Pour the mixture over the flour mixture; mix it thoroughly to combine. Add the shredded coconut and fold in with vanilla extract into batter. Scoop the batter into the lined muffin tin 2/3 full for each liner.
- Let it bake inside the oven for roughly 25 minutes until a toothpick poked in the middle comes out clean. Take it out from the oven and place on a wire rack to cool through.
- Put the chopped chocolate in a bowl.
- Pour the cream in a small saucepan and heat over medium heat until for roughly 5 minutes until edges are bubbling. Put the hot cream over chocolate in the bowl. Stir until ganache turns shiny and smooth. Chill in the fridge until set for about an hour.
- Take the ganache out from the fridge. Beat using an electric mixer set on medium speed for about 3 to 5 minutes until the consistency turns fluffy and the color has slightly lightened. Put the ganache in a piping bag with a round tip fitted in.
- Apply the whipped ganache frosting on cooled cupcakes.

Nutrition Information

- Calories: 301 calories;
- Total Fat: 19.9
- Sodium: 133
- Total Carbohydrate: 29
- Cholesterol: 37
- Protein: 3.1

14. Chocolate Beer Cupcakes With Whiskey Filling And Irish Cream Icing

Serving: 24 | Prep: 30mins | Cook: 20mins | Ready in:

Ingredients

- 1 cup Irish stout beer (such as Guinness®)
- 1 cup butter
- 3/4 cup unsweetened cocoa powder
- 2 cups all-purpose flour
- 2 cups white sugar
- 1 1/2 teaspoons baking soda
- 3/4 teaspoon salt
- 2 large eggs
- 2/3 cup sour cream
- 2/3 cup heavy whipping cream
- 8 ounces bittersweet chocolate, chopped
- 2 tablespoons butter
- 1 teaspoon Irish whiskey, or more to taste
- 1/2 cup butter, softened
- 3 cups confectioners' sugar, or more as needed
- 3 tablespoons Irish cream liqueur (such as Baileys®), or more to taste

Direction

- Set oven to 175°C (350°F) for preheating.
- Arrange 24 muffin cups with paper liners.
- In a saucepan, boil a cup of butter and Irish stout beer. Let it stand, stirring regularly, until the butter melts. Put in cocoa powder until it smoothens.
- In a bowl, whisk baking soda, flour, sugar and salt. Mix until well-combined.
- In a large bowl, use an electric mixer on low speed to beat sour cream with eggs. Mix until thoroughly combined. Gradually beat in the

beer mixture and the flour mixture until the batter becomes smooth.
- Distribute batter among the prepared cupcake cups. Fill each cup 2/3 full.
- In the preheated oven, bake the cupcakes for 17 minutes until toothpick shows up clean after inserting in the middle of the cupcake.
- Let the cupcakes cool fully. Using a sharp paring knife, remove the cores from the middle of each cupcake. Put away the cores.
- In a saucepan, simmer the cream over low heat. Mix in bittersweet chocolate until it melts.
- Stir in Irish whiskey and 2 tablespoons of butter until the butter melts. Allow the mixture to cool in room temperature. As it cools, the filling becomes thick.
- Scoop the filling into the cored cupcakes.
- To make frosting, use electric mixer to whip half cup butter in a bowl. Whip for 2 to 3 minutes until fluffy.
- Adjust the mixer to low speed and gradually beat in confectioners' sugar, a cup at a time. Beat until frosting turns spreadable and smooth. Beat in the Irish cream liqueur. Change the thickness of frosting using more confectioners' sugar, if necessary.
- Apply frosting on filled cupcakes.

Nutrition Information

- Calories: 387 calories;
- Sodium: 253
- Total Carbohydrate: 48.8
- Cholesterol: 61
- Protein: 3.3
- Total Fat: 20.3

15. Chocolate Brownie Cupcake

Serving: 48 | Prep: 20mins | Cook: 23mins | Ready in:

Ingredients

- 2 cups butter
- 1 (8 ounce) package semisweet chocolate (such as Baker's®
- 1 (7 ounce) package shredded coconut (such as Baker's® Angel Flake®)
- 8 eggs
- 3 cups white sugar
- 2 cups all-purpose flour
- 1 tablespoon vanilla extract
- 1/2 teaspoon salt
- 2 cups walnuts, or more to taste

Direction

- Set the oven to 350°F or 175°C for preheating. Grease or line 4 muffin tins using the paper liners.
- In a saucepan, mix the chocolate and butter over medium-low heat. Cook and stir the mixture for 5 minutes until melted. Whisk in the coconut.
- Use an electric mixer to whisk the eggs in a bowl. Stir in the vanilla extract, salt, flour, and sugar. Fold the walnuts into the mixture. Mix in the chocolate mixture. Spread the batter into the prepared muffin tins, filling them up to 2/3 full.
- Let them bake inside the preheated oven for 18-20 minutes until the inserted toothpick into the center will come out clean.

Nutrition Information

- Calories: 225 calories;
- Cholesterol: 51
- Protein: 2.9
- Total Fat: 14.8
- Sodium: 101
- Total Carbohydrate: 21.9

16. Chocolate Chip Cookie Dough + Cupcake = The BEST Cupcake. Ever.

Serving: 24 | Prep: 20mins | Cook: 20mins | Ready in:

Ingredients

- 1 1/2 cups all-purpose flour
- 1/4 teaspoon baking soda
- 1/4 teaspoon sea salt
- 1/2 cup butter, softened
- 1/4 cup white sugar
- 1/2 cup brown sugar
- 1 egg
- 2 teaspoons vanilla extract
- 1 cup miniature semisweet chocolate chips
- 1 (18.25 ounce) box yellow cake mix
- 1 1/3 cups water
- 1/3 cup canola oil
- 3 eggs

Direction

- Whisk sea salt, baking soda and flour; put aside. Beat brown sugar, white sugar and butter with electric mixer till smooth in a big bowl. Add vanilla extract and 1 egg; beat till smooth. Mix in flour mixture just till incorporated. Fold in chocolate chips; mix enough just to combine evenly. Shape dough to tablespoon-sized balls; put onto baking sheet. Freeze for 2 hours till solid.
- Preheat oven to 175°C/350°F; use paper liners to line 24 muffin cups.
- Beat 3 eggs to break up with electric mixer in a big bowl. Add canola oil, water and cake mix; beat on medium speed for 2 minutes. Put into prepped cupcake liners; fill each to 2/3 full. Put frozen cookie dough ball over top center of every cupcake.
- In preheated oven, bake for 20 minutes till inserted toothpick in cupcake's cake portion, not cookie dough ball, exits clean; cool for 10 minutes in pans. Transfer onto wire rack; fully cool.

Nutrition Information

- Calories: 256 calories;
- Total Fat: 12.5
- Sodium: 215
- Total Carbohydrate: 34
- Cholesterol: 42
- Protein: 3.2

17. Chocolate Cornflake Cupcakes

Serving: 24 | Prep: 10mins | Cook: 5mins | Ready in:

Ingredients

- 1 cup semisweet chocolate chips
- 1/2 cup butter
- 3 tablespoons maple syrup
- 8 cups cornflakes cereal

Direction

- In a big saucepan, mix together maple syrup, butter and chocolate chips on moderate heat, then cook and stir for 5-7 minutes, until melted. Take away from the heat and allow to cool, about 5-7 minutes.
- Stir into the chocolate mixture with cornflakes until fully covered. Scoop the mixture into 24 cupcake liners, then chill all for a minimum of an hour, until set.

Nutrition Information

- Calories: 109 calories;
- Sodium: 96
- Total Carbohydrate: 14.4
- Cholesterol: 10
- Protein: 1
- Total Fat: 6.1

18. Chocolate Cupcakes

Serving: 16 | Prep: 15mins | Cook: 15mins | Ready in:

Ingredients

- 1 1/3 cups all-purpose flour
- 1/4 teaspoon baking soda
- 2 teaspoons baking powder
- 3/4 cup unsweetened cocoa powder
- 1/8 teaspoon salt
- 3 tablespoons butter, softened
- 1 1/2 cups white sugar
- 2 eggs
- 3/4 teaspoon vanilla extract
- 1 cup milk

Direction

- Set the oven to 3500F (1750C) and preheat. Use foil liners or paper to line a muffin pan. Sift together salt, cocoa, baking soda, baking powder and flour. Put aside.
- Whisk sugar and butter together in a large bowl until fluffy and light. One at a time, beat in the eggs, whisking well after each addition, then mix in the vanilla. Stir in the flour mixture alternately with the milk; beat well. Fill muffin cups 3/4 full.
- Put in the prepared oven and bake for 15 to 17 minutes, or until when put a toothpick into the cake, it comes out clean. When cool, top with your favorite frosting.

Nutrition Information

- Calories: 158 calories;
- Protein: 3.2
- Total Fat: 3.9
- Sodium: 114
- Total Carbohydrate: 29.8
- Cholesterol: 30

19. Chocolate Cupcakes With Caramel Frosting

Serving: 15 | Prep: 20mins | Cook: 20mins | Ready in:

Ingredients

- 1 cup white sugar
- 2 cups all-purpose flour
- 1/4 cup unsweetened cocoa powder
- 2 teaspoons baking soda
- 1 cup water
- 2 tablespoons grape jelly
- 1 cup mayonnaise
- 1 teaspoon vanilla extract
- 1/4 cup butter, melted
- 1/3 cup half-and-half cream
- 3/4 cup packed brown sugar
- 1/2 teaspoon vanilla extract
- 1 3/4 cups confectioners' sugar

Direction

- Set the oven to 175°C or 350°F and use paper baking cups to line 15 muffin cups or grease them all.
- Stir baking soda, cocoa, flour and white sugar together in a big bowl. Make a well in the center of the flour mixture and add 1 tsp. of vanilla, mayonnaise, grape jelly and water. Mix the flour mixture just until blended, then scoop into the prepared cups, distributing evenly.
- In the preheated oven, bake for 20-25 minutes, until the tops spring back when you press them slightly. Allow to cool in the pan placed over a wire rack. Once cooled, place cupcakes on a serving platter.
- While the cupcakes are cooling, make the frosting. In a medium saucepan, mix together brown sugar, half-and-half, and butter. Bring the mixture to a boil while stirring often. Take away from the heat and stir in vanilla and confectioners' sugar. Place pan over a bowl containing ice water, then use an electric mixer to beat or whisk until fluffy. Once cupcakes are cooled thoroughly, frost them.

Nutrition Information

- Calories: 362 calories;
- Total Fat: 15.7
- Sodium: 279
- Total Carbohydrate: 54.7
- Cholesterol: 16
- Protein: 2.3

20. Chocolate Fudge Cupcakes

Serving: 24 | Prep: 30mins | Cook: 30mins | Ready in:

Ingredients

- 4 (1 ounce) squares semisweet chocolate, chopped
- 1 cup butter
- 1 cup all-purpose flour, sifted
- 1 3/4 cups white sugar
- 4 eggs
- 1 teaspoon vanilla extract
- 2 cups chopped pecans

Direction

- Set the oven to 325°F or 165°C for preheating. Use paper liners to line 24 muffin cups. Combine the butter and chocolate on top of the double broiler. Heat the mixture while occasionally stirring it until smooth and melted. Remove it from the heat and let it cool to lukewarm.
- In a large bowl, sift the sugar and flour. Use a mixer to beat in the eggs on low speed, adding the eggs one at a time. Mix in the vanilla, chocolate mixture, and pecans. Fill the muffin cups with 2/3 full of the mixture.
- Bake them inside the preheated oven for 25 minutes (make sure they are not overbaked). Their tops must be shiny yet give in slightly when touched.

Nutrition Information

- Calories: 242 calories;
- Total Fat: 16.6
- Sodium: 66
- Total Carbohydrate: 22.6
- Cholesterol: 51
- Protein: 2.8

21. Chocolate Hazelnut Cupcakes

Serving: 18 | Prep: 25mins | Cook: 15mins | Ready in:

Ingredients

- 2 cups white sugar
- 1 cup all-purpose flour
- 3/4 cup ground toasted hazelnuts
- 3/4 cup unsweetened cocoa powder
- 1 1/2 teaspoons baking powder
- 1 1/2 teaspoons baking soda
- 1 teaspoon salt
- 2 eggs
- 1/2 cup vegetable oil
- 1 cup milk
- 2 teaspoons vanilla extract
- 1/3 cup water
- 2 cups chocolate-hazelnut spread, such as Nutella®
- 1 cup chopped toasted hazelnuts

Direction

- Set the oven to 350°F or 175°C for preheating. Grease the 18 muffin cups or simply line them using the paper baking cups. Mix the flour, cocoa powder, sugar, baking powder, salt, baking soda, and ground hazelnuts; put aside.
- Use an electric mixer to beat the vegetable oil, vanilla extract, milk, and eggs until smooth. Mix in the flour mixture until the mixture has moistened. Mix in the water until the batter turns smooth (it may be a little bit thin). Distribute the mixture among the prepared muffin cups.

- Bake them inside the preheated oven for 15 minutes until the inserted toothpick into the center will come out clean. Let them cool in the pan for 10 minutes. Transfer them from the pan onto a wire rack and let them cool completely. Frost them with the chocolate-hazelnut spread once cool. Garnish them with a dusting of chopped hazelnuts.

Nutrition Information

- Calories: 391 calories;
- Cholesterol: 22
- Protein: 5.8
- Total Fat: 21.2
- Sodium: 316
- Total Carbohydrate: 48.8

22. Chocolate Muck Muck Cake

Serving: 6 | Prep: 20mins | Cook: 7mins | Ready in:

Ingredients

- 7 (1 ounce) squares finely chopped bittersweet chocolate
- 14 tablespoons unsalted butter
- 4 eggs
- 4 egg yolks
- 1 1/2 cups confectioners' sugar
- 3/4 cup all-purpose flour

Direction

- Set the oven to 425°F or 220°C for preheating. Spray the nonstick cooking spray into the six 3-inches muffin cups lightly.
- In a metal bowl, combine the butter with the chopped chocolate. Place the bowl above the saucepan with lightly simmering water. Melt the mixture until even and smooth. Remove it from the heat. Mix in the yolks and eggs using the whisk. Mix in the flour and powdered sugar at last.

- Let it bake inside the preheated oven for accurately 7 minutes. The cake may look like under-baked. Remove it from the oven and serve it right away.

Nutrition Information

- Calories: 682 calories;
- Total Fat: 44.3
- Sodium: 58
- Total Carbohydrate: 62.5
- Cholesterol: 333
- Protein: 10.1

23. Chocolate Raspberry Cupcakes

Serving: 24 | Prep: 40mins | Cook: 18mins | Ready in:

Ingredients

- Reynolds® StayBrite® Baking Cups
- 2 cups all-purpose flour
- 3/4 cup unsweetened cocoa powder
- 1 teaspoon baking soda
- 3/4 teaspoon baking powder
- 1/2 teaspoon salt
- 3/4 cup butter, softened
- 1 1/2 cups granulated sugar
- 3 eggs
- 2 teaspoons vanilla
- 1 1/2 cups milk
- 1/2 cup seedless raspberry preserves
- Fresh raspberries, for garnish
- Raspberry Frosting:
- 1 (8 ounce) package cream cheese, softened
- 1/2 cup butter, softened
- 6 cups powdered sugar
- 1/4 cup seedless raspberry preserves

Direction

- Preheat an oven to 350°F. Line Reynolds® StayBrite® Baking Cups on muffin pans.

- Mix salt, baking powder, baking soda, cocoa powder and flour in a medium bowl. Beat butter using an electric mixer for 30 seconds on medium – high speed in a big mixing bowl. 1/4 cup at 1 time, add sugar slowly, beating at medium speed till combined. Scrape bowl's sides; beat till fluffy and light for 2 minutes. One by one, add eggs; beat well after each. Beat in vanilla. Add milk and flour mixture to butter mixture alternately, beating at low speed after every addition till combined; beat for 20 seconds on medium – high speed.
- Put batter in prepped muffin cups, filling each to 1/2 - 2/3 full. Smooth batter in cups out using the back of the spoon.
- Bake till inserted wooden toothpick in middle exits clean for 18 minutes. Cool cupcakes for 5 minutes in muffin cups on the wire racks. Remove cupcakes from the muffin pans; fully cool on the wire racks.
- To remove cone-shape cupcake piece, use small paring knife, only going down to 1/3-1/2 of way into cupcake. Use 1 tsp. preserves to fill each. Put removed portion of cupcake over then fresh raspberries and raspberry frosting.
- Raspberry frosting: Beat butter and cream cheese with an electric mixer at medium – high speed till fluffy and light in a big mixing bowl. Add powdered sugar slowly, beating till smooth; fold in raspberry preserves gently.

Nutrition Information

- Calories: 377 calories;
- Total Carbohydrate: 61.3
- Cholesterol: 60
- Protein: 3.7
- Total Fat: 14.3
- Sodium: 228

24. Chocolate Dipped Strawberry Cupcakes

Serving: 24 | Prep: 20mins | Cook: 20mins | Ready in:

Ingredients

- Cupcakes:
- 1 (15.25 ounce) package chocolate cake mix
- 1 1/4 cups water
- 3 large eggs
- 1/3 cup vegetable oil
- 6 strawberries, or more to taste, chopped
- Frosting:
- 2/3 cup unsweetened cocoa powder
- 1/2 cup butter, melted
- 3 cups confectioners' sugar
- 1/3 cup milk
- 1 teaspoon vanilla extract

Direction

- Set the oven to 350°F (175°C) for preheating. Grease or line 24 muffin cups with the paper muffin liners.
- In a bowl, whisk the oil, water, cake mix, and eggs using the electric mixer at medium speed until the batter is well-combined. Distribute the batter among the prepared muffin cups. Sprinkle the batter with pieces of strawberry.
- Let them bake inside the preheated oven for 19-22 minutes until the inserted toothpick into the center will come out clean. Let them cool in the pans for 10 minutes. Remove them onto a wire rack and let them cool completely.
- In a bowl, mix the melted butter with the cocoa powder. Beat in confectioners' sugar gradually, adding it alternately with the milk using the electric mixer at medium speed. Add the vanilla extract. Beat the mixture until the frosting turns smooth. Spread the frosting all over the cooled cupcakes.

Nutrition Information

- Calories: 214 calories;
- Total Carbohydrate: 29.9

- Cholesterol: 34
- Protein: 2.5
- Total Fat: 10.7
- Sodium: 187

25. Chocolate Orange Cupcakes With Pistachio Buttercream

Serving: 12 | Prep: 20mins | Cook: 20mins | Ready in:

Ingredients

- 1 teaspoon shortening, or as needed
- 1 teaspoon all-purpose flour, or as needed
- Cake:
- 1 1/2 cups all-purpose flour, sifted
- 1 cup white sugar
- 3 tablespoons cocoa powder
- 1 teaspoon baking soda
- 1/4 teaspoon salt
- 1 cup cold water
- 1/3 cup olive oil
- 2 tablespoons orange juice
- 1/2 teaspoon vanilla extract
- 1 tablespoon grated orange zest
- Icing:
- 1/2 cup unsalted butter
- 2/3 cup confectioners' sugar, sifted
- 2 tablespoons instant pistachio pudding mix
- 2 tablespoons cold water
- 1 ounce dark chocolate, grated

Direction

- Set the oven to 175°C or 350°F. Use a paper towel to coat 12 muffin cups with shortening, then use paper liners to line cups or dust them with 1 tsp. of flour.
- In the bowl of a stand mixer, mix together salt, baking soda, cocoa powder, white sugar and 1 1/2 cups of flour. Beat vanilla extract, orange juice, olive oil and 1 cup of cold water into the mixture of flour on medium-low speed for 2 minutes, or until the batter is just blended.
- Fold orange zest into the batter, then put batter into prepared muffins cups, to within 2/3 full.
- In the preheated oven, bake for 20 minutes, until a toothpick comes out clean after inserting into the center of cupcake. Turn cupcakes to a wire rack and allow them to cool thoroughly for about a half hour.
- Use an electric mixer to beat butter in a bowl in medium speed for one minute, until fluffy. Pour gradually confectioners' sugar into creamed butter and beat for 2 minutes, or until blended. Beat pudding mixture into the mixture of butter until just mixed. Pour in water until getting the desired consistency of icing, one tablespoon at a time. Ice the cooled cupcakes and decorate with grated chocolate.

Nutrition Information

- Calories: 301 calories;
- Sodium: 190
- Total Carbohydrate: 40.4
- Cholesterol: 20
- Protein: 2.1
- Total Fat: 15.2

26. Chocolate Zucchini Cupcakes

Serving: 24 | Prep: | Cook: | Ready in:

Ingredients

- 2 (1 ounce) squares unsweetened chocolate, melted
- 3 eggs
- 1 3/4 cups packed brown sugar
- 1 cup vegetable oil
- 2 cups all-purpose flour
- 1 teaspoon baking powder
- 1 teaspoon baking soda
- 1/2 teaspoon salt
- 2 cups grated zucchini
- 3/4 cup chopped walnuts

- 1 (16 ounce) package chocolate frosting
- 1/2 cup walnut halves

Direction

- Set the oven to 350°F or 175°C for preheating.
- Beat the eggs and sugar in a large bowl for 10 minutes until pale and thickened. Whisk in cooled chocolate and oil.
- Mix the baking soda, flour, salt, and baking powder in a small bowl. Add the flour mixture into the egg mixture and whisk until just blended. Mix in the chopped nuts and zucchini. Spoon the batter into 24 greased or paper-lined muffin cups using the ice-cream scoop, making sure the cups are filled to 2/3 full.
- Let them bake for 20 minutes until the inserted toothpick or fork into the center of the cupcake comes out clean. Allow them to cool in the pans that are set on a rack for 10 minutes. Remove them from the pans and let them cool completely. Spread the chocolate frosting all over the cupcake and garnish them with pecan or walnut halves.

Nutrition Information

- Calories: 316 calories;
- Total Fat: 18.3
- Sodium: 171
- Total Carbohydrate: 37.8
- Cholesterol: 23
- Protein: 3.4

27. Christmas Santa Cupcakes

Serving: 12 | Prep: 20mins | Cook: | Ready in:

Ingredients

- 12 unfrosted cupcakes, cooled
- 1 1/2 cups vanilla frosting
- 1/2 cup red sprinkles
- 1 (6 ounce) package white chocolate chips
- 24 mini chocolate chips
- 12 red candy-coated chocolate pieces (such as M&M's®)
- 1/2 cup coconut flakes

Direction

- Frost a thin layer of vanilla frosting onto each cupcake. Place the red sprinkles in a small bowl. To make a Santa's hat, dredge the lower third of the frosted cupcake into the sugar. Arrange six white chocolate chips into the edges of the red sugar portion, flat-sides up to make a white rim for Santa's hat. For the pom-pom, insert the top with one white chocolate chip.
- For the eyes, arrange two mini chocolate chips into the face of Santa. For the nose, insert the red candy-coated chocolate piece in the Santa's face. Sprinkle the bottom third of the cupcake with coconut flakes to make a beard.

Nutrition Information

- Calories: 390 calories;
- Total Fat: 18.9
- Sodium: 186
- Total Carbohydrate: 52.6
- Cholesterol: 22
- Protein: 3.2

28. Christmas Tree Mini Cupcakes

Serving: 48 | Prep: 30mins | Cook: 8mins | Ready in:

Ingredients

- Cupcakes:
- 1 1/2 cups pastry flour
- 1 cup white sugar
- 1/3 cup cocoa powder
- 1 cup water
- 1/2 cup vegetable oil

- 1 teaspoon vanilla extract
- Toppings:
- 1 cup vanilla frosting, or as desired
- 1 drop green food coloring, or as desired
- 48 small strawberries, hulled
- 1/4 cup round red candies, or as desired
- star-shaped candies

Direction

- Set the oven to 350°F (175°C), and start preheating. Coat mini muffin cups with oil or line with paper liners.
- In a bowl, combine cocoa powder, white sugar and pastry flour together; put in vanilla extract, oil and water; blend until smooth. Spoon the batter into the prepped muffin cups.
- Bake in the prepped oven for 8 - 12 minutes, till a toothpick put in the middle goes out clean. Allow to cool for 5 minutes in the tin.
- In a bowl, combine green food coloring and frosting together till evenly combined. Place frosting to a plastic bag or pipe bag with a snipped corner; place in the fridge for 5 minutes.
- Squeeze a little bit of frosting onto the hulled side of each strawberry; put each onto a cupcake to make the tree shape. Pipe frosting onto every strawberries to make leaves. Arrange candies onto the "tree" as ornaments and add a star-shaped candy atop each "tree" to complete.

Nutrition Information

- Calories: 77 calories;
- Total Fat: 3.2
- Sodium: 9
- Total Carbohydrate: 12.2
- Cholesterol: 0
- Protein: 0.5

29. Cinco De Chili Chocolate Cupcakes With Chili Cream Cheese Frosting

Serving: 24 | Prep: 30mins | Cook: 18mins | Ready in:

Ingredients

- 1 (18.25 ounce) box devil's food chocolate cake mix
- 1 1/2 teaspoons ground ancho chile pepper
- 1/4 teaspoon cayenne pepper
- 1 1/4 cups water
- 1/3 cup vegetable oil
- 3 eggs
- 1 teaspoon ground ancho chile pepper
- 1/8 teaspoon cayenne pepper
- 1/2 teaspoon ground cinnamon
- 4 cups confectioners' sugar, or more as needed
- 1 (8 ounce) package cream cheese, softened
- 1/2 cup butter, softened
- 1/2 teaspoon clear vanilla extract, or to taste
- 24 small dried red chiles

Direction

- Set the oven to 175°C or 350°F and use paper liners to line 24 cupcake cups.
- In a mixing bowl, add whole boxed cake mix and whisk in 1/4 tsp. cayenne pepper and 1 1/2 tsp. ground ancho chile. Beat in eggs, vegetable oil and water for 2 minutes, with an electric mixer on medium speed. Scoop the batter into the prepared cupcake cups until 2/3 full.
- In the preheated oven, bake for 18-22 minutes, until a toothpick comes out clean after inserting into the center of the cupcake. Take them out and let cool thoroughly before frosting.
- Sift confectioners' sugar, cinnamon, 1/8 tsp. cayenne pepper and 1 tsp. ground ancho chile in a bowl. Use an electric mixer on medium speed to beat in butter and cream cheese until the frosting is smooth, then blend in vanilla extract. Spread frosting over the cooled cupcakes in appealing swirls and decorate by

poking a small dried chile into the frosting, stem-side up.

Nutrition Information

- Calories: 273 calories;
- Sodium: 249
- Total Carbohydrate: 36.1
- Cholesterol: 57
- Protein: 3
- Total Fat: 13.5

30. Coconut Chocolate Chip Cupcakes

Serving: 12 | Prep: 15mins | Cook: 20mins | Ready in:

Ingredients

- 3/4 cup gluten-free all purpose baking flour, like Bell® brand
- 1/4 cup coconut flour
- 3/4 teaspoon baking powder
- 1 teaspoon baking soda
- 1/4 teaspoon salt
- 2 tablespoons chia seeds (mixed with water)*
- 2/3 cup water
- 1 1/3 cups So Delicious® Dairy Free Vanilla Coconut Milk
- 1/2 cup coconut oil, warmed to liquefy
- 1/4 cup agave nectar
- 1 teaspoon apple cider vinegar
- 1 teaspoon vanilla extract
- 1/2 cup mini chocolate chips

Direction

- Preheat oven to 350°.
- Sift dry ingredients together, Gf flour through salt; put aside.
- Make chia seed mixture; put aside.
- Mix all leftover liquid ingredients, water to vanilla extract.
- Put wet ingredients in dry ingredients while rapidly mixing; add chocolate chips and chia seed mixture.
- Rest batter for 15 minutes.
- Put cupcake liners in muffin tin.
- Scoop batter in each liner.
- Bake the cupcakes for 15-20 minutes.

Nutrition Information

- Calories: 180 calories;
- Protein: 1.5
- Total Fat: 12.7
- Sodium: 187
- Total Carbohydrate: 17.8
- Cholesterol: 0

31. Cream Filled Chocolate Cupcakes

Serving: 24 | Prep: 40mins | Cook: 20mins | Ready in:

Ingredients

- 2 1/2 cups all-purpose flour
- 2 cups white sugar
- 1/3 cup unsweetened cocoa powder
- 1 teaspoon baking powder
- 1/4 teaspoon salt
- 1 cup vegetable oil
- 1 cup buttermilk
- 2 eggs
- 1 teaspoon vanilla extract
- 2 teaspoons baking soda
- 1 cup hot water
- 2/3 cup shortening
- 1/2 cup white sugar
- 1/3 cup milk
- 1 tablespoon water
- 1 teaspoon vanilla extract
- 1/4 teaspoon salt
- 1/2 cup confectioners' sugar

Direction

- Set the oven to 175°C or 350°F to preheat. Coat 2 12-cup muffin tins with grease.
- In a big bowl, sift together salt, baking powder, cocoa powder, 2 cups of white sugar and flour. Use an electric hand mixer to beat into flour mixture with 1 tsp. of vanilla extract, eggs, buttermilk and vegetable oil on medium speed for 3 minutes until smooth.
- Stir together in a small bowl with hot water and baking soda, and then blend into batter. Transfer batter into muffin cups until 2/3 full.
- In the preheated oven, bake for 20 minutes, until a toothpick exits clean after being inserted into the center of cupcake. Allow to cool in pans for about 10 minutes prior to transferring to a wire rack to cool thoroughly.
- In a bowl, use an electric hand mixer to beat together salt, 1 tsp. of vanilla extract, 1 tbsp. of water, milk, 1/2 cup of white sugar and shortening for 5-7 minutes. Put in confectioners' sugar, and then beat for 3-5 minutes until blended thoroughly.
- Use a pastry tube fitted with a rosette tip to insert into cupcakes with frosting, and then use leftover frosting to frost cupcakes' tops.

Nutrition Information

- Calories: 284 calories;
- Total Fat: 15.6
- Sodium: 192
- Total Carbohydrate: 34.8
- Cholesterol: 16
- Protein: 2.6

32. Cream Filled Cupcakes

Serving: 36 | Prep: 15mins | Cook: 20mins | Ready in:

Ingredients

- 3 cups all-purpose flour
- 2 cups white sugar
- 1/3 cup unsweetened cocoa powder
- 2 teaspoons baking soda
- 1 teaspoon salt
- 2 eggs
- 1 cup milk
- 1 cup water
- 1 cup vegetable oil
- 1 teaspoon vanilla extract
- 1/4 cup butter
- 1/4 cup shortening
- 2 cups confectioners' sugar
- 1 pinch salt
- 3 tablespoons milk
- 1 teaspoon vanilla extract

Direction

- Preheat oven to 190°C/375°F. Line paper liners in 36 muffin cups.
- Mix 1 teaspoon of salt, baking soda, cocoa, sugar, and flour in a large bowl. Push some of the powder mixture to the sides of the bowl to make a well in the center, pour 1 teaspoon of vanilla, oil, water, 1 cup of milk, and eggs into the well. Mix thoroughly. Pour batter into each muffin cup, filling halfway full.
- Bake until a toothpick pierced down the center of the cake comes out clean with no batter on it, or around 15 to 20 minutes. Let cakes cool.
- For the filling, beat shortening and butter together in a large bowl until smooth. Blend in a pinch of salt and confectioners' sugar, then beat 1 teaspoon of vanilla and 3 tablespoons of milk gradually until fluffy and light. Transfer the filling into a pastry bag with a small tip. In the bottom of paper liner, push the tip through to fill each cupcake.

Nutrition Information

- Calories: 196 calories;
- Total Fat: 9.4
- Sodium: 151
- Total Carbohydrate: 26.9
- Cholesterol: 14

- Protein: 1.9

33. Creamy Chocolate Cupcakes

Serving: 18 | Prep: 20mins | Cook: 25mins | Ready in:

Ingredients

- 1 1/2 cups all-purpose flour
- 1 cup white sugar
- 1/4 cup unsweetened cocoa powder
- 1 teaspoon baking soda
- 1/2 teaspoon salt
- 2 eggs, beaten
- 3/4 cup water
- 1/2 cup vegetable oil
- 1 tablespoon apple cider vinegar
- 1 teaspoon Mexican vanilla extract
- 1 (8 ounce) package cream cheese, softened
- 1/3 cup white sugar
- 1/8 teaspoon salt
- 1 cup semisweet chocolate chips
- 1 cup chopped walnuts

Direction

- Turn the oven to 350°F (175°C) to preheat. Use paper cupcake liners to line 18 muffin cups.
- In a big mixing bowl, combine 1/2 teaspoon salt, baking soda, cocoa powder, 1 cup sugar, and flour. Add vanilla extract, vinegar, vegetable oil, water, and eggs; stir thoroughly. Add the batter to the prepared muffin cups.
- In another bowl, use an electric hand mixer to whisk together 1/8 teaspoon salt, 1/3 cup sugar, and cream cheese until the sugar has completely blended into the cream cheese. Fold the cheese mixture with chocolate chips. Drop into the middle of each cupcake by tablespoonfuls, sprinkle walnuts over.
- Put in the preheated oven and bake for 25-30 minutes until a toothpick will come out clean when you insert it into the middle. Leave in the pans to cool for 10 minutes, and then transfer to a wire rack to fully cool.

Nutrition Information

- Calories: 291 calories;
- Total Fat: 18.3
- Sodium: 197
- Total Carbohydrate: 30.6
- Cholesterol: 34
- Protein: 4.3

34. Cupcake Graveyard

Serving: 24 | Prep: 30mins | Cook: 25mins | Ready in:

Ingredients

- 1 (18.25 ounce) package chocolate cake mix
- 2 (16 ounce) packages vanilla frosting
- 3/4 cup chocolate sandwich cookie crumbs
- 24 chocolate covered graham cracker cookies

Direction

- Prep and bake cake mix following packaging instructions for cupcakes.
- Mix cookie crumbs and a pack of frosting in medium size bowl. Frost the cupcakes that has been cooled.
- Put the rest of white frosting into pastry bag, equipped with plain tip. On every graham cracker cookie covered in chocolate, write R.I.P. On top of each cupcake, stand one decorated cookie, making it looks like tombstone. Put cupcakes on a green paper-lined-big cookie sheet. Put the paper bats and ghosts anywhere through the graveyard. Serve.

Nutrition Information

- Calories: 312 calories;
- Sodium: 284
- Total Carbohydrate: 49.3
- Cholesterol: 0

- Protein: 1.7
- Total Fat: 12.4

- Total Carbohydrate: 25.3
- Cholesterol: 19
- Protein: 2.9
- Total Fat: 10.3

35. Cupcake Surprise

Serving: 24 | Prep: 15mins | Cook: 30mins | Ready in:

Ingredients

- 1 (8 ounce) package cream cheese
- 1/4 cup confectioners' sugar
- 1 egg
- 1 (6 ounce) package chocolate chips
- 1 (18.25 ounce) package chocolate cake mix
- 4 maraschino cherries
- 4 milk chocolate candy kisses
- 4 walnut halves
- 1 (1.4 ounce) bar chocolate covered toffee bars, chopped
- 1/8 cup raisins
- 1/4 cup candy coated peanut butter pieces

Direction

- Preheat the oven to 175°C or 350°F. Line paper liners on 2 dozen muffin cups. Combine sugar, egg and cream cheese in medium size bowl till thoroughly incorporated. Mix chocolate chips in. Put aside.
- Prep cake mix following packaging directions. Fill every cup mid-full. Drop cream cheese mix by heaping teaspoonful in the middle of every cupcake. Force some raisins or pieces of peanut putter, toffee piece, walnut half and a cherry or chocolate kiss into the middle of every cupcake.
- Bake for 25 minutes to half an hour in prepped oven, or till an inserted toothpick in the middle of cake gets out clean. Cool.

Nutrition Information

- Calories: 194 calories;
- Sodium: 218

36. Dark Chocolate Bacon Cupcakes

Serving: 24 | Prep: 15mins | Cook: 25mins | Ready in:

Ingredients

- 12 slices bacon
- 2 cups all-purpose flour
- 3/4 cup unsweetened cocoa powder
- 2 cups white sugar
- 2 teaspoons baking soda
- 1 teaspoon baking powder
- 1/2 teaspoon sea salt
- 2 eggs
- 1 cup cold, strong, brewed coffee
- 1 cup buttermilk
- 1/2 cup vegetable oil
- 1 tablespoon unsweetened cocoa powder, for dusting

Direction

- Set the oven at 375°F (190°c) and start preheating. Place a large, deep skillet over medium-high heat and cook bacon till evenly brown. Drain; crumble; set aside.
- In a large bowl, combine salt, baking powder, baking soda, sugar, 3/4 cup of cocoa powder and flour. In the center, form a well; put in oil, buttermilk, coffee and eggs. Combine just till blended. Stir in 3/4 of the bacon; set aside the rest for garnish. Using a spoon, transfer the batter to the prepared cups, distributing evenly.
- Bake for 20-25 minutes in the preheated oven, till the tops spring back when pressed lightly. Allow to cool in the pan on a wire rack. Once cool, arrange the cupcakes on a serving platter. Use your favorite chocolate frosting to frost;

sprinkle the top with the reserved bacon crumbles. Dust with more cocoa powder.

Nutrition Information

- Calories: 185 calories;
- Total Fat: 7.5
- Sodium: 285
- Total Carbohydrate: 26.8
- Cholesterol: 21
- Protein: 4.2

37. Easter Bird Nest Cupcakes

Serving: 18 | Prep: 30mins | Cook: 10mins | Ready in:

Ingredients

- 1 cup self-rising flour
- 2 tablespoons self-rising flour
- 1/2 cup unsalted butter, at room temperature
- 7 tablespoons white sugar
- 2 eggs
- 2 tablespoons cocoa powder
- Chocolate Buttercream:
- 3/4 cup unsalted butter, softened
- 1 1/2 cups cocoa powder
- 5 cups confectioners' sugar, or more as needed
- 1/2 cup milk
- 2 tablespoons milk, or more as needed
- 1 drop vanilla extract
- Decoration:
- 3 tablespoons chocolate sprinkles, or as needed
- 58 mini chocolate candy-coated Easter eggs

Direction

- Set the oven to 375°F (190°C) for preheating. Use paper liners to line the 18 muffin cups or you can also grease the muffin cups.
- In a bowl, beat a half cup of butter, a cup plus 2 tbsp. of flour, eggs, 2 tbsp. of cocoa powder, and sugar using the electric blender until the batter is well-combined.
- Distribute the batter among the prepared muffin cups, filling them up to 3/4 full.
- Bake them inside the preheated oven for 10-12 minutes until their tops spring back when pressed lightly. Let them cool in the tins for 5 minutes. Place them onto a wire rack and let them cool totally for 20 minutes.
- In the meantime, prepare the buttercream. In a bowl, beat 3/4 cup of butter using the electric blender until fluffy and light. Alternately add the confectioner's sugar and 1 1/2 cups of cocoa powder with 1/2 cup plus 2 tbsp. of milk. Add the vanilla extract and beat the frosting until it reaches into a spreading consistency. If necessary, add more milk or confectioners' sugar.
- Pour the chocolate buttercream into a piping bag with a star tip. Pipe a round nest of frosting onto each cupcake. Sprinkle each nest with the chocolate sprinkles. Arrange 3 mini chocolate eggs into each of the nests.

Nutrition Information

- Calories: 346 calories;
- Total Fat: 15.8
- Sodium: 116
- Total Carbohydrate: 52.3
- Cholesterol: 55
- Protein: 3.6

38. Easter Lamb Cupcakes

Serving: 12 | Prep: 30mins | Cook: | Ready in:

Ingredients

- 12 unfrosted cupcakes, cooled
- 1 (16 ounce) package prepared vanilla frosting
- Lambs:
- 6 large marshmallows, halved lengthwise
- 5 black licorice laces

- 1 (10.5 ounce) package miniature marshmallows
- 24 candy eyeballs

Direction

- With a palette knife or spatula, frost each cupcake with an even layer of frosting.
- In the top end of each marshmallow half, poke 2 holes, using a skewer to make ears. At the bottom of the front side, poke 2 holes to make nostrils.
- Cut the black licorice laces into short lengths: 36 1/3-inch lengths for the tails and ears and 24 small pieces for the nostrils. Stick the shorter licorice pieces into the marshmallows where there are holes for the nostrils. Stick 24 of the longer pieces into the marshmallows where there are holes for the ears. Attach a marshmallow head to each cupcake.
- Use mini marshmallows to cover cupcakes; stick them to the frosting flat-side down. On the opposite side of the head, leave space to attach the tail. Use a skewer to poke a hole there; stick in the rest of licorice pieces to make the tails.
- With a bit of frosting, spread the backs of 2 candy eyeballs. Attach to the marshmallow; position above the nose. Do the same with the rest of eyeballs.

Nutrition Information

- Calories: 400 calories;
- Total Carbohydrate: 70.7
- Cholesterol: 18
- Protein: 2.4
- Total Fat: 12.1
- Sodium: 223

39. Easy Black Bottom Cupcakes

Serving: 24 | Prep: | Cook: | Ready in:

Ingredients

- 1 (18.25 ounce) package devil's food cake mix
- 1 (8 ounce) package cream cheese
- 1 cup white sugar
- 1 cup semisweet chocolate chips

Direction

- Follow package directions to preheat oven. Line paper liners on muffin pans. Follow box directions to prep cake mix. Mix sugar and softened cream cheese till smooth in another bowl; fold in chocolate chips.
- Use chocolate cake mix to fill cupcake papers to 1/3 full; put cream cheese mixture over. Follow box instructions to bake till cream cheese just begins to be light golden color.

Nutrition Information

- Calories: 192 calories;
- Total Fat: 8.3
- Sodium: 187
- Total Carbohydrate: 28.1
- Cholesterol: 15
- Protein: 2.7

40. Easy Chocolate Cupcakes

Serving: 16 | Prep: 10mins | Cook: 20mins | Ready in:

Ingredients

- 10 tablespoons butter
- 1 1/4 cups white sugar
- 4 eggs
- 1/4 teaspoon almond extract
- 1 teaspoon vanilla extract
- 1 1/2 cups all-purpose flour
- 3/4 cup unsweetened cocoa powder
- 2 teaspoons baking powder
- 1/4 teaspoon salt
- 3/4 cup milk

Direction

- Turn oven to 350°F (175°C) to preheat. Butter 2 muffin pans or line them with 20 paper baking cups.
- Beat butter with sugar in a medium bowl using an electric mixer until fluffy and light. Stir in vanilla, almond extract, and eggs. Mix together salt, baking powder, cocoa, and flour; stir alternately with milk into the batter just until incorporated. Fill batter equally into the prepared cups.
- Bake for 20 to 25 minutes in the preheated oven until tops are springy when slightly pressed. Allow cupcakes to cool in the pan on a wire rack. Once cooled, place cupcakes on a serving platter, and top with frosting of your choice.

Nutrition Information

- Calories: 201 calories;
- Sodium: 172
- Total Carbohydrate: 27.6
- Cholesterol: 66
- Protein: 4
- Total Fat: 9.3

41. Everything Cupcakes

Serving: 24 | Prep: 20mins | Cook: 15mins | Ready in:

Ingredients

- 1 (18.25 ounce) package white cake mix (such as Duncan Hines®)
- 1 1/3 cups water
- 1/3 cup canola oil
- 3 large egg whites
- 1 cup miniature marshmallows
- 3/4 cup butterscotch chips
- 1/2 cup chocolate-coated toffee bits
- 1/2 cup miniature chocolate chips
- 1/3 cup sweetened flaked coconut
- 1 1/2 cups creamy peanut butter

Direction

- Set the oven to 350°F or 175°C for preheating.
- Use paper liners to line the 24 muffin cups.
- In a large bowl, beat the water, egg whites, canola oil, and cake mix using an electric mixer at low speed until the mixture has moistened. Adjust the speed of the electric mixer to medium and beat the mixture for 2 minutes longer.
- Fold into cake batter the butterscotch chips, chocolate chips, flaked coconut, marshmallows, and chocolate-covered toffee.
- Distribute batter among the prepared muffin cups, filling the cups 2/3-3/4 full.
- Bake them inside the preheated oven for 15-25 minutes until the cupcakes are set and turn golden brown.
- Allow them to cool in pans for 10 minutes. Transfer them on a wire rack to cool completely.
- Put the peanut butter into the pastry bag with a star tip fitted in it.
- Insert the star tip into each cupcake's center gently. Squeeze in a small amount of peanut butter into each cupcake.

Nutrition Information

- Calories: 303 calories;
- Sodium: 259
- Total Carbohydrate: 30.6
- Cholesterol: 4
- Protein: 5.6
- Total Fat: 18.3

42. Flourless Chocolate Cupcakes

Serving: 12 | Prep: 15mins | Cook: 18mins | Ready in:

Ingredients

- 2 cups rolled oats
- 1/2 cup unsweetened cocoa powder
- 6 tablespoons peanuts
- 1 cup coffee
- 3 eggs
- 1 1/2 banana
- 1/4 cup honey
- 1/4 cup maple syrup
- 1 1/2 teaspoons vanilla extract
- 1 teaspoon baking soda
- 1 teaspoon baking powder

Direction

- Turn on the oven to 375°F (190°C) to preheat. Use cupcake liners to line or grease 12 muffin cups.
- In a blender, add peanuts, cocoa powder and oats; process until well-mixed. Transfer into a large bowl.
- In the blender, mix together vanilla extract, maple syrup, honey, banana, eggs and coffee; puree until smooth. Transfer onto oat mixture and whisk to incorporate the batter. Stir in baking powder and baking soda until just combined.
- Scoop batter into prepped muffin cups.
- Put into the preheated oven to bake for 18-20 minutes until a toothpick comes out clean when inserted into the center.

Nutrition Information

- Calories: 155 calories;
- Total Fat: 4.8
- Sodium: 200
- Total Carbohydrate: 25.8
- Cholesterol: 46
- Protein: 5.2

43. German Chocolate Cupcakes

Serving: 12 | Prep: 25mins | Cook: 25mins | Ready in:

Ingredients

- Reynolds® Cut Rite® Wax Paper
- Chocolate-Pecan Ice Cream "Frosting":
- 1/2 gallon chocolate ice cream
- 3/4 cup toasted pecan pieces, or as needed
- Cupcakes:
- 1 cup all-purpose flour
- 1/2 teaspoon baking soda
- 1/4 teaspoon salt
- 2 (1 ounce) squares sweet baking chocolate
- 1/4 cup water
- 1/2 cup butter, softened
- 1/2 cup sugar
- 2 eggs
- 1/2 teaspoon vanilla
- 1/2 cup buttermilk or sour milk
- Caramel ice cream topping
- 2/3 cup toasted shaved coconut*

Direction

- Chocolate-Pecan Ice Cream: Use Reynolds(R) Cut Rite(R) Wax Paper to line a cookie sheet; set aside. Slice chocolate ice cream into sheets, around 2 in. thick. Cut rounds with a cookie cutter, just larger than the cupcakes from frozen ice cream. Arrange on the prepared sheet. Press toasted pecan pieces into the ice cream, allowing the pecans to protrude from the ice cream. Freeze with a cover for 4 hours or overnight.
- Set the oven at 350°F and start preheating. Use paper baking cups to line twelve 2 1/2-in. muffin cups. Set aside.
- Mix salt, baking soda and flour in a small bowl; set aside.
- Mix water and chocolate in a small saucepan. Cook while stirring over low heat till melted; allow to cool for around 10 minutes.
- Beat butter on medium to high speed in a large bowl using an electric mixer for 30 seconds. Beat in sugar till fluffy. Add in vanilla and eggs; beat on low speed until blended, and then beat on medium speed for 1 minute. Beat in the chocolate mixture. Add buttermilk and the flour mixture alternately into the beaten

mixture, beating properly on low speed after each addition just till well-combined. Pour batter into bake cups, around 2/3 full.
- Bake till a wooden toothpick comes out clean, around 25 minutes. Allow to cool for 10 minutes in the pans on wire racks. Take away from the pans. Allow to cool thoroughly.
- Heat caramel ice cream topping till warm just before serving. Take the wrappers away from the cupcakes; arrange the cupcakes in shallow bowls or on plates. Place one round of chocolate-pecan ice cream frosting on top of each cupcake. Place toasted coconut on top; drizzle warm caramel ice cream topping over.

Nutrition Information

- Calories: 437 calories;
- Protein: 7.1
- Total Fat: 26
- Sodium: 258
- Total Carbohydrate: 48.4
- Cholesterol: 82

44. Gingerbread Cupcakes With Cream Cheese Frosting

Serving: 12 | Prep: | Cook: | Ready in:

Ingredients

- 5 tablespoons unsalted butter, softened
- 1/2 cup white sugar
- 1/2 cup unsulfured molasses
- 1 egg
- 1 egg yolk
- 1 1/4 cups all-purpose flour
- 1 tablespoon Dutch process cocoa powder
- 1 1/4 teaspoons ground ginger
- 1 teaspoon ground cinnamon
- 1/2 teaspoon ground allspice
- 1/2 teaspoon ground nutmeg
- 1/4 teaspoon salt
- 1 teaspoon baking soda
- 1/2 cup hot milk
- 2 tablespoons unsalted butter, softened
- 2 ounces cream cheese, softened
- 2/3 cup sifted confectioners' sugar
- 1/4 teaspoon lemon extract

Direction

- Set the oven to 175°C or 350°F. Butter a 12-cup muffin tin or use paper liners to line them.
- Cream together white sugar and 5 tbsp. butter, then put in egg yolk, egg and molasses.
- Sift salt, nutmeg, allspice, cinnamon, ginger, cocoa powder and flour together. Dissolve baking soda in hot milk. Put flour mixture into creamed mixture and stir until just blended. Stir in the hot milk mixture and pour the batter into prepared tin evenly.
- Bake at 175°C or 350°F until slightly springy to the touch, about 20 minutes. Let it cool for several minutes in the pan and transfer to a rack to cool.
- For making of frosting: Cream together cream cheese and 2 tbsp. butter. Beat in the confectioners' sugar until fluffy, then put in lemon extract and beat. Once the cupcakes are cooled, use frosting to frost the tops and serve.

Nutrition Information

- Calories: 241 calories;
- Cholesterol: 56
- Protein: 3
- Total Fat: 9.6
- Sodium: 185
- Total Carbohydrate: 36.8

45. Gluten Free Chocolate Cupcakes

Serving: 24 | Prep: 15mins | Cook: 20mins | Ready in:

Ingredients

- 1 1/2 cups white rice flour
- 3/4 cup millet flour
- 1/2 cup unsweetened cocoa powder
- 1 teaspoon salt
- 1 teaspoon baking soda
- 1 tablespoon baking powder
- 1 teaspoon xanthan gum
- 4 eggs
- 1 1/4 cups white sugar
- 2/3 cup sour cream
- 1 cup milk
- 2 teaspoons vanilla extract

Direction

- Preheat the oven to 175 degrees C (350 degrees F). Use the paper baking cups to line two 12-in. cup muffin pans or grease the pans.
- In a medium-sized bowl, whisk the xanthan gum, baking powder, baking soda, salt, cocoa, millet flour and rice flour together. In another big bowl, whip vanilla, milk, vanilla, sour cream, sugar and eggs. Whisk in dry ingredients till smooth. Scoop batter into prepped cups, distributing equally.
- Bake in preheated oven for 20-25 minutes or till tops spring back when being pressed gently. Let cool down in pan which is set over the wire rack. Once cooled, arrange cupcakes on the serving platter.

Nutrition Information

- Calories: 130 calories;
- Total Fat: 2.9
- Sodium: 235
- Total Carbohydrate: 23.8
- Cholesterol: 35
- Protein: 3

46. Gluten Free Chocolate Chickpea Cupcakes

Serving: 12 | Prep: 20mins | Cook: 20mins | Ready in:

Ingredients

- 1 1/2 cups semisweet chocolate chips
- 1/4 cup coconut oil
- 1 (15 ounce) can chickpeas (garbanzo beans), drained
- 4 eggs
- 1/2 cup white sugar
- 1 teaspoon baking powder
- 1 teaspoon vanilla extract

Direction

- Turn oven on to 350 degrees F or 175 degrees C and grease or line with paper liners 12 muffin cups.
- Melt together coconut oil and chocolate chips in the top of a double boiler over simmering water, stirring often, while scraping the sides down using a rubber spatula to avoid any scorching.
- In a food processor or blender, blend together vanilla extract, baking powder, sugar, eggs, and chickpeas until it becomes smooth. Add the chocolate mixture and blend till smooth. Pour the batter into the prepped muffin cups.
- Bake in the preheated oven for 20 - 25 minutes, or until a toothpick comes out clean when you insert it into the center.

Nutrition Information

- Calories: 226 calories;
- Total Fat: 12.9
- Sodium: 136
- Total Carbohydrate: 27.1
- Cholesterol: 62
- Protein: 4.1

47. Gluten Free Chocolate Whiskey Bacon Cupcakes

Serving: 24 | Prep: 20mins | Cook: 25mins | Ready in:

Ingredients

- Cupcakes:
- 12 slices bacon
- 2 cups gluten-free all purpose baking flour
- 2 cups white sugar
- 3/4 cup unsweetened cocoa powder
- 2 1/4 teaspoons xanthan gum
- 2 teaspoons baking soda
- 1 teaspoon baking powder
- 1/2 teaspoon sea salt
- 1 cup cold strong-brewed coffee
- 1 cup buttermilk
- 2 eggs
- 1/2 cup canola oil
- 1 fluid ounce whiskey
- Frosting:
- 1 (8 ounce) package cream cheese, softened
- 1 cup confectioners' sugar
- 1 fluid ounce whiskey (such as Jack Daniel's®), divided

Direction

- Start preheating oven to 190 degrees C (375 degrees F). Use paper liners to line 24 muffin cups.
- In a large skillet, add the bacon and cook on medium-high heat for 10 minutes, turning occasionally, until evenly browned. On paper towels, drain the bacon slices.
- In a bowl, combine flour, sea salt, white sugar, baking powder, cocoa powder, baking soda, and xanthan gum together. In a separate large bowl, whisk coffee, 1 fluid ounce whiskey, buttermilk, canola oil and eggs together. Slowly add dry ingredients into wet until it's a well-combined batter.
- In the batter, crumble about half of the cooked bacon and stir; separate batter evenly between the lined muffin cups.
- In the preheated oven, bake for 15 to 20 minutes until a toothpick inserted into the center comes out clean. Let it rest in the pans for 10 minutes and then transfer to a wire rack to cool completely.
- In a small bowl, whisk cream cheese, 1 fluid ounce whiskey and confectioners' sugar together. Sprinkle the mixture over the top of the cooled cupcakes. Fetch remaining bacon, crumble and sprinkle over the frosted cupcakes.

Nutrition Information

- Calories: 285 calories;
- Total Fat: 15.5
- Sodium: 334
- Total Carbohydrate: 33.1
- Cholesterol: 36
- Protein: 4.9

48. Gluten Free Cocoa Coconut Cupcakes

Serving: 15 | Prep: 20mins | Cook: 20mins | Ready in:

Ingredients

- 1 cup self-rising gluten-free flour
- 1/2 cup brown sugar
- 1 tablespoon brown sugar
- 2 tablespoons unsweetened cocoa powder
- 1 teaspoon gluten-free baking powder
- 3 eggs
- 1/2 cup dairy-free margarine
- 2 tablespoons olive oil
- 2 tablespoons lactose-free milk
- 2 tablespoons creamed coconut, roughly chopped (such as Patak's®)

Direction

- Set the oven to 375°F or 190°C for preheating. Grease the 15 muffin cups or line them with some paper liners.
- Combine the cocoa powder, flour, baking powder, and 1/2 cup plus 1 tbsp. of brown sugar in a large bowl. Stir in the margarine, milk, eggs, and olive oil until the batter is

already thick and has no visible lumps. Mix in the chopped creamed coconut.
- Fill the prepared muffin cups with the batter, filling them almost to the top.
- Bake them inside the preheated oven for 20-25 minutes until the tops will spring back once they are pressed lightly.

Nutrition Information

- Calories: 146 calories;
- Total Fat: 9
- Sodium: 107
- Total Carbohydrate: 15.3
- Cholesterol: 33
- Protein: 2.2

49. Gluten Free Dark Chocolate Cupcakes

Serving: 18 | Prep: 15mins | Cook: 20mins | Ready in:

Ingredients

- 1 1/2 cups gluten-free all-purpose flour
- 1 1/2 cups coconut sugar
- 1 cup dark chocolate chips
- 1 cup cocoa powder
- 1/4 cup coconut flour
- 2 teaspoons baking powder
- 1 teaspoon baking soda
- 1 teaspoon xanthan gum
- 1/2 teaspoon salt
- 1 3/4 cups buttermilk
- 4 eggs
- 3/4 cup vegetable oil
- 2 teaspoons vanilla extract

Direction

- Preheat an oven to 175°C/350°F. Line paper liners on muffin pans.
- Mix salt, xanthan gum, baking soda, baking powder, coconut flour, cocoa powder, dark chocolate chips, coconut sugar and gluten-free flour well to combine in a bowl.
- Whisk vanilla extract, vegetable oil, eggs and buttermilk till combined in another big bowl. Add flour mixture; use spatula to fold in till blended completely. Evenly divide batter to muffin cups, filling each cup to halfway.
- In preheated oven, bake cupcakes for 20 minutes till an inserted toothpick in middle exits clean. Cool for 5 minutes in pans; transfer to wire rack. Completely cool.

Nutrition Information

- Calories: 272 calories;
- Total Fat: 13.9
- Sodium: 244
- Total Carbohydrate: 37
- Cholesterol: 42
- Protein: 4.8

50. Gluten Free, Sugar Free Red Velvet Cupcakes With Sugar Free Cream Cheese Frosting

Serving: 8 | Prep: | Cook: | Ready in:

Ingredients

- Cupcakes:
- 1/2 cup coconut flour
- 2 tablespoons natural, unsweetened cocoa powder
- 1/4 teaspoon salt
- 1/4 teaspoon baking soda
- 2 eggs
- 2 egg whites
- 2 tablespoons Melt® Organic Buttery Spread, melted over low heat
- 1/2 cup low fat buttermilk*
- 1/2 cup erythritol, such as NOW Foods
- 1/2 teaspoon vanilla stevia extract
- 7 drops red gel food coloring

- Frosting:
- 4 ounces reduced-fat cream cheese, room temperature
- 2 ounces Melt® Organic Buttery Spread
- 1 cup erythritol, powdered**
- 15 drops vanilla stevia, or to taste

Direction

- Preheat an oven to 350°F. Put cupcake liners in 8 wells of muffin tin.
- Whisk powdered milk (optional), baking soda, salt, cocoa powder and coconut flour in small bowl; put aside.
- Mix stevia, erythritol, water/buttermilk, Melt, egg whites and eggs in bigger bowl; use hand blender to mix on low speed till combined. Add dry ingredients; mix well, starting on low speed then increasing to high for 2 minutes till there are no lumps and well blended. Blend food coloring in till you get desired color.
- Evenly divide batter to cupcake liners. Bake till an inserted toothpick in middle of cupcake exits clean for 20 minutes. Before frosting, completely cool.
- Frosting: Beat Melt and cream cheese till fluffy. You don't have to warm melt to room temperature because it's soft straight out of the fridge. In several additions, add powdered erythritol, beating well till fluffy. Beat liquid vanilla stevia drops in to taste.

Nutrition Information

- Calories: 124 calories;
- Cholesterol: 55
- Protein: 4.8
- Total Fat: 10.9
- Sodium: 266
- Total Carbohydrate: 39.1

51. Grandma Gudgel's Black Bottom Cupcakes

Serving: 24 | Prep: | Cook: |Ready in:

Ingredients

- 1 (8 ounce) package cream cheese
- 1 egg
- 1/3 cup white sugar
- 1/8 teaspoon salt
- 1 cup semisweet chocolate chips
- 1 1/2 cups all-purpose flour
- 1 cup white sugar
- 1/4 cup cocoa
- 1 teaspoon baking soda
- 1/2 teaspoon salt
- 1 cup water
- 1/3 cup vegetable oil
- 1 tablespoon distilled white vinegar
- 1 teaspoon vanilla extract

Direction

- Start preheating the oven to 350°F (175°C). Lightly coat the muffin tins with butter. Put aside.
- Beat salt, sugar, egg and cream cheese together. Mix in the chocolate chips and put aside.
- Sift salt, baking soda, cocoa, sugar and flour together in a separate bowl. Pour in vanilla, vinegar, oil and water. Whisk until they are well combined. The batter should be thin.
- Fill chocolate batter into the muffin cups by 1/3 full. Add a spoonful of cream cheese mixture over the top of each one.
- Bake 30-35 mins.

Nutrition Information

- Calories: 172 calories;
- Total Fat: 8.7
- Sodium: 144
- Total Carbohydrate: 22.4
- Cholesterol: 18

- Protein: 2.5

52. Halloween Cyclops Cupcakes

Serving: 12 | Prep: 30mins | Cook: 10mins | Ready in:

Ingredients

- Cupcakes:
- 9 tablespoons unsweetened cocoa powder
- 5 tablespoons boiling water, or more if needed
- 3/4 cup unsalted butter
- 3/4 cup white sugar
- 2 tablespoons white sugar
- 3 eggs
- 1 cup all-purpose flour
- 2 teaspoons baking powder
- Frosting:
- 1 (8 ounce) package cream cheese, softened and cubed
- 1/4 cup unsalted butter, softened
- 1/2 teaspoon vanilla extract
- 1 cup confectioners' sugar
- 3 drops green food coloring
- Cyclops:
- 1 (.68 oz. tube) black decorating gel
- 12 blue candy-coated milk chocolate pieces
- 4 marshmallows
- 3 dark colored fruit leather
- 2 tablespoons confectioners' sugar
- 1/2 teaspoon lemon juice, or more as needed
- 3 tablespoons silver dragees decorating candy
- 24 sunflower seeds

Direction

- Set the oven to 400°F or 200°C for preheating. Use paper liners to line the cups of the 12-cup muffin tin or you can also grease them.
- In a large bowl, sift the cocoa powder. Add 5 tbsp. of boiling water to the bowl. Whisk the mixture until it forms a thick paste, adding more water if needed, 1 tbsp. at a time. Add 3/4 cup plus 2 tbsp. of sugar and 3/4 cup of butter to the bowl. Whisk the mixture using the electric mixer until creamy and smooth. Whisk in the eggs, one at a time and whisking well after every addition. The batter must be smooth.
- In a bowl, mix the baking powder and flour. Whisk the mixture into the batter until well-mixed. Pour the batter into prepared muffin cups. Fill each cup with the batter to 2/3 to the top using the ice cream scoop.
- Bake them inside the preheated oven for 10-15 minutes until their tops will spring back when pressed lightly and the inserted toothpick will come out clean. Let them cool in the muffin tin for several minutes. Place them on a wire rack. Let them cool fully for 1 hour.
- In a bowl, beat 1/4 cup of butter and cream cheese until creamy. Stir in the vanilla extract. Gradually mix in a cup of confectioners' sugar until the frosting turns smooth. Whisk in the greed food coloring.
- Frost a thin layer of the green frosting into each of the cupcakes. For you to decorate the cupcakes easily, store them inside the fridge for 30 minutes. Frost the cupcakes with a second thin layer of the green frosting.
- For the pupil, use the black decorating gel to create a small dot onto each piece of candy-coated milk chocolate. Use a sharp knife to slice the marshmallows into 4 pieces. Insert a blue pupil into the center of each marshmallow piece.
- For the mouth, use the small sharp scissors to cut the fruit leather into semi-circles or crescent shapes.
- For the icing, mix the lemon juice and 2 tbsp. of confectioners' sugar in a bowl. Dip the toothpick into the icing and use it to stick the silver dragees onto each fruit leather mouth.
- To assemble the cyclops, arrange one marshmallow eye and its mouth onto each of the cupcakes. For the horns, insert two sunflower seeds on the cupcake's top.

Nutrition Information

- Calories: 425 calories;

- Total Fat: 25.2
- Sodium: 276
- Total Carbohydrate: 48.2
- Cholesterol: 102
- Protein: 5.3

53. Jama's Fancy Cakes

Serving: 36 | Prep: | Cook: | Ready in:

Ingredients

- 1 (18.25 ounce) package chocolate cake mix
- 3 cups heavy whipping cream
- 1/3 cup confectioners' sugar
- 1 (21 ounce) can cherry pie filling

Direction

- Preheat the oven as directed for the cupcakes. Line the cupcake pans using cupcake liners. (Make sure to use liners, not just the pan).
- Stir cake according to the directions of the package. Fill the cupcake liners slightly lower than half full. (Cupcake needs to be baked up close to level with the top of the liner).
- Bake according to the directions of the package. Cool entirely.
- Mix the sugar and whipping cream in a chilled medium bowl. Beat on high using an electric mixer until stiff peaks form. Refrigerate until ready for use.
- Frost with 1 level layer of whipped cream frosting after the cupcakes are fully cooled.
- In pastry bag fitted a star decorating tip, spoon the leftover frosting. Pipe around the edges of cupcakes.
- Spoon a small portion of cherry pie filling in the middle of each. Refrigerate then serve!

Nutrition Information

- Calories: 153 calories;
- Sodium: 129

- Total Carbohydrate: 16.8
- Cholesterol: 27
- Protein: 1.3
- Total Fat: 9.6

54. Joey's Mini Cupcakes

Serving: 44 | Prep: 30mins | Cook: 30mins | Ready in:

Ingredients

- Filling:
- 1 (8 ounce) package cream cheese, softened
- 1/2 cup white sugar
- 1 egg
- 1/8 teaspoon salt
- 16 ounces miniature chocolate chips
- Cupcakes:
- 1 1/2 cups all-purpose flour
- 1 cup white sugar
- 1/4 cup unsweetened cocoa powder
- 1 teaspoon baking soda
- 1/2 teaspoon salt
- 1 cup water
- 1/3 cup vegetable oil
- 1 tablespoon vinegar
- 1 teaspoon vanilla extract
- 2 tablespoons white sugar, or as needed

Direction

- Preheat oven to 350°F (175°C). Grease 44 miniature muffin cups or line with paper liners.
- In a bowl, beat 1/8 teaspoon salt, egg, 1/2 cup sugar and cream cheese together till the filling is smooth; then fold in chocolate chips.
- In a bowl, sift 1/2 teaspoon salt, baking soda, flour, cocoa powder and 1 cup of sugar together. Beat in vanilla extract, vinegar, vegetable oil and water till the batter is evenly mixed. Fill batter into muffin cups, each 1/3-full; add about 1 teaspoon of cream cheese filling on top of each. Sprinkle the remaining 2 tablespoons of sugar on top.

- Bake in the preheated oven for 30 - 35 minutes, till a toothpick put in the sides of a cupcake goes out clean.

Nutrition Information

- Calories: 129 calories;
- Total Fat: 6.8
- Sodium: 80
- Total Carbohydrate: 17.6
- Cholesterol: 10
- Protein: 1.5

55. Keto Friendly Brownie Cakes

Serving: 6 | Prep: 10mins | Cook: 19mins | Ready in:

Ingredients

- 1 (1 ounce) square unsweetened chocolate
- 1/2 cup granular sucralose sweetener (such as Splenda®)
- 1/2 cup water, or as needed
- 1/4 cup butter, melted
- 1 egg
- 1/4 cup soy flour
- 1 teaspoon mayonnaise (optional)
- 1/2 teaspoon vanilla extract
- 1/2 teaspoon salt
- 1/4 teaspoon baking soda

Direction

- Set an oven to preheat to 165°C (325°F). Use paper liners to line an 18-cup mini muffin tin.
- In a ceramic bowl or microwave-safe glass bowl, melt the chocolate in 15 second intervals for 1-3 minutes, mixing after each melting.
- In a bowl, mix the egg, butter, water, sweetener and melted chocolate, then mix until the sugar has been dissolved. Add baking soda, salt, vanilla extract, mayonnaise and soy flour and whisk it until no chunks remain. In the muffin cups, pour the batter.

- Let it bake in the preheated oven for 18-21 minutes, until an inserted toothpick in the middle of a brownie cake exits clean.

Nutrition Information

- Calories: 124 calories;
- Total Fat: 11.8
- Sodium: 319
- Total Carbohydrate: 3.5
- Cholesterol: 52
- Protein: 3.4

56. Lemon Daisy Cupcakes

Serving: 24 | Prep: 30mins | Cook: | Ready in:

Ingredients

- 1 package (2-layer size) white cake mix
- 24 NILLA Wafers
- 3 (1 ounce) squares BAKER'S Semi-Sweet Chocolate, melted
- 2 (3.4 ounce) packages JELL-O Lemon Flavor Instant Pudding
- 2 cups milk
- 2 cups thawed COOL WHIP Whipped Topping
- 2 cups JET-PUFFED Miniature Marshmallows

Direction

- Follow the package directions to prepare and bake the cake batter for the 24 cupcakes. Let them cool in pans for 10 minutes. In the meantime, plunge 12 wafers into the chocolate and put them aside.
- In a large bowl, beat the milk and pudding mixes using the whisk for 2 minutes. Mix in 2 cups of the COOL WHIP. Transfer 1 1/2 cups of the mixture into the resealable plastic bag. Seal the bag and cut a small corner from the bottom of the bag.

- Pipe into the center of the cupcake with 1 tbsp. of pudding mixture. Frost the cupcake with the remaining pudding mixture.
- Garnish the cupcakes with marshmallow, wafers, and leftover melted chocolate until they resemble the daisies. Keep the cupcakes refrigerated.

Nutrition Information

- Calories: 195 calories;
- Total Carbohydrate: 34.7
- Cholesterol: 2
- Protein: 2.2
- Total Fat: 5.6
- Sodium: 268

57. Little French Fudge Cakes

Serving: 6 | Prep: 15mins | Cook: 20mins | Ready in:

Ingredients

- 1 (4 ounce) bittersweet chocolate bar, chopped
- 1 1/2 (1 ounce) squares unsweetened chocolate, chopped
- 5 tablespoons unsalted butter
- 1 teaspoon ground cinnamon
- 1 1/2 teaspoons vanilla extract
- 2 eggs
- 1 egg yolk
- 3/4 cup white sugar
- 1/8 teaspoon salt
- 3 tablespoons organic all-purpose flour
- 1/2 (4 ounce) bittersweet chocolate bar, broken into 1/2-inch pieces

Direction

- Preheat the oven to 190 degrees C (375 degrees F). Grease 6 cupcake cups in the dark-colored metal pan for better result.
- Put butter, unsweetened chocolate and 1 chopped bar of the bittersweet chocolate into the microwave-safe bowl; put the bowl into the microwave and cook on the low power for 2-3 minutes or till chocolate softens and butter melts. Check and whisk frequently to prevent chocolate from burning. Whisk till smooth.
- In the mixing bowl, stir the salt, sugar, egg yolk, eggs, vanilla extract, and cinnamon till combined thoroughly, and whisk in flour just till blended. Stir in chocolate mixture, whisk batter several times till smooth, and gently stir in half bar of the bittersweet chocolate broken into half-an-in. pieces. Scoop the batter to prepped cupcake cups, filling them to roughly three-fourth full.
- Bake in preheated oven for roughly 18 minutes or till the knife inserted in the middle of the cake runs out with the streaks of the thick batter. Cakes' tops should be nearly firmed. Let cool down in pan on the rack for 5-10 minutes to serve while warm, or for 20 minutes to serve at the room temperature.

Nutrition Information

- Calories: 427 calories;
- Total Carbohydrate: 47
- Cholesterol: 123
- Protein: 5.9
- Total Fat: 25.3
- Sodium: 78

58. Mexican Chocolate Cupcakes

Serving: 12 | Prep: 20mins | Cook: 15mins | Ready in:

Ingredients

- 1/2 cup white sugar
- 1/2 cup brown sugar
- 1/4 cup butter, at room temperature
- 1 egg
- 1 teaspoon vanilla extract
- 1 1/3 cups all-purpose flour
- 2/3 cup unsweetened cocoa powder

- 1 1/2 teaspoons baking powder
- 1/2 teaspoon instant coffee granules
- 1/4 teaspoon salt
- 1/4 teaspoon baking soda
- 1/4 teaspoon ground cinnamon
- 1 cup milk
- Chocolate Buttercream Frosting:
- 1 cup butter, softened
- 5 cups confectioners' sugar
- 2 tablespoons milk
- 1/2 cup unsweetened cocoa powder
- 1 teaspoon vanilla extract

Direction

- Set the oven to 350°F or 175°C for preheating. Use the paper liners to line 12-cup muffin tin.
- In a bowl of a stand mixer, whisk the butter with brown sugar and white sugar until creamy and well-blended. Add the egg and whisk well. Stir in 1 tsp. of vanilla extract.
- In a separate bowl, mix the baking powder, cinnamon, coffee, flour, baking soda, salt, and 2/3 cup of cocoa powder. Beat the mixture using the whisk until no clumps are visible and the mixture is fluffy. Add the flour mixture and a cup of milk alternately to the butter mixture, whisking well until just blended. Pour the mixture into the muffin cups, filling them to 2/3 full.
- Let them bake inside the preheated oven for 15-17 minutes until the inserted toothpick into the center will come out clean. Place them on a wire rack and let them cool for at least 25 minutes.
- In a bowl of a stand mixer, whisk the butter. Add the confectioners' sugar, 1 cup at a time and whisking well until creamy. Add 2 tbsp. of milk and whisk the mixture until the frosting turns creamy. Stir in 1 tsp. of vanilla extract and 1/2 cup of cocoa powder.
- Insert the coupler and tip in a piping bag. Place the piping bag into a tall glass. Fold the edges of the bag down all around the glass. Pour the frosting into the bag and collect all of its edges. Twist the edges together and start frosting the cupcakes.

Nutrition Information

- Calories: 530 calories;
- Total Fat: 21.4
- Sodium: 292
- Total Carbohydrate: 86
- Cholesterol: 68
- Protein: 4.6

59. Mexican Hot Chocolate Cupcakes (Vegan)

Serving: 12 | Prep: 20mins | Cook: 30mins | Ready in:

Ingredients

- Cupcakes:
- 1 1/2 cups all-purpose flour
- 1 cup raw cane sugar
- 1/4 cup unsweetened cocoa powder
- 1 teaspoon ground cinnamon, or to taste
- 1 teaspoon baking soda
- 1/2 teaspoon cayenne pepper, or to taste
- 1/4 teaspoon coarse kosher salt
- 1 cup water
- 1/3 cup natural unsweetened applesauce
- 1 tablespoon vegetable oil
- 1 teaspoon vanilla extract
- 1 teaspoon distilled white vinegar
- Frosting:
- 1 (6 ounce) package semisweet chocolate chips
- 2 teaspoons vegan margarine (such as Earth Balance®)
- 1 teaspoon ground cinnamon, or to taste
- 1/2 teaspoon cayenne pepper, or to taste

Direction

- Set an oven to preheat to 175°C (350°F). Lightly grease a 12-cup muffin tin or use paper liners to line the cups.
- In a big bowl, stir the salt, 1/2 tsp cayenne pepper, baking soda, 1 tsp cinnamon, cocoa

powder, sugar and flour. Add the vinegar, vanilla extract, vegetable oil, applesauce and water, then stir until the batter becomes smooth.
- Scoop the batter into the prepped muffin cups and fill each 3/4 full.
- Let it bake in the preheated oven for about 25 minutes, until the tops bounce back once pressed lightly. Move to a wire rack and allow it to cool for a minimum of 15 minutes.
- Put the margarine and chocolate on top of a double boiler atop the simmering water. Mix often and use rubber spatula to scrape down the sides to prevent it from scorching, until the chocolate melts, approximately 5 minutes. Stir 1/2 tsp cayenne pepper and 1 tsp cinnamon into the frosting.
- Spoon the frosting on top of the cupcakes and swirl it around to cover the surface.

Nutrition Information

- Calories: 209 calories;
- Total Fat: 6.3
- Sodium: 159
- Total Carbohydrate: 38.7
- Cholesterol: 0
- Protein: 2.6

60. Mini Egg Cupcakes

Serving: 12 | Prep: 20mins | Cook: 20mins | Ready in:

Ingredients

- 12 small solid chocolate Easter eggs, unwrapped and frozen
- 1 1/2 cups all-purpose flour
- 1 3/4 teaspoons baking powder
- 1 cup white sugar
- 1/2 cup butter, softened
- 2 eggs
- 2 teaspoons vanilla extract
- 1/2 cup milk
- 1/2 cup butter, softened
- 2 cups confectioners' sugar
- 1/2 teaspoon vanilla extract
- 1 tablespoon milk, or as needed
- 1 drop food coloring, any color, or as needed
- 12 candy-coated chocolate eggs (such as Cadbury Mini Eggs®)

Direction

- Preheat an oven to 175 degrees C (350 degrees F). Line paper liners onto 12 cupcake cups. Whisk baking powder and flour together in a bowl.
- Beat 1/2 cup butter and white sugar together in a mixing bowl until combined well. Beat in eggs, one by one, and incorporate each egg before you add the next. Mix in two teaspoons vanilla extract. Mix flour mixture into the egg mixture, then add milk and combine to form a smooth batter. Fill about 2/3 full of batter into each lined cupcake cup and then press a frozen solid chocolate egg into batter in the middle of every cupcake such that a small bit of egg sticks out.
- Bake the cupcakes for 20 to 25 minutes in the preheated oven, until the cakes spring back when pressed with a finger and the tops are browned lightly. Leave the cupcakes to cool completely.
- Beat half cup of butter with 1/2 teaspoon of vanilla extract and confectioners' sugar in a bowl. Put in one tablespoon milk, 1 teaspoon at a time, until frosting is smooth, then beat in your desired food color and spread the frosting onto each cupcake. For garnish, place a candy-coated mini egg on top of each cupcake.

Nutrition Information

- Calories: 429 calories;
- Sodium: 208
- Total Carbohydrate: 57.5
- Cholesterol: 76
- Protein: 3.9
- Total Fat: 21

61. Mini OREO Surprise Cupcakes

Serving: 24 | Prep: 10mins | Cook: 19mins | Ready in:

Ingredients

- 1 package (2-layer size) chocolate cake mix
- 1 (8 ounce) package cream cheese, softened
- 1 egg
- 2 tablespoons white sugar
- 48 Mini OREO Bite Size Cookies, divided
- 1 1/2 cups thawed frozen whipped topping

Direction

- Set the oven to 350°F, and start preheating.
- Prepare cake batter following package's instructions. Combine sugar, egg and cream cheese till blended.
- Spoon 1/2 the cake batter into 24 muffin cups lined with paper. Add about 1-1/2 teaspoon cream cheese mixture and 1 cookie on top of each cup; add remaining cake batter over the cream cheese mixture to cover.
- Bake for 19 - 22 minutes or until toothpick put in middles go out clean. Allow to cool for 5 minutes; transfer from pans to wire racks. Let them cool down completely.
- Frost the cupcakes with whipped topping. Add the remaining cookies on top.

Nutrition Information

62. Mini Panda Cupcakes

Serving: 36 | Prep: 1hours | Cook: 10mins | Ready in:

Ingredients

- Mini Chocolate Cupcakes:
- 9 tablespoons unsweetened cocoa powder
- 5 tablespoons boiling water, or as needed
- 3/4 cup unsalted butter
- 3/4 cup white sugar
- 2 tablespoons white sugar
- 1 cup all-purpose flour
- 2 teaspoons baking powder
- 3 eggs
- Cream Cheese Frosting:
- 1 (8 ounce) package cream cheese, softened
- 1/4 cup unsalted butter
- 1/2 teaspoon vanilla extract
- 1 cup confectioners' sugar, sifted
- Panda Face Decoration:
- 1/4 cup white sugar
- 180 miniature semisweet chocolate chips
- 2 tablespoons chocolate sprinkles
- 1 ounce fondant, ready-to-use, white

Direction

- Heat oven to 190°C (375°F) beforehand. Greasing a 12-cup mini muffin tin and a 24-cup mini muffin tin or use paper liners to line cups.
- In a large bowl, sifting cocoa powder and putting in five tablespoons of boiling water. Stirring till forms a thick paste, add extra water if needed, one tablespoon at a time. In an electric mixer, combine 3/4 cup and 2 tablespoons of sugar with 3/4 cup of butter and beat till creamy and smooth. Beating in eggs, 1 egg at a time, after every addition, beat well till batter becomes smooth.
- In a bowl, mixing baking powder and flour; stirring into the batter till well mixed. Use an ice scream scoop to scoop batter into every prepped mini muffin cup till 2/3 full to the top.
- In the preheated oven, allow to bake for 10-12 minutes till an inserted toothpick comes out clean and tops spring back when pressed lightly. Let it cool down for a few minutes in muffin tin; remove to wire rack and let it completely cool down for approximately 30 minutes.

- In a bowl, combine a quarter cup of butter and cream cheese; using an electric mixer to beat till well mixed. Mixing in vanilla extract. Gradually stirring in confectioners' sugar.
- Frosting a layer of white frosting on each cupcake. In a small bowl, adding white sparkling sugar and dunking every frosted cupcakes into the sugar, so that the frosting is covered evenly.
- For the eyes, in the middle of each cupcake, lay 2 chocolate chips, pointy side facing the cupcake. For the nose, lay a chocolate chip, pointy side points down (like an upside-down triangle). For the mouth, lay 3 chocolate sprinkles in an anchor shape. For the ears, on top of the cupcakes, lay 2 chocolate chips.
- For the eyes, rolling fondant to create tiny balls which are smaller compared to the mini chocolate chips; for the pupils, in each ball, sticking a half piece of chocolate sprinkle. Use some frosting to glue eyes onto the 2 eyes made from chocolate chips.

Nutrition Information

- Calories: 135 calories;
- Sodium: 53
- Total Carbohydrate: 14.8
- Cholesterol: 36
- Protein: 1.7
- Total Fat: 8.2

63. Mint Chocolate Cupcakes

Serving: 12 | Prep: 40mins | Cook: 15mins | Ready in:

Ingredients

- Cupcakes:
- 1 cup boiling water
- 1/2 cup unsweetened cocoa powder
- 1 1/3 cups all-purpose flour
- 1 teaspoon baking soda
- 1/4 teaspoon baking powder
- 1/4 teaspoon salt
- 1/2 cup butter, at room temperature
- 1 cup white sugar
- 2 tablespoons white sugar
- 2 eggs
- 1 teaspoon vanilla extract
- 2 tablespoons crushed peppermint candies
- Mint Buttercream:
- 1/2 cup shortening
- 1/2 cup butter, at room temperature
- 1 1/4 teaspoons peppermint extract
- 3 cups confectioners' sugar, divided
- 3 tablespoons milk, divided
- 3 drops green food coloring paste, or as needed

Direction

- Heat oven to 175°C (350°F) beforehand. Using greased liners to line a muffin tin.
- In a small bowl, combine cocoa powder and boiling water; whisking till smooth. Let it cool down for approximately 10 minutes.
- In a bowl, sifting together salt, baking powder, baking soda and flour.
- In a large bowl, combine a cup and two tablespoons of white sugar and half a cup of butter; using an electric mixer to beat together till creamy on medium speed. Beating in one egg at a time till smooth. Mixing in vanilla extract. Mixing in the flour mixture in three additions, alternate with the cocoa mixture. Folding into the batter with peppermint candies.
- In the muffin tin, scooping batter.
- In the preheated oven, allow to bake for 15-18 minutes till cupcakes are firm to the touch or when insert a toothpick into a cupcake's center, it comes out clean. Removing cupcakes from the pan and laying on a rack for approximately 30 minutes for cooling down.
- In a large bowl, combine half a cup of butter and shortening. Using an electric mixer to beat till smooth on medium speed. Adding peppermint extract. Adding confectioners' sugar, half a cup at a time, after every addition, thoroughly beating. Beating in milk

till buttercream gets the desired consistency, adding one tablespoon at a time. Folding in food coloring, a little at a time till reach the shade of green as desired.
- Fitting a star or round tip into a pipping bag; removing buttercream to the piping bag. Using buttercream to frost every cupcakes.

Nutrition Information

- Calories: 488 calories;
- Total Fat: 25.5
- Sodium: 289
- Total Carbohydrate: 64.7
- Cholesterol: 72
- Protein: 3.5

64. Mint Devil's Food Cupcakes

Serving: 12 | Prep: 35mins | Cook: 35mins | Ready in:

Ingredients

- Cupcakes:
- cooking spray
- 1/4 cup unsalted butter
- 2 (1 ounce) squares semisweet chocolate
- 1 cup all-purpose flour
- 2 tablespoons all-purpose flour
- 3/4 teaspoon baking soda
- 1/8 teaspoon salt
- 2 tablespoons milk
- 1/2 teaspoon distilled white vinegar
- 1/2 drop pure peppermint extract
- 1 cup white sugar
- 1 egg
- 1/2 cup boiling water
- Whipped Cream Frosting:
- 2 tablespoons cold water, or more as needed
- 1 (.25 ounce) package unflavored gelatin
- 1 cup heavy whipping cream
- 3 tablespoons heavy whipping cream
- 1/4 cup confectioners' sugar
- 2 teaspoons confectioners' sugar
- 1/2 teaspoon imitation vanilla extract
- 1 drop green food coloring
- 6 chocolate sandwich cookies (such as Oreo®)

Direction

- Set the oven to 350°F (175°C) to preheat. Lightly coat 12 muffin cups with cooking spray.
- In a small saucepan, heat chocolate and butter together over low heat for 5 minutes until melted. Take away from heat, put aside for 5 minutes to cool a bit.
- In a small bowl, mix together salt, baking soda, and 1 cup plus 2 tablespoons flour.
- In a separate small bowl, mix together peppermint extract, vinegar, and milk.
- In a big bowl, use an electric mixer to whisk together eggs and sugar on medium speed for 3 minutes until pale. Add the melted chocolate and whisk thoroughly to blend. Add 1/2 cup boiling water and whisk until the batter fully combines. Add the flour mixture, whisk on low speed until blended. Add the milk mixture and whisk thoroughly. Fill the batter into the muffin cups until 3/4 full.
- Put in the preheated oven and bake for 25-30 minutes until a toothpick comes out clean when you insert in the cupcake. Remove the cupcakes to wire rack and let cool for 45 minutes until they reach room temperature.
- In a small saucepan, mix together gelatin and 2 tablespoons cold water over low heat. Whisk continuously for 5 minutes to dissolve the gelatin. Take away from heat and let cool a bit for 5 minutes without setting.
- In a big bowl, mix together green food coloring, vanilla extract, 1/4 cup plus 2 teaspoons confectioners' sugar, and 1 cup plus 3 tablespoons heavy cream. Use an electric mixer to whip on low speed for 5 minutes until a bit thickened. Gradually whisk in the dissolved gelatin. Raise the speed to high and whisk for 3 minutes until the frosting is stiff.
- Spread the frosting over the cooled cupcakes. Remove the cream filling from chocolate

sandwich cookies and dispose, crush the cookies. Top the cupcakes with cookie crumbs.

Nutrition Information

- Calories: 292 calories;
- Sodium: 145
- Total Carbohydrate: 35.7
- Cholesterol: 58
- Protein: 3.4
- Total Fat: 15.6

65. Molten Chocolate Cakes With Sugar Coated Raspberries

Serving: 8 | Prep: | Cook: | Ready in:

Ingredients

- 1 cup unsalted butter or unsalted margarine*
- 8 ounces semisweet chocolate chips, or bars, cut into bite-size chunks
- 5 large eggs
- 1/2 cup sugar
- Pinch of salt
- 4 teaspoons flour (or matzo meal, ground in a blender to a fine powder)
- 8 extra-large paper muffin cups (or use regular paper muffin cups, which will make 12 cakes)
- Garnish:
- 1 (6 ounce) container raspberries, barely moistened and rolled in about
- 1/2 cup sugar right before serving

Direction

- In a medium heat-proof bowl set over a saucepan filled with simmering water, melting chocolate and butter; removing from the heat. In a medium bowl, using a hand mixer to beat salt, sugar, and eggs till sugar gets dissolved. Beating into chocolate with egg mixture till smooth. Beating in matzo meal or flour till just mixed. (You can make batter a day in advance; before baking, returning to room temperature for one hour or so.)
- Adjusting oven rack to middle position before serving dinner; heating oven to 450°. Using eight extra-large muffin papers for lining a standard-size muffin tin (1/2 cup capacity), make sure the paper extends above cups for facilitating removal). Use vegetable cooking spray to spray muffin papers. Dividing among muffin cups with the batter.
- Allow to bake for 8-10 minutes till batter puffs but center is not set. Lifting cakes from tin carefully and placing on a work surface. Pulling papers away from cakes and removing cakes to dessert plates.
- Place sugared raspberries on top of each and serve right away.

Nutrition Information

- Calories: 494 calories;
- Sodium: 210
- Total Carbohydrate: 46.4
- Cholesterol: 177
- Protein: 5.7
- Total Fat: 34.7

66. Monster Mini Cupcakes

Serving: 24 | Prep: 45mins | Cook: 14mins | Ready in:

Ingredients

- Mini Chocolate Cupcakes:
- 1/2 cup milk
- 1 tablespoon white vinegar
- 1/2 cup unsalted butter, at room temperature
- 10 tablespoons white sugar
- 2 teaspoons vanilla sugar
- 2 large eggs
- 3/4 cup all-purpose flour
- 1 tablespoon all-purpose flour
- 1/2 cup unsweetened cocoa powder
- 1/2 teaspoon baking powder

- 1/4 teaspoon baking soda
- 1 pinch salt
- Cream Cheese Frosting:
- 1 (8 ounce) package cream cheese, softened
- 1/4 cup unsalted butter, at room temperature
- 1 teaspoon vanilla extract
- 1 cup confectioners' sugar, sifted
- 2 drops orange food coloring
- 48 small candy eyeballs
- 2 pieces dried mango

Direction

- In a bowl, combine vinegar and milk. Let rest 5 minutes, or till milk curdles.
- Set oven to 175° C (350° F) and start preheating. Oil a 24-cup mini muffin tin or line paper liners onto cups.
- In a big bowl, combine vanilla sugar, white sugar and 1/2 cup butter; using an electric mixer to beat until creamy and smooth. Put in eggs, an egg at a time, beating thoroughly after each addition.
- In a bowl, mix salt, baking soda, baking powder, cocoa powder and 3/4 cup plus 1 tablespoon flour. Alternately put flour mixture and the curdled milk into creamed butter mixture, whisking till batter is thoroughly combined. Using a spoon to transfer batter into prepared muffin cups, filling 3/4 full of each cup.
- Put into the preheated oven and bake for 14 minutes, or till you insert a toothpick into the center of a cupcake and it comes out clean, and tops spring back as slightly pressed. Allow to cool in the muffin tin for some minutes. Place on the wire rack and let cool for 1 hour, or until completely cooled.
- In a bowl, combine 1/4 cup butter and cream cheese; using an electric mixer to beat until well blended. Blend in vanilla extract. Slowly mix in confectioners' sugar. Using some drops of food coloring, color frosting orange.
- Put orange frosting into a pastry bag fitted with a grass tip. Vertically hold the pastry bag at a 90° angle 1/8 in. from the surface of a cupcake then squeeze bag. Pull tip up and away as the icing strand is about 1/2 in. high to form orange 'fur'. Repeat to evenly cover cupcake with fur.
- Put 2 eyes onto each cupcake. Slice dried mango into small strips then place on the frosting as 'horns'.

Nutrition Information

- Calories: 163 calories;
- Total Fat: 10.2
- Sodium: 67
- Total Carbohydrate: 17
- Cholesterol: 41
- Protein: 2.3

67. Peanut Butter Cup Chocolate Cupcakes With Toasted Peanut Butter Meringue Frosting

Serving: 14 | Prep: 20mins | Cook: 25mins | Ready in:

Ingredients

- 1 cup all-purpose flour
- 1 cup white sugar
- 1/2 cup unsweetened cocoa powder
- 1 teaspoon baking powder
- 1/2 teaspoon baking soda
- 1/2 teaspoon salt
- 1/2 cup milk
- 1/4 cup vegetable oil
- 1 egg
- 1/2 teaspoon vanilla extract
- 1/2 cup boiling water
- 14 miniature peanut butter cup candies
- 4 egg whites
- 1 cup white sugar
- 1 tablespoon peanut butter

Direction

- Set the oven to 165°C or 325°F and use paper muffin liners to line 14 muffin cups.

- In a big bowl, whisk together salt, baking soda, baking powder, cocoa powder, 1 cup of sugar and flour. Put in vanilla extract, an egg, vegetable oil and milk, then use an electric mixer to beat the mixture on low speed until just combined. Turn to medium speed and blend well.
- Lower the mixer speed to low and pour boiling water gradually into the flour mixture. Turn speed to medium and beat about one minute more.
- Fill each muffin cup to within 1/2 full, then put in the center of each with a peanut butter cup.
- In the preheated oven, bake for 20 minutes, or until they turn golden and tops spring back when you press them lightly. Take away from the oven and allow to cool in pan about 5-10 minutes, then cool them on a cooling rack thoroughly before frosting.
- Preheat the oven's broiler and place oven rack approximately six inches from the source of heat.
- In a bowl, whisk together sugar and egg whites until just mixed. Add the egg mixture to a small saucepan and heat on medium heat until sugar is dissolved, then turn egg mixture back to bowl. Whisk egg mixture on high speed until forming still peaks.
- In a microwave-safe bowl, put peanut butter. Heat on high setting at 15-second intervals while stirring in between, until the peanut butter is creamy and thin. Fold melted peanut butter gently into egg whites. Turn the peanut butter frosting to a piping bag.
- Pipe frosting onto cooled cupcakes.
- Under the preheated broiler, toast the cupcakes for one minute, or until browned slightly.

Nutrition Information

- Calories: 293 calories;
- Total Carbohydrate: 47.3
- Cholesterol: 13
- Protein: 5.3

- Total Fat: 10.7
- Sodium: 246

68. Peanut Butter And Chocolate Chip Cupcakes

Serving: 12 | Prep: 10mins | Cook: 20mins | Ready in:

Ingredients

- 1 cup all-purpose flour
- 1 1/2 teaspoons baking powder
- 1 pinch salt
- 1/2 cup brown sugar
- 1/4 cup chunky peanut butter
- 3 tablespoons unsalted butter, softened
- 1 egg
- 1/2 teaspoon vanilla extract
- 1/2 cup milk
- 1/2 cup semisweet chocolate chips

Direction

- Start preheating the oven to 350°F (175°C). Line paper liners on a muffin tin.
- In a bowl, whisk together salt, baking powder, and flour.
- In another bowl, combine butter, peanut butter and brown sugar. Using electric mixer, beat together until creamy. Beat in vanilla extract and egg. Mix in milk and flour mixture; beat until they become smooth. Then fold chocolate chips into batter.
- Spoon the batter into prepared muffin tin.
- Bake in prepared oven for 20-25 mins or until a toothpick comes out clean when inserted into middle. Place on a wire rack to cool for half an hour.

Nutrition Information

- Calories: 175 calories;
- Total Fat: 8.4
- Sodium: 114

- Total Carbohydrate: 23.2
- Cholesterol: 24
- Protein: 3.6

69. Peppermint Cupcakes With Marshmallow Fluff White Chocolate Frosting

Serving: 24 | Prep: 15mins | Cook: 15mins | Ready in:

Ingredients

- Cupcakes:
- 2 cups white sugar
- 1 cup butter, softened
- 2 eggs
- 1 teaspoon peppermint extract
- 1/8 teaspoon almond extract
- red food coloring (optional)
- 2 cups all-purpose flour
- 1 teaspoon baking powder
- 1/2 teaspoon salt
- 3/4 cup milk
- Frosting:
- 1 (6 ounce) package white chocolate chips
- 1 (7 ounce) jar marshmallow fluff
- 1/2 cup butter, softened
- 2 cups confectioners' sugar
- 1 teaspoon milk, or as needed

Direction

- Preheat an oven to 175°C/350°F; line paper liners on 24 muffin cups.
- Use electric mixer to beat 1 cup butter and white sugar till creamy and smooth in bowl; one by one, add eggs, beating well after every addition. Mix food coloring, almond extract and peppermint extract into creamed butter mixture.
- Whisk salt, baking powder and flour in another bowl. Alternating with 3/4 cup milk, mix flour mixture into creamed butter mixture, finishing with flour mixture till batter just combined. Put batter in prepped muffin cups using spoon.
- In preheated oven, bake for 15-20 minutes till an inserted toothpick in center exits clean.
- In microwave-safe glass/ceramic bowl, melt white chocolate chips for 1-3 minutes in 15-sec intervals, mixing with every melting. Cool melted white chocolate to room temperature.
- Mix 1/2 cup butter and marshmallow fluff till smooth in bowl; mix melted white chocolate into marshmallow mixture. 1-2 tbsp. at a time, add confectioners' sugar into marshmallow mixture till incorporated fully. Add enough milk to get preferred consistency; put frosting in resealable plastic bag with corner cut/piping bag. Pipe frosting on every cupcake.

Nutrition Information

- Calories: 322 calories;
- Sodium: 174
- Total Carbohydrate: 45.9
- Cholesterol: 48
- Protein: 2.5
- Total Fat: 14.7

70. Raspberry White Chocolate Buttercream Cupcakes

Serving: 24 | Prep: 30mins | Cook: 25mins | Ready in:

Ingredients

- 1 (18.25 ounce) package vanilla cake mix
- 1 cup water
- 1/3 cup vegetable oil
- 3 eggs
- 8 ounces fresh raspberries
- 1 tablespoon water
- 3 tablespoons white sugar
- 1 tablespoon cornstarch
- 1/4 cup water
- 2 cups white chocolate chips

- 1 cup butter
- 5 cups confectioners' sugar
- 2 tablespoons milk, or as needed

Direction

- Preheat an oven to 175°C/350°F.
- Grease/line paper liners on 24 muffin cups.
- Use electric mixer to mix eggs, vegetable oil, 1 cup water and vanilla cake mix on low speed till cake mix is moist in mixing bowl; put mixer speed on medium. Beat for 2 minutes till batter is smooth.
- Put batter in prepped muffin cups with spoon; fill to about 2/3 full.
- In preheated oven, bake for 18-23 minutes till an inserted toothpick in middle of cupcake exits clean and cupcakes are browned very lightly.
- Cool cupcakes for 5 minutes in pans; put cupcakes on cooling rack to complete cooling.
- Pulse white sugar, 1 tbsp. water and raspberries a few times to chop raspberries in blender; blend for about 30 seconds till pureed.
- Whisk 1/4 cup water and cornstarch till combined thoroughly; put mixture in raspberry mixture in blender. Blend again till smooth.
- Put raspberry mixture in saucepan; simmer for about 5 minutes on low heat till thickened. Cool raspberry filling.
- Cut core out of every cupcake, about 1-in. in diameter and 1 1/2-in. long.
- Put 2 tsp. raspberry filling in every cupcake using spoon.
- Heat white chocolate chips in microwave-safe bowl for about 1 minute, in 30-sec intervals till chips start to melt; mix and repeat. Heat chips till thoroughly melted, about 10 seconds at a time; mix till there is no lumps and chocolate is smooth.
- Use electric mixer to beat butter on medium speed till fluffy in mixing bowl; beat milk, melted white chocolate chips and 1/2 confectioner's sugar in till mixture is creamy and smooth.
- Beat leftover confectioners' sugar in slowly till smooth; 1 tsp. at a time, beat more milk in if frosting is too stiff.
- Pipe/spread white chocolate frosting on cupcakes to cover raspberry filling. Pipe/drizzle leftover raspberry filling on cupcakes.

Nutrition Information

- Calories: 393 calories;
- Cholesterol: 47
- Protein: 3
- Total Fat: 19
- Sodium: 222
- Total Carbohydrate: 54.1

71. Red Velvet Cupcakes

Serving: 20 | Prep: 30mins | Cook: 20mins | Ready in:

Ingredients

- 1/2 cup butter
- 1 1/2 cups white sugar
- 2 eggs
- 1 cup buttermilk
- 1 fluid ounce red food coloring
- 1 teaspoon vanilla extract
- 1 1/2 teaspoons baking soda
- 1 tablespoon distilled white vinegar
- 2 cups all-purpose flour
- 1/3 cup unsweetened cocoa powder
- 1 teaspoon salt

Direction

- Set oven to preheat at 350°F (175°C). Put 20 paper baking cups into pans, or grease two 12-cup muffin pans.
- Beat sugar and butter in a bowl, using an electric mixer, until fluffy and light. Beat in the eggs, vanilla, buttermilk and red food coloring. Mix in the vinegar and baking soda.

Mix salt, flour, and cocoa powder together, then mix it into the batter. Stir well. Pour batter into the muffin cups, spooning evenly.
- Bake for 20-25 minutes, until they spring back when you touch them. Let it cool on a wire rack. Once cooled, arrange the cakes on a platter. Apply frosting as desired.

Nutrition Information

- Calories: 160 calories;
- Total Fat: 5.5
- Sodium: 264
- Total Carbohydrate: 26
- Cholesterol: 31
- Protein: 2.7

72. Rice Flour Mexican Chocolate Cupcakes (Gluten Free)

Serving: 12 | Prep: 15mins | Cook: 18mins | Ready in:

Ingredients

- 1/2 cup unsalted butter, softened
- 1/2 cup white sugar
- 2 eggs
- 2 teaspoons vanilla extract
- 1 1/2 cups rice flour
- 1/4 cup dark cocoa powder
- 1 teaspoon baking powder
- 1 teaspoon ground cinnamon
- 1 teaspoon cayenne pepper
- 1/4 teaspoon baking soda
- 1/4 cup milk

Direction

- Preheat an oven to 175°C/350°F; line paper liners on 12 muffin cups.
- Beat sugar and butter till fluffy and creamy with electric hand mixer/stand mixer bowl on high speed. One by one, add eggs; beat well after each addition. Add vanilla extract; mix well.
- Mix baking soda, cayenne pepper, cinnamon, baking powder, cocoa powder and rice flour into creamed butter mixture; mix till flour is moist on low speed. Put speed on medium; mix till there are no lumps. Lower mixer speed to low. Add milk; mix till batter is blended well. Use 3 tbsp. batter to fill each prepped muffin cup.
- In preheated oven, bake for 18-20 minutes till inserted toothpick in middle exits clean.

Nutrition Information

- Calories: 194 calories;
- Total Fat: 9.2
- Sodium: 82
- Total Carbohydrate: 25.9
- Cholesterol: 52
- Protein: 2.8

73. Salad Dressing Cupcakes

Serving: 12 | Prep: 30mins | Cook: 25mins | Ready in:

Ingredients

- 1 1/2 cups all-purpose flour
- 1 1/2 teaspoons baking soda
- 1/3 cup unsweetened cocoa powder
- 3/4 cup creamy salad dressing
- 1 cup white sugar
- 1 cup warm water
- 1 teaspoon vanilla extract

Direction

- Set the oven to 350°F or 175°C for preheating. Grease or line the 12 muffin cups with paper liners. Sift the cocoa, all-purpose flour, and baking soda; put aside.
- Whip the vanilla, white sugar, salad dressing, and water until well-blended. Gradually add

- the flour mixture. Whisk the mixture using the electric mixer at medium speed for 2 minutes. Distribute the batter among the prepared pans.
- Bake them inside the preheated oven for 15-25 minutes.

Nutrition Information

- Calories: 173 calories;
- Total Fat: 4.5
- Sodium: 283
- Total Carbohydrate: 31.9
- Cholesterol: 5
- Protein: 2.1

74. Self Filled Cupcakes I

Serving: 12 | Prep: | Cook: |Ready in:

Ingredients

- 1 (8 ounce) package cream cheese, softened
- 1/2 cup white sugar
- 1 egg
- 1 cup semisweet chocolate chips
- 1 (18.25 ounce) package chocolate cake mix

Direction

- Set the oven to 175°C to 350°F to preheat or to the recommended temperature on the package of cake mix.
- Following package directions to prepare chocolate cake mix without baking. Cream sugar and cream cheese together in another bowl until the mixture is smooth. Beat in egg until the mixture is well-combined, then stir in chocolate chips.
- Use cupcake papers to line cupcake tins, then fill chocolate cake batter into the tins until 2/3 full. Put into the center with 1 tsp. of cream cheese mixture and put additional cake batter on top.
- Following package directions to bake cupcakes, then allow to cool and frost together with cream cheese or chocolate frosting.

Nutrition Information

- Calories: 355 calories;
- Total Fat: 17.8
- Sodium: 418
- Total Carbohydrate: 49.1
- Cholesterol: 36
- Protein: 5.1

75. Simple 'N' Delicious Chocolate Cake

Serving: 8 | Prep: 15mins | Cook: 35mins |Ready in:

Ingredients

- 1 cup white sugar
- 1 1/8 cups all-purpose flour
- 1/2 cup unsweetened cocoa powder
- 1 teaspoon baking soda
- 1 teaspoon salt
- 1/2 cup butter
- 1 egg
- 1 teaspoon vanilla extract
- 1 cup cold, strong, brewed coffee

Direction

- Set the oven to 350°F or 175°C for preheating. Grease the 8-inches pan, and then dust it with flour. Sift the cocoa, salt, baking soda, and flour; put aside.
- Cream the sugar and butter in a medium bowl until fluffy and light. Add the vanilla and egg. Beat the mixture well, and then add the flour mixture alternately with coffee. Whisk the mixture until incorporated.
- Bake it inside the preheated oven for 35-45 minutes until the inserted toothpick into the

cake will come out clean. Let the cake cool before frosting it.

Nutrition Information

- Calories: 282 calories;
- Protein: 3.7
- Total Fat: 13
- Sodium: 541
- Total Carbohydrate: 40.7
- Cholesterol: 54

76. Spider Cupcakes

Serving: 24 | Prep: 1hours | Cook: 30mins | Ready in:

Ingredients

- 1 (18.25 ounce) package chocolate cake mix
- 1 pound black shoestring licorice
- 1 (16 ounce) can white frosting
- 48 pieces candy corn
- 48 cinnamon red hot candies
- 1/4 cup orange decorator sugar

Direction

- Follow the package instructions in making the cupcakes. Allow the cupcakes to fully cool down.
- Cut the licorice into smaller pieces that are 3 inches in size. Frost 1 or 2 pieces of cupcakes at a time with the white frosting, do this by batch so that the frosting does not set before you even start putting decorations on the cupcakes. For the spider legs, poke licorice pieces into the outside edges of each cupcake, only 3 pieces per side because 4 pieces will overcrowd the cupcake. Put 2 candy corn pieces on the front part of the cupcake to make the fangs and 2 red hots to make the eyes of the spider. Finish it off with a sprinkle of decorator sugar. Do the same process for the rest of the undecorated cupcakes.

Nutrition Information

- Calories: 260 calories;
- Protein: 1.7
- Total Fat: 6.4
- Sodium: 241
- Total Carbohydrate: 49.8
- Cholesterol: 0

77. Strawberry Chocolate Cream Cheese Cupcakes

Serving: 24 | Prep: 15mins | Cook: 20mins | Ready in:

Ingredients

- 1 (18.25 ounce) package chocolate cake mix with pudding
- 1 (8 ounce) container sour cream
- 1/2 cup vegetable oil
- 1/2 cup water
- 2 eggs
- 1 (12 ounce) package whipped cream cheese
- 1/4 cup strawberry preserves
- 1 (16 ounce) container whipped cream cheese frosting
- 12 strawberries, sliced

Direction

- Heat oven to 350°F (175°C) to preheat.
- Line 24 muffin cups with cupcake liners.
- In a large bowl, mix eggs, water, vegetable oil, sour cream and chocolate cake mix together.
- Spoon batter evenly into lined muffin cups.
- Put a small spoonful of whipped cream cheese in each cup.
- In a bowl, mix strawberry preserves until smooth; scoop about a quarter teaspoon per cupcake on top of the cream cheese.
- Push strawberry preserves and cream cheese down lightly into the batter with a spoon.
- Bake in heated oven 18 to 20 minutes until cupcake tops spring back when lightly pressed.

- Cool in the pans for 10 minutes before taking out to cool entirely on a wire rack.
- Arrange cream cheese frosting evenly over cooled cupcakes and top with sliced strawberries.

Nutrition Information

- Calories: 295 calories;
- Sodium: 294
- Total Carbohydrate: 30.9
- Cholesterol: 33
- Protein: 2.8
- Total Fat: 18.9

78. Super Easy Chocolate Cupcakes

Serving: 18 | Prep: 15mins | Cook: 20mins | Ready in:

Ingredients

- 3/4 cup shortening
- 1 2/3 cups white sugar
- 2 eggs
- 1 teaspoon vanilla extract
- 1 teaspoon instant coffee granules
- 1 pinch cayenne pepper
- 2 1/4 cups all-purpose flour
- 2/3 cup unsweetened cocoa powder
- 1/4 teaspoon baking powder
- 1/2 teaspoon baking soda
- 1 teaspoon salt
- 1 1/2 cups water

Direction

- Set the oven to 350°F or 175°C for preheating. Grease the 2 12-cup muffin pans or line them with 18 paper baking cups.
- Beat the sugar and shortening in a medium bowl using the electric mixer until fluffy and light. Stir in eggs, one at a time. Mix in the vanilla, cayenne pepper, and instant coffee. Mix the flour, baking soda, salt, cocoa, and baking powder, and then mix the mixture into the batter, adding it alternately with water until just blended. Fill the prepared cups with batter, dividing it evenly.
- Bake it inside the preheated oven for 20-25 minutes until the tops spring back when pressed lightly. Let them cool in the pan that is set over the wire rack. Once cool, place the cupcakes onto the serving platter. If desired, frost the cupcakes.

Nutrition Information

- Calories: 220 calories;
- Total Carbohydrate: 32.3
- Cholesterol: 21
- Protein: 2.9
- Total Fat: 9.7
- Sodium: 180

79. Toasted Marshmallow Cupcakes

Serving: 12 | Prep: 20mins | Cook: 15mins | Ready in:

Ingredients

- 1 1/2 cups all-purpose flour
- 1 1/2 cups white sugar
- 3/4 cup unsweetened cocoa powder
- 1 1/2 teaspoons baking soda
- 3/4 teaspoon baking powder
- 1/4 teaspoon salt
- 3/4 cup warm water
- 2 large eggs, lightly beaten
- 1/2 cup whole milk
- 1/3 cup unsalted butter, melted
- 1/4 cup sour cream
- 3/4 teaspoon pure vanilla extract
- 12 large marshmallows

Direction

- Set the oven to 350°F or 175°C for preheating. Use paper liners to line the 12 muffin cups.
- In a large bowl, mix the cocoa powder, salt, baking powder, sugar, flour, and baking soda. Mix in butter, vanilla extract, eggs, warm water, milk, and sour cream until the batter turns smooth. Distribute the batter among the muffin cups, filling them halfway.
- Let them bake inside the preheated oven for 15-18 minutes until the inserted toothpick into the center of each cupcake comes out clean. Allow the cupcakes to cool for 5 minutes.
- Switch the oven's broiler on.
- Position 1 marshmallow into the center of each cupcake vertically.
- Place the cupcakes inside the oven. Broil them for 10-30 seconds, watching them carefully until the marshmallows are puffed slightly and turn golden brown. Use the back of a spoon to press the marshmallows into the cupcakes, making the entire top covered.

Nutrition Information

- Calories: 263 calories;
- Total Carbohydrate: 46.5
- Cholesterol: 48
- Protein: 4.4
- Total Fat: 8.2
- Sodium: 263

80. White Chococonut Cupcakes

Serving: 12 | Prep: 15mins | Cook: 16mins | Ready in:

Ingredients

- 1 teaspoon butter, or as needed
- 2 cups baking mix
- 1 cup milk
- 1/3 cup white sugar
- 1 egg, beaten
- 2 tablespoons vegetable oil
- 1 cup sweetened flaked coconut
- 3/4 cup white chocolate chips, divided

Direction

- Set the oven to 400 0 F (200 0 C) and preheat. Coat a muffin tin with butter.
- In a bowl, mix together vegetable oil, egg, sugar, milk and baking mix. Stir well. Fold in 1/4 cup of chocolate chips and 3/4 cup of coconut flakes. Fill the buttered tin with batter; add the rest of coconut flakes to scatter on top.
- Put in the prepared oven and bake cupcakes for 15 to 18 minutes until when you insert a toothpick into the center, it should come out clean. Let it cool for about 10 minutes.
- In a microwave-safe glass or ceramic bowl, melt the remaining half a cup chocolate chips in 15-second intervals, stirring after each melting, about 1 minute. Drizzle over cooled cupcakes with melted chocolate.

Nutrition Information

- Calories: 234 calories;
- Sodium: 298
- Total Carbohydrate: 28.4
- Cholesterol: 20
- Protein: 3.6
- Total Fat: 12.1

81. White Chocolate Cranberry Poke Cupcakes

Serving: 24 | Prep: 30mins | Cook: | Ready in:

Ingredients

- 1 package (2-layer size) white cake mix
- 1 cup boiling water
- 1 (3 ounce) package JELL-O Brand Cranberry Flavor Gelatin
- 6 ounces BAKER'S White Chocolate, broken into pieces

- 1 (8 ounce) package PHILADELPHIA Cream Cheese, softened
- 1/4 cup butter or margarine, softened
- 1 teaspoon vanilla
- 2 1/2 cups powdered sugar
- 1/2 cup dried cranberries

Direction

- Follow package directions to prep cake batter for 24 cupcakes; cool for 10 minutes in pans. Use fork to pierce tops.
- Mix gelatin mix and boiling water in small bowl for 2 minutes till fully dissolved. Put on cupcakes; refrigerate for 30 minutes.
- As directed on package, melt chocolate. Use mixer to beat butter and cream cheese till blended in big bowl. Add vanilla and chocolate; stir well. Add sugar slowly, beating well with every addition till fluffy and light.
- Spread frosting on cupcakes; put cranberries on top.

Nutrition Information

- Calories: 247 calories;
- Cholesterol: 18
- Protein: 2.4
- Total Fat: 9.2
- Sodium: 213
- Total Carbohydrate: 39.4

82. Zucchini Chocolate Chip Cupcakes

Serving: 18 | Prep: 30mins | Cook: 30mins | Ready in:

Ingredients

- 2 cups all-purpose flour
- 1 teaspoon baking soda
- 1/2 teaspoon salt
- 1/2 teaspoon ground cinnamon
- 1/2 teaspoon ground nutmeg
- 4 tablespoons instant hot chocolate mix
- 1/2 cup butter
- 1/2 cup olive oil
- 1 3/4 cups white sugar
- 2 eggs
- 1/2 cup sour milk
- 1 teaspoon vanilla extract
- 2 1/2 cups grated zucchini
- 1 cup chocolate chips

Direction

- Set the oven to 325°F or 165°C for preheating. Grease 18 muffin cups and flour them or use the paper liners to line the muffin cups. Mix the salt, nutmeg, hot chocolate mix, cinnamon, flour, and baking soda. Put the mixture aside.
- Cream the butter, sugar, and olive oil in a large bowl until fluffy and light. Mix in the eggs, one at a time. Mix in vanilla and sour milk. Whisk into butter mixture with flour mixture until incorporated. Mix in the chocolate chips and grated zucchini. Spread the batter into the prepared pan.
- Let them bake inside the preheated oven for 25-30 minutes until the tops of each of the cupcakes spring back once pressed lightly. Let them cool in the pans that are set on a wire rack for at least 10 minutes. Remove them from the baking cups and serve while they are fresh from the oven.

Nutrition Information

- Calories: 291 calories;
- Total Fat: 14.8
- Sodium: 198
- Total Carbohydrate: 38.5
- Cholesterol: 34
- Protein: 3.1

83. Zucchini Raspberry Cupcakes

Serving: 24 | Prep: 15mins | Cook: 20mins | Ready in:

Ingredients

- 2 1/2 cups all-purpose flour
- 1/4 cup unsweetened cocoa powder
- 1 1/2 teaspoons baking soda
- 3/4 cup butter, softened
- 1 cup white sugar
- 2 eggs
- 1 teaspoon vanilla extract
- 1/2 cup buttermilk
- 2 cups shredded zucchini
- 1 1/4 cups fresh raspberries
- 1 cup chocolate chips

Direction

- Set the oven to 350°F or 175°C for preheating. Grease or line 24 muffin cups with the paper muffin liners.
- Mix the baking soda, flour, and cocoa; put aside. Use an electric mixer to whisk the sugar and butter in a large bowl until fluffy and light-colored. Add 1 egg at a time and let each egg incorporate into the butter mixture before adding the next one. Whisk in vanilla together with the last egg. Add the flour mixture alternately with the buttermilk. Make sure to whisk the mixture until incorporated. Fold in the chocolate chips, zucchini, and raspberries and whisk just until well-combined. Pour the batter into the prepared muffin cups, filling the cups to 3/4 full.
- Let them bake inside the preheated oven for 20 minutes until the inserted toothpick into the center will come out clean. Let them cool in the pans for 10 minutes. Remove them from the pans and let them cool on a wire rack completely.

Nutrition Information

- Calories: 179 calories;
- Total Fat: 8.6
- Sodium: 133
- Total Carbohydrate: 24.6
- Cholesterol: 31
- Protein: 2.8

Chapter 2: Cheesecake Cupcake Recipes

***

84. Bite Sized Cheesecake Cupcakes

Serving: 12 | Prep: 15mins | Cook: 20mins | Ready in:

Ingredients

- 12 vanilla wafer cookies
- 2 (8 ounce) packages cream cheese, softened
- 1/2 cup white sugar
- 2 eggs, beaten
- 1/2 teaspoon vanilla extract
- 3/4 cup cherry pie filling, or to taste (optional)

Direction

- Set oven to 175°C (or 350°F) and start preheating. Prepare 12 muffin cups lined with foil cupcake liners.
- Put a vanilla wafer cookie to the bottom of each cupcake liner.
- In a bowl, beat vanilla extract, eggs, sugar and cream cheese until smoothened; fill about 3/4 of each liner with the creamed mixture.
- Bake in prepared oven for about 20 minutes until the middle is almost set and collapsed a little.
- Leave cupcakes in the fridge for 2 hours or overnight. Spread each cupcake with cherry pie filling.

Nutrition Information

- Calories: 223 calories;
- Sodium: 144
- Total Carbohydrate: 18.4
- Cholesterol: 72
- Protein: 4.2
- Total Fat: 15

85. Brownie Cheesecake Cupcakes

Serving: 12 | Prep: 20mins | Cook: 20mins | Ready in:

Ingredients

- Brownies:
- 1 (18.25 ounce) package brownie mix (such as Pillsbury®)
- 2/3 cup oil
- 2 eggs
- 1/4 cup water
- Cheesecake:
- 1 (8 ounce) package cream cheese, softened
- 1/2 cup white sugar
- 3 tablespoons butter, softened
- 2 tablespoons all-purpose flour
- 1 teaspoon vanilla extract

Direction

- Set the oven to 350°F or 175°C for preheating. Use the paper liners to line 12-muffin cups.
- In a bowl, combine the eggs, oil, brownie mix, and water and stir until well-blended. In a separate bowl, mix the sugar, vanilla extract, cream cheese, flour, and butter.
- Pour the brownie mix into each of the muffin cups, filling them half-full. Top the brownie mix with the cream cheese mixture. Spread the brownie mix all over the cream cheese mixture.
- Let them bake inside the preheated oven for 20-25 minutes until the inserted toothpick into the center of the brownie portion will come out clean.

Nutrition Information

- Calories: 435 calories;
- Sodium: 218
- Total Carbohydrate: 43
- Cholesterol: 59
- Protein: 4.3
- Total Fat: 28.8

86. Cheesecake Cupcakes

Serving: 18 | Prep: | Cook: | Ready in:

Ingredients

- 3 (8 ounce) packages cream cheese
- 1 cup white sugar
- 5 eggs
- 1 teaspoon vanilla extract
- 8 ounces sour cream
- 1 cup white sugar
- 1 teaspoon vanilla extract

Direction

- Preheat the oven to 350°F or 175°C. Use the paper cupcake liners to line the cupcake pans.
- Cream a cup of sugar and cream cheese in a medium bowl. Mix in the eggs, one at a time. Whisk in the vanilla. Pour the mixture into the cupcake pans, filling them to 2/3-3/4 full.
- Let them bake in preheated oven for half an hour until golden brown. Remove them from the oven and allow them to cool for 5-10 minutes.
- For the sour cream topping, whisk the vanilla, sour cream, and a cup of sugar until smooth. Spread the mixture into the well of the cupcake's top.
- Place them back into the oven and bake for 5-7 more minutes until set. Place the cupcake pans on racks and let them cool. Make sure not to remove the cupcakes from the pan if they are

not yet fully cool. To finish the cupcakes, place a dollop of your desired pie filling on top of each cupcake.

Nutrition Information

- Calories: 265 calories;
- Total Fat: 17
- Sodium: 137
- Total Carbohydrate: 23.9
- Cholesterol: 98
- Protein: 5

87. Cheesecake Cups

Serving: 16 | Prep: 20mins | Cook: 15mins | Ready in:

Ingredients

- 16 vanilla wafer cookies
- 1 (8 ounce) package cream cheese, softened
- 3/4 cup white sugar
- 2 eggs
- 1 teaspoon vanilla extract

Direction

- Set the oven to 350°F (175°C), and start preheating. Line cupcake liners on 16 muffin tin cups.
- In the bottom of each cupcake liner, arrange 1 cookie.
- In a medium bowl, beat sugar and cream cheese together with an electric mixer till creamy. Beat in vanilla extract and eggs until smooth. In the cupcake liners, pour batter over the wafers.
- Bake in the prepped oven for about 15 minutes, until set and golden.

Nutrition Information

- Calories: 123 calories;
- Cholesterol: 39
- Protein: 2.1
- Total Fat: 6.7
- Sodium: 69
- Total Carbohydrate: 14.1

88. Cherry Cheesecake Cupcakes

Serving: 24 | Prep: 15mins | Cook: 10mins | Ready in:

Ingredients

- Crust:
- 1 cup graham cracker crumbs
- 3/4 cup butter, melted
- 2 tablespoons white sugar
- Filling:
- 1 pound whipped cream cheese
- 3/4 cup sugar
- 2 eggs
- 1 teaspoon vanilla extract
- Topping:
- 1 (21 ounce) can cherry pie filling

Direction

- Set the oven to 350°F or 175°C for preheating. Use foil liners to line the 24 muffin cups.
- In a bowl, mix the melted butter with 2 tbsp. of sugar and graham cracker crumbs. Press the crumbs into the prepared muffin cups' bottoms.
- In a bowl, whisk the vanilla extract, cream cheese, eggs, and 3/4 cup of sugar until the filling is smooth. Distribute the filling among the muffin cups.
- Bake them inside the preheated oven for 10 minutes until around the edges of the top are golden and cracked slightly. Let them cool completely. Place the cherry pie filling onto the top of each cupcake.

Nutrition Information

- Calories: 182 calories;

- Total Carbohydrate: 17.9
- Cholesterol: 49
- Protein: 1.8
- Total Fat: 11.9
- Sodium: 152

89. Chocolate Chip Cheesecake Cupcakes

Serving: 24 | Prep: 20mins | Cook: 25mins | Ready in:

Ingredients

- 1 (18.25 ounce) package chocolate cake mix (such as Duncan Hines® Moist Deluxe®)
- 1 1/4 cups water
- 4 eggs, divided
- 1/2 cup oil
- 1 (8 ounce) package cream cheese, at room temperature
- 2/3 cup white sugar
- 3/4 teaspoon Mexican vanilla extract
- 3/4 cup miniature chocolate chips, or more to taste, divided
- 1 (16 ounce) container cream cheese frosting

Direction

- Set the oven to 350°F (175°C) for preheating. Use paper liners to line the 24 muffin cups.
- In a bowl, mix 3 eggs with oil, water, and cake mix using the electric mixer for 2 minutes until it forms a smooth batter. Scoop the batter into the prepared muffin cups.
- In a blender, blend 1 egg, vanilla extract, sugar, and cream cheese until the cheesecake filling is already smooth. Mix in a half cup of chocolate chips. Stuff each cupcake with 1 tbsp. of the cheesecake filling.
- Bake them inside the preheated oven for 25 minutes until the inserted toothpick into the cupcake will come out clean. Let them cool on a wire rack.
- Use the cream cheese frosting to frost each cupcake. Sprinkle each cupcake with the remaining chocolate chips.

Nutrition Information

- Calories: 309 calories;
- Total Fat: 18.1
- Sodium: 263
- Total Carbohydrate: 36.3
- Cholesterol: 41
- Protein: 3.3

90. Chocolate Cupcakes With Pumpkin Cheesecake Filling

Serving: 12 | Prep: 15mins | Cook: 25mins | Ready in:

Ingredients

- Filling:
- 1 (8 ounce) package cream cheese, at room temperature
- 1/3 cup white sugar
- 1 egg
- 2 tablespoons 100% pure pumpkin
- 6 drops yellow food coloring (optional)
- 3 drops red food coloring (optional)
- 1/8 teaspoon salt
- 1/2 cup semisweet chocolate chips, or more to taste
- Cake:
- 1 1/2 cups all-purpose flour
- 1 cup white sugar
- 1/4 cup unsweetened cocoa powder
- 1 teaspoon baking soda
- 1/2 teaspoon salt
- 1/3 cup vegetable oil
- 1 cup water
- 1 teaspoon white vinegar
- 1 teaspoon vanilla extract

Direction

- Preheat an oven to 175 degrees C (350 degrees F). Line paper liners onto a muffin tin.
- In a bowl, put salt, red food coloring, yellow food coloring, pumpkin, egg, 1/3 cup sugar, and cream cheese. Then beat with an electric mixer until and no lumps remain and combined thoroughly. Mix in chocolate chips.
- In a large bowl, whisk together the 1/2 teaspoon salt, baking soda, cocoa powder, 1 cup sugar and flour. Stir in vanilla extract, vinegar, oil and water until the batter is blended well.
- Add batter into muffin cups until 1/2-full. Add 1 tablespoon of cream cheese mixture on top. Scatter some chocolate chips at the top.
- Bake for about 25 minutes in the prepped oven until a toothpick comes out clean when inserted into the center.

Nutrition Information

- Calories: 306 calories;
- Protein: 4.2
- Total Fat: 15.5
- Sodium: 289
- Total Carbohydrate: 40.1
- Cholesterol: 36

91. Chocolate Peppermint Cheesecake Bites

Serving: 18 | Prep: 15mins | Cook: 27mins | Ready in:

Ingredients

- 2 cups chocolate wafer crumbs
- 1/2 cup butter, melted
- 1 (8 ounce) package cream cheese, softened
- 1 (14 ounce) can chocolate-flavored sweetened condensed milk
- 2 eggs
- 1 teaspoon vanilla extract
- 1/2 teaspoon peppermint extract
- 1/2 cup semisweet chocolate chips
- 3 teaspoons vegetable oil
- 2 tablespoons crushed peppermint candies

Direction

- Heat oven to 165°C (325°F) beforehand. Use foil baking cups to line 18 muffin cups.
- In a medium bowl, mixing butter and chocolate wafer crumbs; evenly divide mixture among the prepared muffin cups, firmly press to shape crusts.
- In the preheated oven, allow to bake for approximately 6 minutes till set. Allow to cool down completely for approximately 30 minutes. Keeping oven on.
- In a bowl, using an electric mixer to beat cream cheese on medium speed till fluffy. Beating in peppermint extract, vanilla extract, eggs, and sweetened condensed milk till a smooth filling formed. On top of the cooled crusts, evenly distribute filling.
- In the preheated oven, allow to bake for 20-25 minutes till filling sets. Allow to cool down completely for approximately an hour. Gently removing foil baking cups.
- In a ceramic or microwave-safe glass bowl, melting chocolate chips in 15-second intervals, after every melting, stir well, for 1-3 minutes. Use melted chocolate to drizzle over cheesecake bites and use peppermint candies to scatter on top. Let it chill for an hour in the refrigerator.

Nutrition Information

- Calories: 257 calories;
- Cholesterol: 54
- Protein: 3.8
- Total Fat: 15.4
- Sodium: 194
- Total Carbohydrate: 26.9

92. Decadent Cheesecake Cups

Serving: 18 | Prep: 15mins | Cook: 25mins | Ready in:

Ingredients

- 1/2 (13.5 ounce) package graham crackers
- 4 tablespoons butter, melted
- 2 tablespoons brown sugar
- 2 (8 ounce) packages cream cheese, softened
- 1/2 cup confectioners' sugar
- 2 eggs
- 1 cup sour cream
- 1 teaspoon vanilla extract
- 1/2 cup heavy cream
- 2/3 cup chocolate chips
- 18 strawberries

Direction

- Heat the oven to 325°F (165°C). Line 18 muffin cups with cupcake liners.
- Put graham crackers in a resealable plastic bag and with a rolling pin, smash into fine crumbs. Put into a bowl. Put in brown sugar and butter; mix together until it looks like wet sand. Put a tablespoon on each cupcake liner. Push firmly to make the shells.
- Bake in the heated oven 8 to 10 minutes until slightly brown on the edges. Take out of the oven and cool.
- In the meantime, whip confectioners' sugar and cream cheese until well combined. Scrape down the sides of the bowl and whip in eggs, one at a time. Scrape down the sides of the bowl and whip in vanilla extract and sour cream. Split the mixture evenly between the 18 crusts.
- Bake in the heated oven for about 15 minutes until centers jiggle slightly and tops look dry. Refrigerate 2 hours to overnight until set.
- Microwave cream for about a minute until it starts to simmer. Put in chocolate chips and let stand about 1 minute until softened. Mix until chocolate melts and ganache becomes glossy.
- Scoop ganache on top of each cheesecake and put a whole strawberry over top.

Nutrition Information

- Calories: 268 calories;
- Sodium: 174
- Total Carbohydrate: 19.8
- Cholesterol: 70
- Protein: 4.3
- Total Fat: 19.9

93. Maille® Mini Cheesecakes

Serving: 12 | Prep: | Cook: | Ready in:

Ingredients

- Cake:
- 2 cups cream cheese
- 3/4 cup sugar
- 2 tablespoons flour
- 3 eggs
- 1 cup creme fraiche
- 2 tablespoons Maille® Honey Dijon Mustard
- Pinch of orange zest
- Crust:
- 2 cups crushed vanilla cookies
- 1 stick butter, melted
- Pinch of orange zest

Direction

- Mix melted butter, orange zest and cookies. Cover cookie mixture over the bottom of cupcake molds, packing down using the back of a spoon. Place in the fridge. Whisk Maille Honey Dijon mustard, sugar and eggs. Put in orange zest, crème fraiche, cream cheese and flour. Stir well. Fill the cupcake molds with mixture. Bake at 350° for 35 minutes till firm. Chill in the fridge for 2 hours, add fresh berries on top to decorate and serve.

Nutrition Information

- Calories: 484 calories;
- Total Fat: 35.7
- Sodium: 285
- Total Carbohydrate: 36.6
- Cholesterol: 137
- Protein: 6.7

94. Mini Cheesecake Cups With Sour Cream Topping

Serving: 6 | Prep: 10mins | Cook: 30mins | Ready in:

Ingredients

- Crust:
- 2/3 cup chocolate graham cracker crumbs
- 2 tablespoons butter, melted
- 1 1/2 tablespoons white sugar
- Filling:
- 1 (8 ounce) package cream cheese, at room temperature
- 1/4 cup white sugar
- 1 egg
- 1 tablespoon lemon juice
- 1 tablespoon milk
- 1 tablespoon all-purpose flour
- 1 teaspoon vanilla extract
- Topping:
- 1/2 cup sour cream
- 1 tablespoon white sugar
- 1/2 teaspoon vanilla extract

Direction

- Turn on the oven to 350°F (175°C) to preheat. Coat a 6-cup muffin tin with butter. Use parchment paper cut into circles to line bottoms.
- In a small bowl, combine sugar, butter and graham cracker crumbs. Divide the mixture into cups evenly; press firmly to form crusts.
- Put into the oven to bake for 5 minutes. Leave oven on; allow to cool for 5 minutes.
- At the same time, in a medium bowl, beat together vanilla extract, flour, milk, lemon juice, egg, sugar and cream cheese until fluffy and light. Stir in egg; transfer the batter into muffin cups.
- Put into the oven to bake for 15 minutes.
- In a small bowl, combine vanilla extract, sugar and sour cream. Add a small dollop of the mixture on cake tops and bake for another 10 minutes for the topping to set.
- Let it cool at room temperature completely for 1 hour at least, then take it out of the tin. Put into the refrigerator.

Nutrition Information

- Calories: 304 calories;
- Cholesterol: 91
- Protein: 5.2
- Total Fat: 22.4
- Sodium: 207
- Total Carbohydrate: 21.5

95. Mini Cheesecakes

Serving: 48 | Prep: 15mins | Cook: 15mins | Ready in:

Ingredients

- 1 (12 ounce) package vanilla wafers
- 2 (8 ounce) packages cream cheese
- 3/4 cup white sugar
- 2 eggs
- 1 teaspoon vanilla extract
- 1 (21 ounce) can cherry pie filling

Direction

- Set oven to 350°F (175°C), and start preheating. Line miniature paper liners on tassie pans (miniature muffin tins).
- Crush the vanilla wafers then add 1/2 tablespoon of the crushed wafers into the prepared miniature muffin tins.

- Cream vanilla, eggs, sugar and cream cheese together with an electric mixer. Fill the mixture into each miniature muffin liner, almost to the top.
- Bake for 15 minutes at 350°F (175°C). Allow to cool down; then add a teaspoonful of cherry (or any flavor you want) pie filling on top.

Nutrition Information

- Calories: 95 calories;
- Sodium: 54
- Total Carbohydrate: 11.8
- Cholesterol: 18
- Protein: 1.3
- Total Fat: 4.8

96. Mini Cheesecakes II

Serving: 12 | Prep: 20mins | Cook: 25mins | Ready in:

Ingredients

- 12 vanilla wafers
- 2 (8 ounce) packages cream cheese, softened
- 1/2 cup white sugar
- 1 teaspoon vanilla extract
- 2 eggs

Direction

- Set the oven to 325°F (165°C), and start preheating.
- Line foil liners on muffin tin. Add 1 vanilla wafer into each liner.
- With an electric mixer on medium speed, combine sugar, vanilla and cream cheese together till well blended. Put in eggs; mix well. Pour the mixture over wafers, about 3/4 full.
- Bake in the prepped oven until set, about 25 minutes. Take off from pan once cool. Refrigerate before serving.

Nutrition Information

- Calories: 204 calories;
- Total Carbohydrate: 13.7
- Cholesterol: 72
- Protein: 4.1
- Total Fat: 15
- Sodium: 141

97. Mini Cheesecakes III

Serving: 6 | Prep: 20mins | Cook: 25mins | Ready in:

Ingredients

- Crust:
- 1/3 cup graham cracker crumbs
- 1 tablespoon white sugar
- 1 tablespoon margarine, melted
- Filling:
- 1 (8 ounce) package cream cheese, softened
- 1/4 cup white sugar
- 1 1/2 teaspoons lemon juice
- 1/2 teaspoon grated lemon zest
- 1/4 teaspoon vanilla extract
- 1 egg

Direction

- Heat oven to 165°C (325°F) beforehand. Greasing one 6-cup muffin pan.
- Mix margarine, sugar, and graham cracker crumbs in a medium bowl using a fork till mixed. In the bottom of each muffin cup, add a rounded tablespoon of the mixture, firmly pressing. In the preheated oven, allow to bake for 5 minutes, then take out for cooling down. Keeping the oven on.
- Beating vanilla, lemon zest, lemon juice, sugar, and cream cheese together till fluffy. Mixing in the egg.
- In each muffin cup, fill the cream cheese mixture till 3/4 full. Allow to bake for 25 minutes at 165°C (325°F). Before removing, let

it sit in pan till completely cool down. Chill in the refrigerator till serving time.

Nutrition Information

- Calories: 219 calories;
- Sodium: 171
- Total Carbohydrate: 15.2
- Cholesterol: 72
- Protein: 4.2
- Total Fat: 16.1

98. Mini Cherry Cheesecakes

Serving: 24 | Prep: 15mins | Cook: 15mins | Ready in:

Ingredients

- 24 vanilla wafer cookies
- 2 (8 ounce) packages cream cheese, softened
- 3/4 cup white sugar
- 2 eggs
- 2 1/2 tablespoons lemon juice
- 1 teaspoon vanilla extract
- 1 (12 ounce) can cherry pie filling

Direction

- Preheat oven to 350°F (175°C). Line paper liners on 24 muffin cups.
- In the bottom of each muffin cup, add a vanilla wafer.
- In a bowl, beat vanilla extract, lemon juice, eggs, sugar and cream cheese until fluffy. Spoon the mixture into muffin cups, about 2/3 full.
- Bake in the prepped oven for 15 - 20 minutes, until cheesecake filling is set. Allow to cool completely, about 1 1/2 hours. Spoon 2 - 3 cherries from pie filling and place over each cheesecake.

Nutrition Information

- Calories: 141 calories;
- Sodium: 82
- Total Carbohydrate: 15.1
- Cholesterol: 36
- Protein: 2.2
- Total Fat: 8.1

99. Mini Chocolate Hazelnut Cheesecakes

Serving: 12 | Prep: 30mins | Cook: 20mins | Ready in:

Ingredients

- 1 1/2 cups crushed chocolate wafers
- 1/3 cup butter, melted
- 2 (8 ounce) packages cream cheese, softened
- 1/3 cup sugar
- 2 tablespoons Pillsbury BEST® All Purpose Flour
- 2 large eggs
- 1 1/2 teaspoons vanilla extract
- 3/4 cup Jif® Mocha Cappuccino Flavored Hazelnut Spread, divided
- 1 tablespoon unsweetened cocoa powder

Direction

- Preheat oven to 325°F. Line foil bake cups on 12 muffin cups. In a medium bowl, mix melted butter and crushed wafers until thoroughly moistened. Spoon 2 tablespoons of the mixture into each baking cup; press on bottoms and 1/2 inch up sides of the bake cups. Allow to chill for 15 minutes.
- In a large bowl, beat flour, sugar and cream cheese using an electric mixer set on medium speed until fluffy. Put in vanilla and eggs, beating just until blended. Take away 2 cups of cheesecake filling from the bowl; put aside. Put 1/2 cup of cappuccino hazelnut spread to the rest of cheesecake filling, beating until smooth.
- Fill each crust with about 1 1/2 tablespoons cappuccino hazelnut filling with a spoon. Add

plain cheesecake filling evenly on top. (The bake cups will be very full.) Bake until the filling is set, about 16 - 18 minutes. Allow to cool for half an hour in pan on wire rack. Cover up and place in the fridge to chill 1 hour or overnight.

- Remove the cheesecakes from pan; discard the foil bake cups. Sprinkle cocoa powder on the surface of cheesecakes. Add the remaining 1/4 cup cappuccino hazelnut spread into a small heavy-duty resealable plastic bag. Microwave on HIGH to soften slightly, for 10 - 15 seconds. Cut very small corner from the bag bottom. Drizzle over cheesecakes.

Nutrition Information

- Calories: 392 calories;
- Total Fat: 28
- Sodium: 260
- Total Carbohydrate: 28.5
- Cholesterol: 86
- Protein: 6.1

100. Mini Pumpkin Cheesecake

Serving: 24 | Prep: 30mins | Cook: 30mins | Ready in:

Ingredients

- 1 1/2 cups white sugar
- 1/2 teaspoon ground cinnamon
- 1/8 teaspoon ground nutmeg
- 1/8 teaspoon ground cloves
- 1/8 teaspoon pumpkin pie spice
- 2 tablespoons all-purpose flour
- 3 (8 ounce) packages cream cheese, softened
- 4 eggs
- 1 (15 ounce) can pumpkin puree
- 1/4 cup sour cream
- 1 teaspoon vanilla extract
- 1/4 teaspoon almond extract
- 24 mini graham cracker pie crusts (such as Keebler®)
- 1 1/2 cups whipped cream
- 1 pinch ground cinnamon, or more to taste

Direction

- Heat an oven to 175°C (350°F) beforehand. In a small bowl, mix flour, pumpkin pie spice, cloves, nutmeg, cinnamon, and sugar.
- In a large bowl, beating cream cheese till fluffy. Beating in spice mixture, sugar, almond extract, vanilla extract, sour cream, pumpkin puree, and eggs; mixing till thoroughly mixed and smooth. In the mini pie crusts, evenly scoop the mixture.
- In preheated oven, allow to bake for approximately 30 minutes till cheesecakes are set. Place on wire racks and allow to cool down for 10 minutes. Before serving, let it sit for 90 minutes in the refrigerator.
- For serving, place whipped cream on top of every mini cheesecake and add a pinch of cinnamon on top.

Nutrition Information

- Calories: 296 calories;
- Total Carbohydrate: 31.1
- Cholesterol: 66
- Protein: 4.8
- Total Fat: 17.5
- Sodium: 286

101. Mini Pumpkin Cheesecakes From Reddi Wip®

Serving: 12 | Prep: 20mins | Cook: | Ready in:

Ingredients

- 1 cup chopped walnuts
- 4 teaspoons granulated sugar
- 1 tablespoon butter, melted

- 1 (8 ounce) package cream cheese, softened
- 1/2 cup granulated sugar
- 1/2 cup canned solid-pack pumpkin
- 1 tablespoon sour cream
- 1/2 teaspoon vanilla extract
- 1/2 teaspoon ground cinnamon
- 1 dash ground cloves
- 1 dash ground nutmeg
- 1 egg, beaten
- Reddi-wip® Original Dairy Whipped Topping
- Ground cinnamon (optional)

Direction

- Preheat an oven to 325 °F, or incase using dark no-stick pan, to 300 °F. Line 2 dozen of mini muffin cups with paper liners.
- Crust: in a food processor, put 4 teaspoons of sugar and walnuts; pulse till ground finely. Put melted butter and pulse till incorporated. Into the bottom of each prepped muffin cup, press a teaspoon of walnut mixture firmly. Let it bake for 5 minutes. Allow to cool.
- Filling: in a big bowl, put the leftover half cup of sugar and the cream cheese. Using an electric mixer, whip on medium speed till creamy. Put nutmeg, cloves, cinnamon, vanilla, sour cream and pumpkin; whip till well incorporated. Put in the egg, whipping on low speed just till incorporated. Scoop evenly on top of crusts.
- Bake till middles are almost set or for 20 minutes. Cool completely for approximately half an hour in pan. Chill for a minimum of 2 hours or till chilled. Just prior to serving, put Reddi-wip on top. Scatter with more cinnamon, if wished.

Nutrition Information

- Calories: 190 calories;
- Total Carbohydrate: 12.8
- Cholesterol: 40
- Protein: 3.6
- Total Fat: 14.7
- Sodium: 94

102. Miniature Cheesecakes

Serving: 24 | Prep: 20mins | Cook: 20mins | Ready in:

Ingredients

- 24 vanilla wafer cookies
- 3 (8 ounce) packages cream cheese, softened
- 1 cup white sugar
- 3 eggs
- 1 teaspoon vanilla extract
- 1/4 teaspoon ground nutmeg
- 1 (12 ounce) can cherry pie filling (optional)

Direction

- Heat oven to 165°C (325°F) beforehand. Use foil baking liners or pepper to line 24 muffin cups. In each cup, add 1 vanilla wafer.
- Beating sugar and cream cheese till smooth in large bowl. Beating in one egg at a time, then stirring in vanilla and nutmeg. In each prepared muffin cup, evenly pouring mixture till 2/3 full.
- In preheated oven, allow to bake till set or for 20 minutes. Let cool down completely, then place cherry pie filling on top. Refrigerate, covered, till serving time.

Nutrition Information

- Calories: 184 calories;
- Total Fat: 11.6
- Sodium: 113
- Total Carbohydrate: 17.3
- Cholesterol: 54
- Protein: 3.2

103. Morgan's Reduced Fat Cheesecake Cups

Serving: 8 | Prep: 10mins | Cook: 15mins | Ready in:

Ingredients

- 8 reduced-fat vanilla wafers
- 1 (8 ounce) package 1/3-less-fat cream cheese, softened
- 1/4 cup white sugar
- 2 tablespoons white sugar
- 1 egg
- 1/4 teaspoon vanilla extract
- 1/4 teaspoon lemon extract
- 1 (16 ounce) can blueberry pie filling, or to taste (optional)

Direction

- Start preheating the oven to 350°F (175°C). Use cupcake liners to line 8 muffin cups.
- Put on the bottom of each cupcake liner with 1 wafer.
- In a bowl, combine 2 tablespoons plus 1/4 cup of sugar and cream cheese until the sugar dissolves. Add lemon extract, vanilla extract, and egg. Whisk until the batter is smooth.
- Put batter in each muffin cup lined with wafer until 1/2-2/3 full.
- Put in the preheated oven and bake for 15 minutes until set. Put blueberry pie filling on top each.

Nutrition Information

- Calories: 231 calories;
- Sodium: 112
- Total Carbohydrate: 39.2
- Cholesterol: 41
- Protein: 4.2
- Total Fat: 6.2

104. OREO Mini PHILLY Cheesecakes

Serving: 12 | Prep: 10mins | Cook: 20mins | Ready in:

Ingredients

- 2 (250 g) packages PHILADELPHIA Brick Cream Cheese, softened
- 1/2 cup sugar
- 2 eggs
- 12 OREO Cookies
- 3 (1 ounce) squares BAKER'S Semi-Sweet Baking Chocolate
- 1 cup thawed COOL WHIP Whipped Topping

Direction

- Heat the oven to 350°F.
- In large bowl, beat sugar and cream cheese with a mixer until well mixed. Put in eggs, 1 at a time; after each, beating on low speed just until combined.
- In the bottom of each of 12 paper-lined muffin cups, add 1 cookie. Fill with batter.
- Bake until the middles are almost set, about 20 minutes. Cool. Chill in the fridge for 3 hours. Melt chocolate as manufacturer's instruction; drizzle over the cheesecakes. Add COOL WHIP on top.

Nutrition Information

- Calories: 269 calories;
- Cholesterol: 78
- Protein: 4.6
- Total Fat: 18.4
- Sodium: 253
- Total Carbohydrate: 24

105. Oreo® Mini Cheesecakes

Serving: 24 | Prep: 10mins | Cook: 15mins | Ready in:

Ingredients

- 2 (8 ounce) packages cream cheese, softened
- 2 eggs, beaten
- 1/2 cup white sugar
- 24 chocolate sandwich cookies (such as Oreo®)

Direction

- Set the oven to 175°C or 350°F to preheat and place oven rack on the middle tier. Use miniature paper liners to line 24 mini-muffin cups.
- In a bowl, beat together sugar, eggs and cream cheese until smooth.
- Put into the bottom of each paper liner with a cookie, then scoop on top of cookies with the cream cheese mixture.
- In the preheated oven, bake for 15 minutes, until almost set in the center.
- Transfer tins to a wire rack to let them cool a bit prior to chilling for 3 hours, until the cheesecake layers are set firmly.

Nutrition Information

- Calories: 134 calories;
- Total Fat: 8.8
- Sodium: 109
- Total Carbohydrate: 11.9
- Cholesterol: 36
- Protein: 2.5

106. Pumpkin Cheesecake Cupcakes

Serving: 24 | Prep: 25mins | Cook: 15mins | Ready in:

Ingredients

- Crust:
- 1 (4.8 ounce) package graham crackers
- 2 tablespoons ground ginger
- 6 tablespoons butter, melted
- Filling:
- 3 (8 ounce) packages cream cheese, softened
- 1/2 cup white sugar
- 1/2 cup packed brown sugar
- 1 (15 ounce) can pumpkin puree
- 1 tablespoon ground cinnamon
- 1 tablespoon ground ginger
- 2 teaspoons ground nutmeg
- 1 teaspoon ground cloves
- 1/4 teaspoon salt
- 3 eggs
- Topping:
- 1 cup sour cream
- 3 tablespoons confectioners' sugar, or to taste
- 1 tablespoon vanilla extract
- 1 pinch ground cinnamon, for garnish

Direction

- Heat oven to 175°C (350°F) beforehand. Use foil liners to line 24 muffin cups.
- In a resealable plastic bag, crushing two tablespoons of ground ginger and graham crackers together; pouring into a bowl. Adding into graham cracker mixture with butter and using a pastry blender or fork to mix till blended.
- In a large bowl, beat together brown sugar, white sugar, cream cheese till creamy; beating in pumpkin puree. Adding salt, cloves, nutmeg, a tablespoon of ginger, and cinnamon; adding in eggs, one egg at a time, after every addition, beating well.
- Pressing a tablespoon of graham cracker mixture into the base of each prepared muffin cup, slightly pressing mixture up the liners' sides. Filling cream cheese mixture into every cup.
- In the preheated oven, allow to bake for approximately 15 minutes till cupcakes slightly jiggle when moved and tops are smooth. Before removing to a wire rack for completely cooling down, let it sit for 10 minutes in the pans to cool first.
- In a bowl, stirring together vanilla extract, confectioners' sugar and sour cream till

frosting becomes smooth. Use topping to top every cheesecake and use cinnamon to scatter on.

Nutrition Information

- Calories: 226 calories;
- Total Fat: 16
- Sodium: 220
- Total Carbohydrate: 17.6
- Cholesterol: 66
- Protein: 3.9

107. RITZ New York Style Mini Crumb Cheesecakes

Serving: 24 | Prep: 20mins | Cook: 30mins | Ready in:

Ingredients

- For the crust:
- 24 RITZ Crackers
- 1/2 cup hot fudge topping
- For the filling:
- 2 (8 ounce) packages 1/3-less-fat cream cheese (Neufchatel)
- 1/2 cup granulated sugar
- 1 egg yolk
- 3 eggs
- 1/4 cup sour cream
- 1 teaspoon lemon juice
- 1 teaspoon vanilla extract
- 1 tablespoon butter, melted
- For the crumb topping:
- 1 cup RITZ Bits Peanut Butter crackers, crushed
- 2 tablespoons flour
- 2 tablespoons light brown sugar
- 1/2 teaspoon ground cinnamon
- 4 tablespoons unsalted butter, melted
- For the caramel topping:
- 1/4 cup creamy peanut butter
- 1/4 cup caramel sauce

Direction

- Let oven warm up to 325°F. Use cupcake liners and line two pieces of muffin containers.
- Arrange 24 crackers and ladle one teaspoon of cold hot fudge sauce on top of it. In the lined cups, transfer the crackers with fudge side up.
- In a big bowl, blend sugar and cream cheese until it becomes creamy. Mix in the eggs and egg yolk one by one, stirring thoroughly each time. Add vanilla extract, lemon juice, butter and sour cream; stir until well-blended.
- Fill muffin cups with batter until 3/4 full, about 2 heaping tablespoons each cup.
- Mix flour, light brown sugar, dissolved butter, cinnamon and crushed RITZ Bits peanut butter sandwich crackers to make crumb topping. Then put aside.
- Let cheesecake bake in a warmed up oven for 15 minutes.
- Take away cheesecakes and even out crumb topping on top of each.
- Put back cheesecake in the oven and let it bake for another 15 minutes until the inserted toothpick comes out clean and topping becomes brown.
- Take out cheesecake from the oven and let it stand to cool fully. Then place in a container with cover and chill up to 2 hours.
- In a microwaveable bowl, mix caramel sauce and peanut butter and heat for 30 seconds. Gently take off dish from the microwave and then stir. Sprinkle peanut butter caramel sauce on the cheesecake and then serve.
- Store in the refrigerator remaining cheesecake.

Nutrition Information

- Calories: 225 calories;
- Total Carbohydrate: 21
- Cholesterol: 53
- Protein: 5
- Total Fat: 13.6
- Sodium: 212

108. S'mores Cheesecake Cupcakes

Serving: 24 | Prep: 45mins | Cook: 20mins | Ready in:

Ingredients

- Filling:
- 1/2 cup semisweet chocolate chips
- 1 cup mini marshmallows
- Crust:
- 1 (14.4 ounce) package graham cracker crumbs
- 1 cup butter, melted
- Cheesecake:
- 2 (8 ounce) packages cream cheese, softened
- 1/4 cup white sugar
- 1/2 cup milk
- 2 eggs
- 1/4 cup sour cream
- 1/4 cup all-purpose flour
- 1/2 teaspoon vanilla extract
- Frosting:
- 1 (7 ounce) jar marshmallow cream
- 1 teaspoon ground cinnamon
- 1 teaspoon cocoa powder

Direction

- Stuff each marshmallow with a chocolate chip. Make sure to use the hot metal spoon to allow the marshmallow to stick to the chocolate and create a tiny ball. Arrange them on a wax paper-lined plate. Place the plate inside the freezer.
- Set the oven to 350°F or 175°C for preheating. Grease the two muffin tins.
- In a bowl, combine the melted butter and graham crumbs.
- Use the back of your spoon to fill the muffin tins with the graham cracker mixture until the bottom of each cup creates a crust.
- In a bowl, beat the sugar and cream cheese using the electric mixer until smooth. Whisk in the milk. Mix in the eggs, adding them one at a time and whisking well until incorporated. Mix in the vanilla extract, flour, and sour cream until the batter turns smooth.
- Pour the batter into the muffin cups, filling them halfway. Stuff the center of the batter with the frozen marshmallow ball. Cover the ball with the remaining batter.
- Let them bake inside the preheated oven for 15-20 minutes until set. Allow them to cool fully for half an hour.
- Pour the marshmallow cream into the small pot and heat it for 5 minutes over low heat until softened. Stir in the cocoa powder and cinnamon. Use this to frost the cooled cupcakes.

Nutrition Information

- Calories: 283 calories;
- Protein: 3.8
- Total Fat: 18
- Sodium: 231
- Total Carbohydrate: 27.5
- Cholesterol: 58

109. Samoa® Cheesecake Cupcakes

Serving: 12 | Prep: 15mins | Cook: 30mins | Ready in:

Ingredients

- 2/3 cup sweetened flaked coconut
- 1 (7 ounce) box caramel and toasted coconut cookies (such as Girl Scout Samoas®)
- 1 (8 ounce) package cream cheese, at room temperature
- 1/2 cup white sugar
- 1 tablespoon coconut extract
- 1/2 teaspoon vanilla extract
- 1/2 teaspoon amaretto liqueur
- 1/4 teaspoon almond extract
- 2 eggs, at room temperature, lightly beaten
- 1/2 cup sour cream
- 1 pinch salt

- 1 cup whipped cream

Direction

- Over medium heat, heat a skillet; cook and stir coconut about 5 minutes, until toasted and fragrant. Discard the skillet from heat.
- Set oven to 275°F (135°C), and start preheating. Line paper liners on 12 muffin cups. In the bottom of each muffin cup, add 1 cookie.
- In a bowl, beat cream cheese with an electric mixer until creamy and smooth. Slowly beat in almond extract, amaretto liqueur, vanilla extract, coconut extract and sugar until smooth. Pour in eggs, a little at a time, and beat until smooth, scraping sides after each adding. Beat salt and sour cream into cream cheese mixture; add in the muffin cups until almost reach the top.
- Bake in the prepped oven for 11 minutes; rotate the pan and keep cooking for 11 - 14 more minutes, until cheesecake is set. Allow to cool in pan on a wire rack for 15 minutes. Remove cheesecakes to a plate and chill in the fridge in at least 4 hours.
- Add toasted coconut and whipped cream on top of each cheesecake.

Nutrition Information

- Calories: 244 calories;
- Total Fat: 16.1
- Sodium: 137
- Total Carbohydrate: 22.3
- Cholesterol: 60
- Protein: 3.6

---

110. Triple Strawberry Cheesecake Cupcakes

Serving: 24 | Prep: 15mins | Cook: 15mins | Ready in:

Ingredients

- Cupcakes:
- 1/4 cup strawberries in syrup, undrained
- 1 (18.25 ounce) package golden butter cake mix (such as Pillsbury®) Moist Supreme®)
- 2/3 cup vegetable oil
- 1/3 cup milk
- 4 eggs
- Icing:
- 2 tablespoons strawberries in syrup, undrained
- 2 (8 ounce) packages cream cheese, softened
- 1/2 cup butter, softened
- 2 cups confectioners' sugar
- 1/2 teaspoon strawberry extract
- 24 fresh strawberries, hulled and sliced

Direction

- Set oven to preheat at 175 o C (350 o F). Use paper liners to line 12 muffin cups.
- In a bowl with syrup, add 1/4 cup strawberries; use an electric mixer to beat until smooth. Add milk, vegetable oil, and cake mix; mix for about 2 minutes until well incorporated on low speed. Beat eggs into cake mix mixture, one by one, until each egg is completely mixed into the batter after each addition. Spoon about 1/4 cup batter into each muffin cup.
- In the preheated oven, bake for about 15 minutes until a toothpick comes out clean when inserted in the center of a cupcake. Transfer cupcakes to a wire rack to let cool thoroughly.
- In a bowl, use an electric mixer to blend 2 tablespoons strawberries in syrup until smooth in a bowl. On low speed, beat butter and cream cheese into strawberries to make the mixture creamy and smooth. On low speed, beat confectioners' sugar into strawberry mixture gradually until the icing becomes smooth; put in strawberry extract and beat for 2 minutes on medium speed.
- Scoop icing into a resealable plastic bag with a cut corner or a piping bag with a star-shaped tip. Frost each cupcake with the icing using the

piping bag or plastic bag. Place strawberry slices on top of each cupcake.

Nutrition Information

- Calories: 301 calories;
- Total Fat: 18.9
- Sodium: 230
- Total Carbohydrate: 30.8
- Cholesterol: 62
- Protein: 3.2

Chapter 3: Lemon Cupcake Recipes

***

111. Frosted Pink Lemonade Cupcakes

Serving: 24 | Prep: 20mins | Cook: 25mins | Ready in:

Ingredients

- Cupcakes:
- 1 (18.25 ounce) package white cake mix
- 3/4 cup frozen lemonade pink concentrate, thawed
- 4 egg whites
- 1/2 cup water
- 1/3 cup vegetable oil
- Icing:
- 3 cups confectioners' sugar
- 1/2 cup unsalted butter, at room temperature
- 2 tablespoons frozen lemonade pink concentrate, thawed
- 1 pinch salt
- 1 dash red food coloring, or desired amount

Direction

- Preheat an oven to 175°C/350°F; line paper cupcake liners on 24 cupcake cups.
- Beat vegetable oil, water, egg whites, 3/4 cup lemonade concentrate and cake mix with an electric mixer on low speed for 30 seconds in a bowl. Put speed on medium; beat for 1 minute till batter is smooth. Put batter in liners to 2/3 full.
- In preheated oven, bake for 25 minutes till inserted toothpick in middle exits clean. Cool for 10 minutes in pans. Transfer onto wire rack; fully cool.
- Beat red food coloring, salt, 2 tbsp. lemonade concentrate, butter and confectioners' sugar with a mixer till even in color and smooth in a bowl; spread on cooled cupcakes.

Nutrition Information

- Calories: 233 calories;
- Total Fat: 9.2
- Sodium: 152
- Total Carbohydrate: 36.9
- Cholesterol: 10
- Protein: 1.6

112. Gluten Free Lemon Cupcakes

Serving: 12 | Prep: 10mins | Cook: 20mins | Ready in:

Ingredients

- 5/8 cup milk, at room temperature
- 3 3/4 teaspoons lemon juice
- 1/4 cup vegetable oil
- 2 egg whites, room temperature
- 2 lemons, zested
- 1 1/2 teaspoons vanilla extract
- 1 1/8 cups gluten-free flour (such as Jeanne's Gluten-Free All-Purpose Flour Mix; recipe in footnotes)

- 3/4 cup white sugar
- 2 teaspoons double-acting baking powder
- 1/4 teaspoon salt

Direction

- Begin preheating oven to 175°C (350°F). Prepare 12 muffin cups lined with paper liners.
- In a bowl, combine lemon juice and milk. Beat vanilla extract, lemon zest, egg whites and vegetable oil into milk mixture.
- In a big bowl, blend salt, baking powder, sugar and gluten-free baking flour together. Pour milk mixture into flour mixture; using an electric mixer, beat for about 2 minutes over medium speed until a well-combined batter is formed. Fill about 3/4 of each lined cup with the batter.
- Bake in the prepared oven for 18-20 minutes until tops turn light golden-brown and a toothpick pierced into the middle comes out with no streaks of batter. Let cupcakes cool for 10 minutes in muffin tin, then move to a wire rack to cool thoroughly.

Nutrition Information

- Calories: 100 calories;
- Sodium: 144
- Total Carbohydrate: 13.6
- Cholesterol: 1
- Protein: 1
- Total Fat: 4.8

113. Lemon Cream Cupcakes

Serving: 24 | Prep: 20mins | Cook: 15mins | Ready in:

Ingredients

- Cream Filling:
- 1/4 cup white sugar
- 3/4 cup cream cheese, softened
- 1 tablespoon lemon juice
- 1 teaspoon lemon zest
- Cupcake Batter:
- 2 1/4 cups all-purpose flour
- 1 1/2 teaspoons baking powder
- 1/2 teaspoon salt
- 3/4 cup butter
- 1 1/4 cups white sugar
- 6 eggs at room temperature
- 1/4 cup fresh lemon juice
- 2 teaspoons lemon zest

Direction

- Set the oven to 350°F (175°C) for preheating. Line the 24 muffin cups with the paper muffin liners or you can simply grease the cups.
- For the filling, whisk 1 tbsp. of lemon juice, 1 tsp. of lemon zest, 1/4 cup of sugar, and cream cheese using the electric mixer until the mixture turns smooth. Pour the filling into the pastry bag; put aside. In a mixing bowl, mix the baking powder, flour, and salt; put aside.
- In a large bowl, whisk 1 1/4 cups of sugar and butter using the electric mixer until fluffy and light. The mixture must have a lighter color. Add the eggs, one at a time and letting each egg incorporate to the mixture before adding the next. Mix in 2 tsp. of lemon zest and 1/4 cup of lemon juice with the last egg. Mix in the flour mixture until just incorporated.
- Spread the batter into the prepared pans, making sure to fill the muffin cups half full. Pipe the center of each cupcake with 1 tbsp. of the filling. Top the filling with the rest of the batter until the cups are 3/4 full.
- Bake them inside the preheated oven for 15 minutes until the tops turn light golden brown. Let them cool on a wire rack completely.

Nutrition Information

- Calories: 186 calories;
- Total Carbohydrate: 22.1
- Cholesterol: 70
- Protein: 3.4

- Total Fat: 9.6
- Sodium: 159

114. Lemon Cupcake With Blackberry Buttercream

Serving: 24 | Prep: 30mins | Cook: 20mins | Ready in:

Ingredients

- 1 cup white sugar
- 1/2 cup butter
- 2 eggs
- 1 1/2 teaspoons vanilla extract
- 1 1/2 cups all-purpose flour
- 1 3/4 teaspoons baking powder
- 1/2 cup low-fat milk
- 1 lemon, juice and zest
- 1 cup butter, softened
- 1 teaspoon vanilla extract
- 1/4 teaspoon salt
- 4 cups confectioners' sugar
- 1/2 cup seedless blackberry jam

Direction

- Set oven to 350°F (175°C) and start preheating.
- Line 24 muffin cups with the paper liners.
- In the bowl of a stand mixer, cream half a cup of butter and sugar until fluffy. Beat in eggs, one by one, and combine 1 1/2 teaspoons of vanilla extract into the mixture along with the second egg.
- Beat in baking powder and flour until thoroughly blended; beat in lemon zest, lemon juice and milk to make a smooth batter.
- Scoop the batter into the prepared muffin cups.
- Bake in the prepared oven for 20-25 minutes until a toothpick pricked into center of a cupcake comes out clean and the cupcake edges are slightly golden brown. Allow the cupcakes to cool completely.
- To make a creamy frosting, beat 1 cup of butter with salt and 1 teaspoon of vanilla extract until creamy and smooth then beat in confectioners' sugar, 1 cup at one time. Beat in the blackberry jam. Spread the frosting over the cooled cupcakes.

Nutrition Information

- Calories: 272 calories;
- Total Fat: 12.1
- Sodium: 151
- Total Carbohydrate: 40.7
- Cholesterol: 46
- Protein: 1.7

115. Lemon Cupcakes With Lemon Frosting

Serving: 12 | Prep: 15mins | Cook: 15mins | Ready in:

Ingredients

- Cupcakes:
- 3/4 cup white sugar, or more to taste
- 1/2 cup butter, softened
- 2 eggs
- 2 teaspoons lemon extract
- 1/2 teaspoon baking powder
- 1/4 teaspoon salt
- 1 1/2 cups all-purpose flour
- 2/3 cup cold milk
- Frosting:
- 3 tablespoons butter, softened
- 2 teaspoons lemon extract
- 1 teaspoon milk, or more as needed
- 1 cup confectioners' sugar, or more as needed

Direction

- Start preheating the oven to 350°F (175°C). Oil 12 muffin cups or use paper liners to line them.
- In a bowl, use an electric mixer to beat together 2 teaspoons lemon extract, eggs, 1/2 cup butter, and white sugar until creamy and

smooth; add salt and baking powder and beat until smooth. Gradually stir flour, switching with cold milk, into the butter mixture until the batter has barely combined. In the prepared muffin cups, add the batter.
- Put in the preheated oven and bake for 15-20 minutes until a toothpick comes out clean when you insert one into the middle of a cupcake.
- Beat together milk, 2 teaspoons lemon extract, and 3 tablespoons butter until smooth. Beat confectioners' sugar into the butter mixture until reaching the consistency you want, then spread onto the cupcakes.

Nutrition Information

- Calories: 262 calories;
- Total Carbohydrate: 35.6
- Cholesterol: 60
- Protein: 3.2
- Total Fat: 11.8
- Sodium: 162

116. Lemon PHILLY Cupcakes

Serving: 24 | Prep: 10mins | Cook: 25mins | Ready in:

Ingredients

- 1 package (2-layer size) white cake mix
- 1 pkg. (4 serving size) Jell-O Lemon Instant Pudding
- 1 cup water
- 4 egg whites
- 2 tablespoons oil
- 3 3/4 cups icing sugar
- 1 (250 g) package Philadelphia Light Brick Cream Cheese, softened
- 1/4 cup butter, softened
- 2 tablespoons lemon juice

Direction

- Preheat the oven to 175 ° C or 350 ° F. In big bowl, whip oil, egg whites, water, dry pudding mix and cake mix on low speed using electric mixer to moisten. The batter will become thick. Whip for 2 minutes on moderate speed. Evenly scoop batter to 2 dozen muffin cups lined with paper.
- Bake till inserted wooden toothpick in middles gets out clean for 21 to 24 minutes. Cool for 10 minutes in pans; transfer onto wire racks. Cool fully.
- Meantime, use an electric mixer to whip juice, butter, cream cheese and sugar on low speed till thoroughly incorporated. Frost the cupcakes.

Nutrition Information

- Calories: 235 calories;
- Total Fat: 7
- Sodium: 265
- Total Carbohydrate: 40.9
- Cholesterol: 10
- Protein: 2.6

117. Lemon Pineapple Daisy Bites

Serving: 48 | Prep: 20mins | Cook: 12mins | Ready in:

Ingredients

- 1 (8 ounce) can DOLE® Crushed Pineapple
- 1 (18.25 ounce) package white cake mix
- 1 (3 ounce) package lemon flavored gelatin
- 2 eggs
- 3/4 cup water
- 1/3 cup vegetable oil
- 1 (16 ounce) can prepared vanilla frosting
- Multi-colored sprinkles, as needed

Direction

- Set the oven to 350°F to preheat. Use mini-cupcake paper with diameter of 1 1/2 inches to line mini-muffin pan.
- In a big bowl, stir oil, water, eggs, gelatin, cake mix and pineapple with juice together, then scoop into each cupcake paper with level tablespoon.
- Bake until a toothpick stuck in the center exits clean, about 10-12 minutes.
- Allow to cool thoroughly on wire racks, then pipe on top of each cake bite with frosting to make a small flower, use sprinkles to garnish.

Nutrition Information

- Calories: 108 calories;
- Total Carbohydrate: 16.4
- Cholesterol: 8
- Protein: 1
- Total Fat: 4.6
- Sodium: 96

118. Lemon Cream Cheese Cupcakes

Serving: 24 | Prep: 15mins | Cook: | Ready in:

Ingredients

- 1 (18.25 ounce) package (2-layer size) white cake mix
- 1 (3.4 ounce) package Jell-O Lemon Instant Pudding
- 1 cup water
- 4 egg whites
- 2 tablespoons vegetable oil
- 1 (250 g) package Philadelphia Brick Cream Cheese, softened
- 1/4 cup butter, softened
- 2 tablespoons lemon juice
- 3 3/4 cups icing sugar

Direction

- Preheat the oven to 350°F.
- Whip the first 5 ingredients in the big bowl using the mixer on low speed till the dry ingredients become moistened or for 60 seconds. The batter will be thick. Whip on medium speed for 2 minutes. Scoop into 24 muffin cups which are lined with paper.
- Bake till the toothpick inserted into middle comes out clean or for 21-24 minutes. Let cool down in the pans for 10 minutes; transfer onto the wire racks. Let cool down totally.
- Whip the lemon juice, butter and cream cheese in the big bowl using the mixer till well-blended. Slowly put in the sugar, whip well after each addition. Spread onto the cupcakes.

Nutrition Information

- Calories: 242 calories;
- Protein: 2.3
- Total Fat: 8.4
- Sodium: 257
- Total Carbohydrate: 40.8
- Cholesterol: 17

119. Lemon Lime Cupcakes

Serving: 24 | Prep: 15mins | Cook: 20mins | Ready in:

Ingredients

- 1 1/2 cups butter
- 3 cups white sugar
- 5 eggs
- 2 tablespoons lemon extract
- 3 cups all-purpose flour
- 3/4 cup lemon-lime soda (e.g. 7-Up™)

Direction

- Start preheating the oven to 350°F (175°C). Oil two 12 cup muffin pans and use paper baking cups to line.

- In a big bowl, use an electric mixer to whisk sugar and butter for 15 minutes until fluffy and light. Stir in 1 egg each time, stir each until well combined. Mix in lemon extract. Mix in flour switching with lemon-lime soda until the batter is just smooth. Put the batter in the prepared cups, splitting evenly.
- Put in the preheated oven and bake for 20-25 minutes until the top will spring back when you gently press it. Put the pan with the cakes on a wire rack to cool down. Once cool, put the cupcakes on a serving dish.

Nutrition Information

- Calories: 276 calories;
- Total Carbohydrate: 37.9
- Cholesterol: 69
- Protein: 3
- Total Fat: 12.7
- Sodium: 98

120. Mattie's Strawberry Lemonade Cupcakes

Serving: 24 | Prep: 10mins | Cook: 19mins | Ready in:

Ingredients

- 1 (15.25 ounce) package classic white cake mix
- 3 large eggs
- 1/2 cup water
- 1/3 cup vegetable oil
- 1/2 cup strawberry jam
- 2 teaspoons lemon juice
- 1 (16 ounce) container prepared strawberry frosting

Direction

- Preheat the oven to 190°C or 375°F. Line paper liners on 2 dozen muffin cups.
- Use an electric mixer to combine vegetable oil, water, eggs and cake mix in bowl; gradually combine in strawberry jam till completely incorporated into batter. Into batter, whip the lemon juice till smooth. Scoop batter to prepped muffin cups.
- Bake for 19 minutes in prepped oven till an inserted toothpick into the middle gets out clean. Let cupcakes cool for half an hour on wire rack.
- Smear strawberry frosting on every cupcake.

Nutrition Information

- Calories: 215 calories;
- Protein: 1.6
- Total Fat: 10.2
- Sodium: 174
- Total Carbohydrate: 30
- Cholesterol: 23

121. One Bowl Lemon Cupcakes

Serving: 24 | Prep: 20mins | Cook: 15mins | Ready in:

Ingredients

- Dry Ingredients:
- 2 1/8 cups all-purpose flour
- 2 cups white sugar
- 1 1/2 teaspoons baking powder
- 1 1/2 teaspoons baking soda
- 1 teaspoon salt
- Wet Ingredients:
- 1 cup milk
- 2 eggs
- 1/2 cup vegetable oil
- 1 teaspoon vanilla extract
- 1 teaspoon lemon extract
- 1 cup strained fresh lemon juice

Direction

- Preheat an oven to 175°C/350°F; line paper liners on 24 muffin cups.

- Mix salt, baking soda, baking powder, sugar and flour in big mixing bowl; use electric mixer on medium speed to beat lemon extract, vanilla extract, vegetable oil, eggs and milk into dry ingredients for 2 minutes.
- In a small saucepan, boil lemon juice. Beat into the batter immediately using the electric mixer on low speed.
- Use batter to fil cupcake liners to 2/3 full.
- In preheated oven, bake for 15-17 minutes till inserted toothpick in middle exits clean; cool for 10 minutes in pans. Transfer to wire rack; fully cool.

Nutrition Information

- Calories: 160 calories;
- Sodium: 216
- Total Carbohydrate: 26.6
- Cholesterol: 16
- Protein: 2
- Total Fat: 5.3

---

122. Pink Lemonade Cupcakes

Serving: 24 | Prep: 15mins | Cook: 25mins | Ready in:

Ingredients

- Cupcakes:
- 1 (18.25 ounce) package white cake mix
- 3/4 cup frozen pink lemonade concentrate, thawed
- 1/2 cup water
- 1/3 cup vegetable oil
- 4 egg whites
- 4 drops red food coloring, or as desired
- Frosting:
- 4 cups confectioners' sugar
- 1/3 cup butter, softened
- 1/4 cup frozen pink lemonade concentrate, thawed
- 2 drops yellow food coloring, or as desired (optional)

Direction

- Preheat the oven to 175°C or 350 °F. Line paper muffin liners on 2 dozen muffin cups.
- Use an electric mixer to whip 4 drops of red food coloring, egg whites, vegetable oil, water, 3/4 cup of pink lemonade concentrate and white cake mix on low speed in bowl for half a minute. Raise the speed to moderate and whip till batter becomes smooth, for an additional of one minute. Put the batter in prepped muffin cups.
- In prepped oven, let cupcakes bake for 25 minutes, till an inserted toothpick into the middle of one cupcake gets out clean. Turn the cupcakes onto wire racks to fully cool.
- Use an electric mixer to whip yellow food coloring, quarter cup of pink lemonade concentrate, butter and confectioners' sugar in bowl till frosting is the preferred consistency and light. Smear the frosting on cooled cupcakes.

Nutrition Information

- Calories: 246 calories;
- Total Fat: 8
- Sodium: 170
- Total Carbohydrate: 43.2
- Cholesterol: 7
- Protein: 1.6

---

123. Raspberry Lemonade Cupcakes

Serving: 24 | Prep: 20mins | Cook: 15mins | Ready in:

Ingredients

- Cupcakes:
- 1 (18.25 ounce) package white cake mix

- 1 1/4 cups water
- 1 (3 ounce) package lemon-flavored gelatin mix (such as Jell-O®)
- 3 egg whites
- 1/3 cup canola oil
- Filling:
- 2 cups milk
- 1 (3.4 ounce) package cheesecake-flavored pudding mix (such as Jell-O®)
- Frosting:
- 7 cups confectioners' sugar
- 1 cup butter, softened
- 1/2 cup frozen raspberry lemonade concentrate, thawed

Direction

- Preheat the oven to 350°F or 175°C. Use the paper liners to line 24 muffin cups.
- In a bowl, mix the lemon-flavored gelatin mix, canola oil, egg whites, water, and white cake mix using the electric mixer at low speed for 30 seconds. Adjust the speed to medium and whisk the batter for 2 more minutes. Pour the batter into the prepared muffin cups, filling them half-full.
- Let them bake inside the preheated oven for 15 minutes or until the inserted toothpick into the cupcake's center comes out clean. Let the cupcakes cool fully for at least 30 minutes.
- In a bowl, whisk the cheesecake-flavored pudding mix with milk using the electric mixer for 2 minutes until thickened and smooth. Pour the pudding mixture into the pastry bag that has an icing tip fitted into it. Use the icing tip to crack an opening into each cupcake. Squeeze the pudding mixture gently into the cupcake until it starts to swell.
- Use an electric mixer to beat the lemonade concentrate, butter, and confectioners' sugar in a bowl until the frosting has thickened and smooth. Spread the frosting all over the cupcakes.

Nutrition Information

- Calories: 381 calories;
- Total Fat: 13.9
- Sodium: 260
- Total Carbohydrate: 63.1
- Cholesterol: 22
- Protein: 2.7

124. Too Much Lemon Lemon Meringue Cupcakes

Serving: 8 | Prep: 20mins | Cook: 15mins | Ready in:

Ingredients

- 3 1/2 tablespoons butter, softened
- 3 1/4 tablespoons superfine sugar
- 2 large eggs
- 1 cup all-purpose flour
- 3/4 teaspoon baking powder
- 1 dash salt
- 1/2 cup lemon juice
- 2 tablespoons sour cream
- 2 teaspoons finely grated lemon zest
- 1/2 cup lemon curd, divided
- 8 plain meringue cookies

Direction

- Turn the oven to 350°F (175°C) to preheat. Use paper liners to line 8 muffin cups or brush them with oil.
- In a big bowl, mix together sugar and butter; beat until creamy. Add eggs, beat until smooth.
- In a bowl, combine salt, baking powder, and flour. Slowly beat into the butter mixture. Stir lemon zest, sour cream, and lemon juice into the batter.
- Distribute the batter between the prepared muffin cups, filling each until nearly full.
- Put in the preheated oven and bake for 15-18 minutes until a toothpick will come out clean when you insert it into the middle and the edges turn light brown. Let stay in the pan to cool for 30 minutes.

- Put 1 meringue cookie and 1 heaping teaspoon of lemon curd on top of each cupcake.

Nutrition Information

- Calories: 233 calories;
- Total Carbohydrate: 37.9
- Cholesterol: 74
- Protein: 3.7
- Total Fat: 8
- Sodium: 169

Chapter 4: Brownie Cupcake Recipes

***

125. Brownie Cups

Serving: 24 | Prep: 15mins | Cook: 25mins | Ready in:

Ingredients

- 14 tablespoons unsweetened cocoa powder
- 3/4 cup butter, melted
- 3 tablespoons vegetable oil
- 2 cups white sugar
- 3 eggs
- 2 teaspoons vanilla extract
- 1 cup all-purpose flour
- 1 cup chopped walnuts (optional)
- 1 1/2 cups finely crushed animal cracker cookies
- 1/3 cup white sugar
- 6 tablespoons butter, melted

Direction

- Start preheating the oven to 350°F (180°C). Lightly oil 24 muffin cups.
- In a large bowl, use an electric mixer to whisk 2 cups of sugar, oil, 3/4 cup of butter, and cocoa powder until smooth. Add the eggs, 1 egg at a time; only add the next egg once the previous one has combined with the butter mixture. Whisk in the vanilla extract together with the final egg. Stir the flour mixture into the egg mixture until barely blended. Fold in walnuts, stirring just until evenly blended.
- In a bowl, mix 6 tablespoons of butter, 1/3 cup of sugar, and animal cracker crumbs; stir until well-combined. Into the bottom of each prepared muffin cup, press the cracker mixture. Pour the brownie mixture into the muffin cups, filling them up to 3/4 full.
- Bake them for 25-35 minutes in the preheated oven until the toothpick will come out clean once you insert it into the center.

Nutrition Information

- Calories: 270 calories;
- Sodium: 107
- Total Carbohydrate: 31.5
- Cholesterol: 46
- Protein: 3.3
- Total Fat: 15.8

126. Brownie Ice Cream Cones

Serving: 2 dozen. | Prep: 20mins | Cook: 20mins | Ready in:

Ingredients

- 4 ounces German sweet chocolate, chopped
- 1/4 cup butter, cubed
- 3/4 cup sugar
- 2 large eggs
- 1/2 cup all-purpose flour
- 1/2 cup chopped walnuts, optional
- 1 teaspoon vanilla extract
- 24 ice cream cake cones (about 3 inches tall)

- 24 scoops ice cream
- Colored sprinkles

Direction

- Melt butter and chocolate in a microwave, then stir until smooth. Let cool lightly; transfer to a big bowl. Put in eggs and sugar, whisk to thoroughly combine. Fold in vanilla, walnuts (optional) and flour.
- In muffin cups, lay ice cream cones; pour in batter until 1/2 full. Bake for 20-22 minutes at 350 degrees until brownies are set on the surface and a toothpick comes out with moist crumbs when inserting in the middle (make sure to not overbake). Let cool completely.
- Scoop ice cream on top and decorate with sprinkles, then serve.

Nutrition Information

- Calories: 228 calories
- Protein: 4g protein.
- Total Fat: 11g fat (7g saturated fat)
- Sodium: 83mg sodium
- Fiber: 0 fiber
- Total Carbohydrate: 30g carbohydrate (21g sugars
- Cholesterol: 52mg cholesterol

127. Brownie Kiss Cupcakes

Serving: 9 cupcakes. | Prep: 10mins | Cook: 20mins | Ready in:

Ingredients

- 1/3 cup butter, softened
- 1 cup sugar
- 2 eggs
- 1 teaspoon vanilla extract
- 3/4 cup all-purpose flour
- 1/2 cup baking cocoa
- 1/4 teaspoon baking powder
- 1/4 teaspoon salt
- 9 milk chocolate kisses

Direction

- Cream sugar and butter in a big bowl until fluffy and light. Whisk in vanilla and eggs. Mix together salt, baking powder, cocoa, and flour; slowly add to the creamed mixture and stir thoroughly.
- Fill muffin cups lined with foil or paper until 2/3 full. Put in the middle of each with a chocolate kiss with the tip end turning down.
- Bake at 350° until the top of the brownie will spring back when you gently touch it, or about 20-25 minutes.

Nutrition Information

- Calories: 239 calories
- Fiber: 1g fiber)
- Total Carbohydrate: 36g carbohydrate (24g sugars
- Cholesterol: 66mg cholesterol
- Protein: 4g protein.
- Total Fat: 10g fat (5g saturated fat)
- Sodium: 163mg sodium

128. Brownie Tarts

Serving: 2 dozen. | Prep: 20mins | Cook: 30mins | Ready in:

Ingredients

- 1/2 cup butter, softened
- 3 ounces cream cheese, softened
- 1 cup all-purpose flour
- FILLING:
- 1/2 cup semisweet chocolate chips
- 2 tablespoons butter
- 1/2 cup sugar
- 1 large egg, lightly beaten
- 1 teaspoon vanilla extract

- 1/2 cup chopped pecans, optional
- Maraschino cherry halves, optional

Direction

- Start preheating the oven to 350°. Whisk cream cheese and butter until smooth; slowly whisk in flour. Put a cover on and chill in the fridge for 60 minutes until firm enough to shape.
- Split and form the dough into twenty-four 1-inch balls. Evenly press up the sides and onto the bottom of a non-oiled mini-muffin cups. To prepare the filling, melt butter and chocolate chips in a microwave; whisk until smooth. Mix in vanilla, egg, and sugar. Mix in pecans if you want. Scoop into the cups.
- Bake for 30-35 minutes until a toothpick will come out clean when you insert it into the middle. Let cool for 10 minutes in the pans. Transfer onto wire racks to cool. Put cherries on top if you want.

Nutrition Information

- Calories: 110 calories
- Protein: 1g protein.
- Total Fat: 7g fat (4g saturated fat)
- Sodium: 62mg sodium
- Fiber: 0 fiber)
- Total Carbohydrate: 10g carbohydrate (6g sugars
- Cholesterol: 26mg cholesterol

129. Brownie Turtles

Serving: 8 servings. | Prep: 15mins | Cook: 25mins | Ready in:

Ingredients

- 1 package brownie mix (13-inch x 9-inch pan size)
- 1/2 cup chopped pecans
- 32 pecan halves
- 16 butterscotch chips
- Caramel ice cream topping

Direction

- Follow instructions on the package to prepare brownie mix. Add chopped pecans and whisk. Pour batter into 8 miniature muffin cups and 8 regular-size muffin cups, all greased, filling them about 2/3 full.
- Bake at 350 degrees for 10-12 minutes for miniature brownies and 23-25 minutes for regular-size brownies or until a toothpick has moist crumbs when coming out of the brownies (remember not to overbake). Let cool totally in pans on wire racks.
- To make turtle brownies, on 8 dessert platters, arrange one small brownie above one regular-sized brownie to mimic turtle's head and body. Place 4 pecan halves around each body to resemble feet. Attach butterscotch chips to make eyes. Spread caramel topping on top of the turtles.

Nutrition Information

- Calories:
- Total Carbohydrate:
- Cholesterol:
- Protein:
- Total Fat:
- Sodium:
- Fiber:

130. Brownies In A Cone

Serving: 17 servings. | Prep: 10mins | Cook: 25mins | Ready in:

Ingredients

- 1 package fudge brownie mix (13-inch x 9-inch pan size)
- 17 ice cream cake cones (about 3 inches tall)
- 1 cup (6 ounces) semisweet chocolate chips
- 1 tablespoon shortening

- Colored sprinkles

Direction

- Make brownie batter as instructed on the package, use 3 eggs. Put into ice cream cones in muffin cups; use a spoon to pour 3 tablespoons of batter into each cone.
- Bake for 25-30 minutes at 350° or until tops are dry and a toothpick exits clean (don't over bake). Allow to cool thoroughly.
- In a microwave, melt shortening and chocolate chips; mix until smooth. Dip brownies tops into the melted chocolate; let the excess drip off. Garnish with sprinkles.

Nutrition Information

- Calories: 279 calories
- Sodium: 152mg sodium
- Fiber: 2g fiber)
- Total Carbohydrate: 35g carbohydrate (22g sugars
- Cholesterol: 34mg cholesterol
- Protein: 4g protein.
- Total Fat: 15g fat (4g saturated fat)

131. Caramel Blondie Cups

Serving: 10 blondie cups. | Prep: 20mins | Cook: 20mins | Ready in:

Ingredients

- 1 cup packed brown sugar
- 1/2 cup butter, melted
- 1 large egg
- 1 teaspoon vanilla extract
- 1 cup all-purpose flour
- 1 teaspoon baking powder
- 1/4 teaspoon salt
- 1/2 cup chopped pecans
- TOPPING:
- 20 caramels
- 2 tablespoons whole milk
- 2 tablespoons butter
- 1/2 cup semisweet chocolate chips
- 1/4 cup finely chopped pecans

Direction

- Beat the butter and brown sugar in a small bowl until light and fluffy. Whip in vanilla and egg. Mix the salt, baking powder and flour; put to butter mixture slowly. Mix in pecans.
- Scoop batter into muffin cups coated with grease or lined with paper, about 2/3 full. Bake for 20 to 25 mins at 350° or until a toothpick inserted in the middle comes out clean (centers won't rise).
- Over low heat, melt the butter, milk and caramels in a small saucepan; mix until smooth.
- Scatter chocolate chips on top of centers of hot blondies; garnish with caramel mixture. Scatter pecans over. Let cool for 10 minutes prior to taking out from the pan to cool completely on a wire rack. Put in an airtight container to store.

Nutrition Information

- Calories: 418 calories
- Protein: 4g protein.
- Total Fat: 23g fat (10g saturated fat)
- Sodium: 247mg sodium
- Fiber: 2g fiber)
- Total Carbohydrate: 53g carbohydrate (40g sugars
- Cholesterol: 53mg cholesterol

132. Cherry Brownie Cups

Serving: 5 dozen. | Prep: 25mins | Cook: 20mins | Ready in:

Ingredients

- 3/4 cup butter, cubed
- 2 ounces unsweetened chocolate, chopped
- 2 cups sugar
- 4 large eggs
- 1 teaspoon vanilla extract
- 1 cup all-purpose flour
- FUDGE FILLING:
- 3 ounces cream cheese, softened
- 1 teaspoon vanilla extract
- 1/4 cup corn syrup
- 1-1/2 ounces unsweetened chocolate, melted and cooled
- 1 cup confectioners' sugar
- 1 jar (10 ounces) maraschino cherries with stems, drained and patted dry

Direction

- Microwave chocolate and butter to melt. Whisk in sugar until dissolved. Put mixture in a big bowl. Pour in eggs, one at a time and beat thoroughly between additions. Mix in vanilla. Slowly mix in flour and stir thoroughly.
- Line mini muffin cups with paper liners and pour in batter to 2/3 full. Bake in 350-degree oven until a toothpick exits clean when inserted into a muffin's center, about 20 to 22 minutes. Allow to cool for 5 minutes.
- Indent the top of each brownie, about 1/2 inch using the end of a wooden spoon handle; take brownies out of the pan and place onto a wire rack until fully cool.
- To make the filling, beat vanilla and cream cheese in a big bowl until smooth. Mix in melted chocolate and corn syrup until fully combined. Beat in confectioners' sugar until smooth. Place a teaspoon of filling into the center of each indented brownie. Place a cherry on top. Keep refrigerated to store.

Nutrition Information

- Calories: 172 calories
- Total Fat: 7g fat (4g saturated fat)
- Sodium: 67mg sodium
- Fiber: 0 fiber
- Total Carbohydrate: 27g carbohydrate (22g sugars
- Cholesterol: 44mg cholesterol
- Protein: 2g protein.

133. Chocolate Cherry Brownie Cups

Serving: 1-1/2 dozen. | Prep: 15mins | Cook: 20mins | Ready in:

Ingredients

- 1 cup butter
- 4 ounces semisweet chocolate, chopped
- 4 eggs
- 1-1/2 cups sugar
- 1 teaspoon vanilla extract
- 1 cup all-purpose flour
- 1-1/2 cups chopped walnuts
- 3/4 cup chopped maraschino cherries

Direction

- In a microwave, melt chocolate and butter; mix until smooth.
- Let cool 10 minutes.
- In a large bowl, beat sugar and eggs until incorporated. Beat in the chocolate mixture and vanilla. Add the flour. Mix in cherries and walnuts.
- Fill three-fourths of paper-lined muffin cups with the batter. Bake for 20-25 minutes at 350° or until tested done with a toothpick. Let cool for 5 minutes before transferring from pans to wire racks.

Nutrition Information

- Calories: 282 calories
- Cholesterol: 74mg cholesterol
- Protein: 5g protein.
- Total Fat: 18g fat (7g saturated fat)

- Sodium: 122mg sodium
- Fiber: 1g fiber)
- Total Carbohydrate: 28g carbohydrate (19g sugars

134. Chocolate Hazelnut Brownie Bites

Serving: 3 dozen. | Prep: 25mins | Cook: 20mins | Ready in:

Ingredients

- 1 package (11-1/2 ounces) milk chocolate chips, divided
- 5 tablespoons butter
- 2 eggs, lightly beaten
- 1/3 cup packed brown sugar
- 1 teaspoon vanilla extract
- 1-1/4 cups ground hazelnuts, toasted
- 1/2 cup all-purpose flour
- 1 teaspoon baking powder
- 1/8 teaspoon salt
- TOPPING:
- 3/4 cup Nutella
- 36 whole blanched hazelnuts, toasted

Direction

- Dissolve butter and 1 cup chocolate chips in a microwave; mix until smooth. Whisk brown sugar and eggs in a large bowl. Mix in vanilla. Mix in a small bowl the salt, baking powder, flour and ground hazelnuts; slowly stir to chocolate mixture. Add in remaining chips then fold.
- Then stuff mini muffin cups lined with paper, three-fourths full. Bake in the oven for 18-22 minutes at 350°F or until a toothpick pricked in the middle comes out clean. Fully cool. Then spread with Nutella; place a hazelnut on each top.

Nutrition Information

- Calories: 134 calories
- Protein: 2g protein. Diabetic Exchanges: 1-1/2 fat
- Total Fat: 9g fat (3g saturated fat)
- Sodium: 45mg sodium
- Fiber: 1g fiber)
- Total Carbohydrate: 13g carbohydrate (10g sugars
- Cholesterol: 18mg cholesterol

135. Coconut Almond Fudge Cups

Serving: 4 dozen. | Prep: 30mins | Cook: 10mins | Ready in:

Ingredients

- 1 package chocolate fudge cake mix (regular size)
- 1/2 cup butter, melted
- 1 large egg
- FILLING:
- 1/4 cup sugar
- 1/4 cup evaporated milk
- 7 large marshmallows
- 1 cup sweetened shredded coconut
- TOPPING:
- 3/4 cup semisweet chocolate chips
- 1/4 cup evaporated milk
- 2 tablespoons butter
- 1/2 cup sliced almonds

Direction

- Whisk egg, butter and cake mix in a large bowl until thoroughly blended. Roll the mixture into 1" balls and arrange on miniature muffin cups lined with foil. Bake for 8 minutes at 350 degrees.
- Dig a 1/2" deep hollow in the middle of each cup using the end of a wooden spoon handle. Bake for another 2-3 minutes or until cake is slightly springy to the touch. Take out of pans and let cool on wire racks.

- In a microwave-safe bowl, heat milk and sugar, stirring often for 2 minutes on high to make fillings. Put in marshmallows and whisk until they melt. Mix in coconut. Pour the mixture into cooled cups.
- In another microwave-safe bowl, mix together butter, milk and chocolate chips to make topping. Melt the mixture in 10 to 20 second intervals in the microwave, then stir until it becomes smooth. Mix in almonds. Spread on top of the filling. Place in a fridge to store.

Nutrition Information

- Calories: 104 calories
- Protein: 1g protein. Diabetic Exchanges: 1 starch
- Total Fat: 5g fat (3g saturated fat)
- Sodium: 107mg sodium
- Fiber: 1g fiber)
- Total Carbohydrate: 14g carbohydrate (9g sugars
- Cholesterol: 12mg cholesterol

136. Cupcake Brownies

Serving: about 1-1/2 dozen. | Prep: 15mins | Cook: 20mins | Ready in:

Ingredients

- 1 cup butter, cubed
- 4 ounces semisweet chocolate
- 4 eggs
- 1-3/4 cups sugar
- 1 teaspoon vanilla extract
- 1 cup all-purpose flour
- 1-1/2 cups chopped pecans

Direction

- Microwave chocolate and butter until melted; whisk until smooth. Allow to cool for 10 minutes.
- Blend sugar and eggs in a big bowl until incorporated. Mix in chocolate mixture and vanilla; slowly whisk in nuts and flour.
- Prepare muffin cups by greasing or lining with paper; pour batter into each cup to 2/3 full. Bake in 350-degree oven until a toothpick comes out clean when pierced into a muffin's center, about 18 – 20 minutes. Allow to cool.

Nutrition Information

- Calories: 283 calories
- Fiber: 1g fiber)
- Total Carbohydrate: 27g carbohydrate (20g sugars
- Cholesterol: 74mg cholesterol
- Protein: 3g protein.
- Total Fat: 19g fat (8g saturated fat)
- Sodium: 117mg sodium

137. Frosted Walnut Brownie Cups

Serving: 32 brownie cups. | Prep: 30mins | Cook: 20mins | Ready in:

Ingredients

- 2 cups (12 ounces) semisweet chocolate chips
- 1 cup butter, cubed
- 1-1/3 cups sugar
- 4 large eggs
- 2 teaspoons vanilla extract
- 1 cup all-purpose flour
- 1 cup chopped walnuts
- GANACHE:
- 2 cups (12 ounces) semisweet chocolate chips
- 3/4 cup heavy whipping cream

Direction

- In a microwave, melt together butter and chocolate chips; whisk till smooth. Allow to slightly cool down.

- In a large bowl, beat together eggs and sugar. Mix in chocolate mixture and vanilla. Add flour slowly; mix in walnuts. Fill the mixture almost full into miniature muffin cups lined with paper.
- Bake for 20-23 minutes at 350° until tested done with a toothpick. Allow to cool for 5 minutes before transferring from pans to wire racks to let cool fully.
- In a small bowl, add chocolate chips. In a small saucepan, heat cream until just boiling. Add on top of chocolate; whisk till smooth. Let cool for 30 minutes or until ganache is spreadable, stirring sometimes. Spread on top of brownies.

Nutrition Information

- Calories: 353 calories
- Total Carbohydrate: 39g carbohydrate (32g sugars
- Cholesterol: 49mg cholesterol
- Protein: 4g protein.
- Total Fat: 24g fat (13g saturated fat)
- Sodium: 56mg sodium
- Fiber: 3g fiber)

---

138. Mint Brownie Cheesecake Cups

Serving: 2-1/2 dozen. | Prep: 20mins | Cook: 25mins | Ready in:

Ingredients

- 1/2 cup crushed chocolate cream-filled chocolate sandwich cookies (about 7 cookies)
- 1 package (4.67 ounces) Andes mint candies or 1 cup Andes creme de menthe baking chips
- 1 package (8 ounces) cream cheese, softened
- 1/4 cup sugar
- 1 egg
- 1/2 teaspoon vanilla extract
- Additional Andes mint candies or Andes creme de menthe baking chips, melted

Direction

- Line or grease miniature muffin cups. Put 1 tsp. of cookie crumbs onto each muffin cup bottom, and then set it aside.
- For 30 seconds to 1 minute, heat the candies in a microwave-safe bowl, mixing it every 15 seconds, until it's completely melted. Let it cool to room temperature.
- Mix, until smooth, sugar and cream cheese in a small bowl. Stir in vanilla and egg. Mix the melted candies in.
- In each muffin cup, put 1 tbsp. of the mixture. Let it bake at 350°F 25 to 30 minutes until each top begins to crack and looks dry. Let muffins rest for about 60 seconds before removing from pan and putting them on wire racks to completely cooling. Sprinkle some more melted candies before storing in the fridge.

Nutrition Information

- Calories: 67 calories
- Sodium: 35mg sodium
- Fiber: 0 fiber)
- Total Carbohydrate: 6g carbohydrate (5g sugars
- Cholesterol: 14mg cholesterol
- Protein: 1g protein.
- Total Fat: 5g fat (3g saturated fat)

---

139. Peanut Butter Brownie

Serving: 2 dozen. | Prep: 30mins | Cook: 15mins | Ready in:

Ingredients

- 1/2 cup peanut butter
- 1/4 cup packed brown sugar
- 2 tablespoons plus 1-1/2 cups all-purpose flour, divided

- 3 ounces unsweetened chocolate, chopped
- 1/2 cup butter, cubed
- 3 eggs
- 1-1/2 cups sugar
- 2 tablespoons water
- 1 teaspoon vanilla extract
- 1 teaspoon baking powder

Direction

- In a small bowl, beat 2 tablespoons flour, brown sugar and peanut butter together until incorporated; put aside.
- In a microwave-safe bowl, melt butter and chocolate; mix until smooth; allow to cool down slightly. In a large bowl, beat together the water, sugar and eggs; mix in vanilla and chocolate mixture. Combine the remaining flour and baking powder; add to chocolate mixture slowly.
- Fill one-fourth of paper-lined muffin cups with the batter. Place about 1 teaspoon of peanut butter mixture on top of each cup. Spoon the rest of the batter on top. Bake for 13-15 minutes at 350° or until their centers set (be careful not to overbake). Let cool for 5 minutes before transferring from pans to wire racks.

Nutrition Information

- Calories: 169 calories
- Total Carbohydrate: 23g carbohydrate (15g sugars
- Cholesterol: 37mg cholesterol
- Protein: 3g protein.
- Total Fat: 8g fat (3g saturated fat)
- Sodium: 89mg sodium
- Fiber: 1g fiber)

140. Peanut Butter Brownie Bites

Serving: 3-1/2 dozen. | Prep: 20mins | Cook: 20mins | Ready in:

Ingredients

- 1 package fudge brownie mix (13x9-inch pan size)
- Frosting:
- 1/2 cup creamy peanut butter
- 3 ounces cream cheese, softened
- 2 cups confectioners' sugar
- 4 teaspoons 2% milk
- 1 teaspoon vanilla extract
- Chopped salted peanuts, optional

Direction

- Start preheating the oven to 350°. Use foil or paper liners to line the 42 mini-muffin cups.
- For the brownie mix batter, prepare it by following the package instructions. Fill the prepared cups until 2/3 full. Bake until a toothpick will come out clean once you insert it into the center, about 18-22 minutes (make sure not to overbake it).
- Put the pans on wire racks. In the middle of each brownie, make a 1/2-inch deep indentation using the end of a wooden spoon handle. Let them cool for 10 minutes, and then take them out from the pans.
- To prepare the frosting, whisk cream cheese and peanut butter in a large bowl until combined. Slowly whisk in vanilla, milk, and confectioners' sugar until smooth. Pipe or spoon the frosting into the indentations. If you want, sprinkle chopped peanuts over. Chill any leftovers.

Nutrition Information

- Calories:
- Total Fat:
- Sodium:
- Fiber:
- Total Carbohydrate:
- Cholesterol:
- Protein:

141. Peanut Butter Brownie Cups

Serving: about 1-1/2 dozen. | Prep: 20mins | Cook: 20mins | Ready in:

Ingredients

- 1 package (21-1/2 ounces) fudge brownie mix
- 15 to 18 miniature peanut butter cups

Direction

- Mix brownie batter as instructed on the package. Fill two-thirds full into muffin cups lined with paper or foil.
- Take wrappers off of peanut butter cups; place one into each muffin cup and push down until the batter reaches the candy's top edge. Bake for 20-25 minutes at 350°. Allow to cool for 5 minutes in the pan before taking out to a wire rack to cool thoroughly.

Nutrition Information

- Calories:
- Total Fat:
- Sodium:
- Fiber:
- Total Carbohydrate:
- Cholesterol:
- Protein:

142. Peppermint Brownie Cups

Serving: 4 dozen. | Prep: 40mins | Cook: 15mins | Ready in:

Ingredients

- 1 cup butter, cubed
- 1 cup plus 3 tablespoons milk chocolate chips
- 3 ounces unsweetened chocolate, chopped
- 3 large eggs
- 1-1/4 cups sugar
- 1 tablespoon instant coffee granules
- 2 teaspoons vanilla extract
- 1/2 teaspoon peppermint extract
- 2/3 cup all-purpose flour
- 1-1/2 teaspoons baking powder
- 1/2 teaspoon salt
- FROSTING:
- 1-1/2 cups confectioners' sugar
- 1 cup butter, softened
- 1 teaspoon peppermint extract
- 1 jar (7 ounces) marshmallow creme
- Peppermint crunch baking chips

Direction

- Set oven to 350° to preheat. Line 48 mini-muffin tins with foil or paper liners.
- Melt unsweetened chocolate, chocolate chips and butter in a metal bowl over simmering water; mix until smooth. Let cool slightly.
- Whip coffee granules, sugar and eggs in a big bowl until combined. Mix in chocolate mixture and extracts. Whip salt, baking powder and flour in the other bowl; put to chocolate mixture gradually, stirring well.
- Put batter in lined cups 3/4 full. Bake until a toothpick inserted in the middle comes out clean, 12-14 minutes (don't overbake). Let cool in pans 5 minutes before taking out to wire racks to cool completely.
- To make the frosting, whip extract, butter and confectioners' sugar in a small bowl until smooth. Fold in marshmallow creme. Spread or pipe frosting on top of brownie cups; garnish with peppermint baking chips.

Nutrition Information

- Calories: 160 calories
- Sodium: 116mg sodium
- Fiber: 0 fiber)
- Total Carbohydrate: 17g carbohydrate (14g sugars
- Cholesterol: 33mg cholesterol
- Protein: 1g protein.

- Total Fat: 10g fat (6g saturated fat)

Chapter 5: Cake Mix Cupcake Recipes

***

---
143. Apple Upside Down Cakes

Serving: 12 | Prep: 12mins | Cook: 22mins | Ready in:

Ingredients

- 1 cup Marzetti's® Old Fashioned Caramel Dip
- 4 Golden Delicious apples, peeled, cored, and sliced into 1/2-inch pieces
- 1/2 teaspoon ground cinnamon
- 2 tablespoons water
- 1 (18.25 ounce) package spice cake mix
- 1 (3.4 ounce) package instant vanilla pudding mix
- 1/4 cup vegetable oil
- 1/4 cup sour cream
- 4 large eggs

Direction

- To preheat: Set oven to 350°F. Grease 2 large six-cup muffin tins.
- Mix water, cinnamon, and apples in a microwave safe bowl then microwave for 3 to 4 minutes. The apples should become slightly soft. Drain apples then toss with a cup of Marzetti Old Fashioned Caramel Dip.
- Put the same amount of apples into each cup.
- Put eggs, sour cream, oil, pudding, cake mix in a large bowl and mix on medium speed till the mixture becomes smooth. Spoon the batter evenly over apples.
- Put into the oven and bake for 15 to 18 minutes till you get a clean toothpick after inserting it into the center of each cake.
- Allow cakes to cool for 8 minutes. Turn pan upside down. A couple of apple slices may need to be placed back into their positions. Let cakes cool.
- Put the remaining Marzetti Old Fashioned Caramel Dip in a microwave safe container then microwave for 10 to 30 seconds, remember stir every 10 seconds. Spoon the warm caramel over cakes. Serve cakes with ice cream or whipped cream.

Nutrition Information

- Calories: 401 calories;
- Cholesterol: 67
- Protein: 5
- Total Fat: 16.6
- Sodium: 481
- Total Carbohydrate: 59.6

---
144. Autumn Harvest Cupcakes

Serving: 21 | Prep: 30mins | Cook: 1hours | Ready in:

Ingredients

- 1 (18.25 ounce) package white cake mix (with pudding)
- 1 (15 ounce) can pumpkin puree
- 1 cup Mott's® Natural Applesauce
- 1 teaspoon ground cinnamon
- 1/2 teaspoon ground nutmeg
- 1/2 teaspoon ground ginger
- 1/4 teaspoon ground cloves
- 1/4 teaspoon ground allspice
- Frosting:
- 1 (8 ounce) package cream cheese, room temperature
- 4 tablespoons butter, room temperature
- 1 1/2 teaspoons vanilla extract

- 3 cups confectioners' sugar
- 1 vanilla bean, seeds removed and set aside
- Candy:
- 1 1/2 cups white sugar
- 1/2 cup water
- 1/2 cup Mott's® Natural Applesauce
- 1/4 teaspoon cinnamon
- 1 pinch nutmeg
- 1/4 cup confectioners' sugar
- 2 tablespoons chopped pecans (optional)

Direction

- Set an oven to 175°C (350°F) and started preheating. Use paper liners to prepare the cupcake pans.
- In a large bowl, mix 1/4 teaspoon of ground allspice, 1/4 teaspoon of ground cloves, 1/2 teaspoon of ground ginger, 1/2 teaspoon of ground nutmeg, a teaspoon of ground cinnamon, applesauce, pumpkin and cake mix. Mix with an electric mixer until the thick cake batter is formed.
- Distribute into each prepared cupcake tins with 2 tablespoons for each. Bake until the tops start to brown and a toothpick comes out clean for 15 to 20 minutes.
- For frosting: Whip the butter and cream cheese using an electric mixer fitted with a whisk attachment until mixed thoroughly and scrape the sides the bowl as needed. Add vanilla, then whip until it is incorporated.
- Add 3 cups of powdered sugar, one cup at a time, whipping the frosting to incorporate each cup fully before adding the next. Add the vanilla seeds and whip one last time. Spread or pipe onto cupcakes.
- For candy, use aluminum foil to line a baking sheet. If desired, scatter with pecan pieces and powdered sugar.
- Mix nutmeg, cinnamon, Mott's® Natural Applesauce, water and sugar into a large saucepan. Heat until the mixture begins to boil on medium heat. Stir frequently until candy audibly crackles when they are dropped into a cup of cold water or the candy achieves the hard-crack phase (a candy thermometer reach 300 degrees F).
- Pour on the pecan pieces and powdered sugar with the prepared candy. Let it cool completely and harden, then break into pieces. Scatter over the frosted cupcakes.

Nutrition Information

- Calories: 313 calories;
- Total Fat: 9.2
- Sodium: 258
- Total Carbohydrate: 57.1
- Cholesterol: 18
- Protein: 2.2

145. Brownie Batter + Cupcake = The SECOND BEST Cupcake. Ever

Serving: 48 | Prep: 10mins | Cook: 40mins | Ready in:

Ingredients

- 1 (19.5 ounce) package brownie mix
- 2 eggs
- 1/2 cup canola oil
- 1/4 cup water
- 1 (18.25 ounce) package white cake mix
- 2 tablespoons canola oil
- 1 1/3 cups water
- 3 egg whites

Direction

- Set the oven to 350°F (175°C), and start preheating. Line paper liners on 48 muffin cups.
- In a bowl, whisk 1/4 cup water, 1/2 cup canola oil, 2 eggs and brownie mix together. Stir just until fully blended, about 50 strokes; put aside.
- In a large bowl, combine 3 egg whites, 1 1/3 cup water, 2 tablespoon canola oil and cake

mix together with an electric mixer on low speed until blended. Mix for 2 minutes on medium speed.
- Spoon the brownie batter into prepped muffin cups, filling 1/3 of each cup. Spoon the cake batter over the brownie batter, till each muffin cup is 2/3 full.
- Bake in the preheated oven for about 20 minutes, until golden and the tops spring back if pressed lightly.

Nutrition Information

- Calories: 125 calories;
- Total Fat: 6
- Sodium: 112
- Total Carbohydrate: 17.2
- Cholesterol: 8
- Protein: 1.4

146. Cake In A Mug

Serving: 8 | Prep: | Cook: |Ready in:

Ingredients

- 1 (18.25 ounce) package yellow cake mix
- 1 (3.4 ounce) package instant vanilla pudding mix
- 2 2/3 cups confectioners' sugar
- 1/4 cup powdered lemonade mix

Direction

- To be sure each one can hold 1 1/2 cups of water, check your coffee mugs.
- Whisk dry pudding mix and dry cake mix to blend well in a big bowl; this makes 4-4 1/2 cups dry mix that creates 8 coffee cup cake mixes. To 8 small plastic bags, divide mix, 1/2 cup each. Put mix in corner of every bag; use a twist tie to tie it there.
- Glaze mix: Mix powdered flavoring mix and confectioners' sugar in a medium bowl. Divide to 8 small plastic bags; use a twist tie to close bag. Attach every glaze mix to cake mix bags along with a twist tie. Put one of every bag into every cup.
- To each cup, attach the following instructions: Spray cooking spray inside of cup generously. Empty cake mix packet's contents in cup. Add 1 tbsp. water, 1 tbsp. oil and 1 egg to dry mix; mix, mixing in all the dry mix carefully, for 15 seconds. Microwave for 2 minutes on full powder. Put ingredients from the glaze mix into very small container as cake cooks; add 1 1/2 tsp. water then stir well. Put glaze on cake in cup when cake is done; eat while warm.

Nutrition Information

- Calories: 504 calories;
- Protein: 2.8
- Total Fat: 7.6
- Sodium: 598
- Total Carbohydrate: 108.1
- Cholesterol: 1

147. Classic Red Velvet Cupcakes

Serving: 24 | Prep: 15mins | Cook: 20mins |Ready in:

Ingredients

- 1 package Duncan Hines® Red Velvet Cake Mix
- 1 1/4 cups water
- 1/3 cup vegetable oil
- 3 large eggs
- 1 (16 ounce) container Duncan Hines® Creamy Home-Style Cream Cheese Frosting
- Sprinkles or additional garnishes

Direction

- Preheat the oven to 350°F. Oil or line muffin pans using paper baking cups.

- In big bowl, combine eggs, oil, water and dry mix on low speed to moisten, for half a minute. Whip for 2 minutes at moderate speed. Scoop batter to paper cups or muffin pan.
- Let cupcakes bake for 19 to 22 minutes. Extend baking time 3 to 5 minutes for coated or dark pans. Once an inserted toothpick in middle gets out clean, cupcakes are done.
- Cool for 15 minutes in pan on the wire rack. Cool fully prior to frosting.
- Decorate and serve.

Nutrition Information

- Calories: 203 calories;
- Total Fat: 9
- Sodium: 177
- Total Carbohydrate: 30.2
- Cholesterol: 23
- Protein: 1.8

148. Filled Cupcakes With Cherry Flavored Filled DelightFulls™

Serving: 24 | Prep: 1hours | Cook: 18mins | Ready in:

Ingredients

- 1 (16.5 ounce) package white cake mix
- 1 1/4 cups water*
- 1/3 cup vegetable oil*
- 4 egg whites*
- 7 cups powdered sugar
- 1 cup butter, softened
- 2 tablespoons milk, or as needed
- 3/4 teaspoon vanilla extract
- 1 cup NESTLE® TOLL HOUSE® Delightfulls Cherry Flavored Morsels, coarsely chopped, divided

Direction

- Preheat the oven to 350°F. Line 2 dozen of muffin cups with paper.
- Prep cake batter following packaging instructions. Scoop to prepped cups of muffins. Bake as instructed or till inserted wooden pick into cupcakes gets out with no crumbs. Cool for 5 minutes in pans; transfer to wire racks for full cooling.
- In big mixer bowl, whip vanilla extract, 2 tablespoons milk, butter and powdered sugar till fluffy and light. If necessary, put one more tablespoon of milk. Transfer a cup of frosting into a small bowl. Mix half cup of chopped DelightFulls morsels in. Scoop mixture of filling in pastry bag equipped with big pastry tip or in storage bag for food with half-inch cut from corner of the bag.
- Use a sharp knife to cut a one-inch round and one-inch deep from every cupcake. Cautiously take pieces of cake and reserve for other use like crumbling on top of ice cream. Pipe mixture of filling in every cupcake. Filling must be even with cupcake top.
- Use leftover frosting in bowl to frost the cupcakes. Scatter leftover half cup of chopped DelightFulls morsels on cupcakes.

Nutrition Information

- Calories: 377 calories;
- Sodium: 196
- Total Carbohydrate: 51.6
- Cholesterol: 20
- Protein: 1.6
- Total Fat: 15.9

149. Frog Cupcakes

Serving: 24 | Prep: 25mins | Cook: 20mins | Ready in:

Ingredients

- 1 (18.25 ounce) package white cake mix
- 1 (16 ounce) can prepared vanilla frosting

- 6 drops green food coloring, or as needed
- 1/4 cup green decorator sugar
- 12 large marshmallows
- 48 semisweet chocolate chips
- 1 drop red food coloring

Direction

- Bake cupcakes as directed on the package. Let cool completely.
- Spoon 2/3 of the frosting into a small bowl; combine with green food coloring. Frost the cupcakes. Top with some green sugar.
- Cut marshmallows in 1/2 to create 2 circles. Coat each marshmallow piece with water, then dunk into green sugar to make eyelids. The rest of white will be eyes. Put on the cupcakes. Attach a chocolate chip into each eye's center with a little bit of white icing for the pupil.
- Combine the rest of frosting with red food coloring to create pink color. Draw smiling mouths and nostrils or tongues on the frogs with pink icing.

Nutrition Information

- Calories: 342 calories;
- Total Carbohydrate: 54.5
- Cholesterol: 0
- Protein: 2.4
- Total Fat: 15
- Sodium: 182

150. Grad Cupcakes

Serving: 24 | Prep: 1hours | Cook: 20mins | Ready in:

Ingredients

- 1 (18.25 ounce) package white cake mix
- 1 cup water
- 3 eggs
- 1/3 cup vegetable oil
- 12 graham crackers
- 1 (16 ounce) container white buttercream frosting
- 1 drop food coloring in school colors, or as desired
- 6 chewy lemon candy squares (such as Starburst®), or as needed
- 24 candy-coated milk chocolate pieces (such as M&M's®) in school colors

Direction

- Preheat an oven to 175°C/350°F.
- Line paper cupcake liners that are in school colors on 24 muffin cups.
- Put white cake mix into big mixing bowl; beat in vegetable oil, eggs and water with electric mixer at low speed till just moist. Put mixer speed on medium; beat it for 2 minutes.
- Put batter in prepped muffin cups; fill to 2/3 full.
- In preheated oven, bake cupcakes for 18-22 minutes till inserted toothpick in middle of cupcake exits clean.
- Thoroughly cool cupcakes; put cupcakes, bottom sides facing up, onto platter.
- Decorate cupcakes: To get 24 2 1/2-in. squares, break the graham crackers in half. Put frosting dab centered on bottom of every cupcake; stick square to frosting to make graduation's cap mortarboard part.
- Put opened frosting container into microwave oven; heat for 10 seconds till frosting is workable, soft and warmed. Should be smooth yet not runny. Use food coloring to color frosting as desired.
- Frost sides and top of graham cracker squares.
- Unwrap the lemon candies; put 2 candies onto waxed paper piece. Microwave candies as needed or for 5 seconds till soft and warm.
- Roll candies out to make thin candy squares on waxed paper; cut small tassel shapes with small scissors or sharp knife from each square. Put aside when tassels are made; microwave 2 extra candies. Repeat steps till you get 24 small candy tassels.
- Put tassel in middle of every graham cracker

square; tassel should slightly hang on square's edge.
- Dip candy-coated chocolate piece's marked side into frosting; put piece into middle of graham cracker square with frosted side up so end of candy tassel string is covered.
- To set frosting, refrigerate decorated cupcakes; keep covered.

Nutrition Information

- Calories: 228 calories;
- Total Carbohydrate: 33.6
- Cholesterol: 23
- Protein: 2
- Total Fat: 9.6
- Sodium: 207

151.   Ice Cream Cone Treats

Serving: 30 | Prep: | Cook: | Ready in:

Ingredients

- 1 (18.25 ounce) package yellow cake mix
- 1 (16 ounce) package vanilla frosting
- 1 ounce colored candy sprinkles

Direction

- Following package directions to prepare cake mix batter or you can make any basic cake recipe batter such as white, chocolate, etc.
- Put in the cups of a regular muffin pan with flat-bottomed ice cream cones, then fill into each cone with enough amount of batter, until 1/2 to 2/3 full.
- Following the recommended baking temperature and time for cupcakes to bake. After they are cooled, use you preferred canned or home-prepped frosting to frost your cupcakes. Use sprinkles or other decorations of your choice to garnish.

Nutrition Information

- Calories: 143 calories;
- Sodium: 142
- Total Carbohydrate: 24.6
- Cholesterol: < 1
- Protein: 0.8
- Total Fat: 4.7

152.   Maharani Cupcakes

Serving: 24 | Prep: 30mins | Cook: 20mins | Ready in:

Ingredients

- Sweet Basil Cream:
- 1 1/2 cups heavy whipping cream
- 1 bunch fresh basil, washed and dried
- Sweet Curry Lemon Curd:
- 1 cup white sugar
- 2 eggs, lightly beaten
- 2 tablespoons mild curry powder
- 3/4 cup fresh lemon juice
- 3 lemons, zested
- 1/4 cup unsalted butter, melted
- Coconut Cupcakes:
- 1 (18.25 ounce) package white cake mix
- 1 cup sweetened flaked coconut
- 1 1/4 cups water
- 3 eggs
- 1/3 cup vegetable oil
- 2 tablespoons coconut extract
- 6 cups confectioners' sugar, divided
- 1/2 (8 ounce) package cream cheese, room temperature
- 1 tablespoon silver dragees decorating candy

Direction

- In a saucepan, heat whipping cream until hot but not boiling to make the sweet basil cream; take off heat. Steep basil with stems and all for an hour in the heated cream. Chill for 3hrs or overnight. Filter then remove the basil.

- In the meantime, prepare the sweet curry lemon curd. Cook curd in a big microwaveable bowl, it will expand to twice its size while cooking. Combine curry powder, 2 eggs, and white sugar until smooth. Mix in butter, lemon zest, and lemon juice. Microwave while mixing at 1min intervals until thick enough to cover the back of a metal spoon. Sieve the cooked curd then chill for at least 3hrs or until set. The mixture will be soft like a pudding.
- Preheat the oven to 175°C or 350°Fahrenheit. Line cupcake liners into 24 muffin cups.
- In a mixing bowl, mix coconut flakes and white cake mix. Mix in coconut extract, water, vegetable oil, and 3 eggs. To produce a very light texture, separate the yolks and whites. Whisk the egg whites until it forms into medium-stiff peaks; fold into the cake batter.
- Spoon the cake batter into the lined cups until 2/3 full. Bake for 20mins in the preheated oven until golden brown on the edges and an inserted toothpick in the middle comes out without residue. Completely cool the cupcakes.
- Whip three cups confectioners' sugar and the cold basil-infused cream in a chilled bowl until it forms into stiff peaks; chill. Whisk the remaining three cups confectioners' sugar and cream cheese until soft and smooth. Fold in whipped cream and gently stir until well blended.
- Slather 1tbsp of lemon curd over each cupcake then a dollop of basil cream on top to decorate. Top with dragees.

Nutrition Information

- Calories: 393 calories;
- Sodium: 193
- Total Carbohydrate: 60
- Cholesterol: 65
- Protein: 3.1
- Total Fat: 16.3

153. Margarita Cupcakes

Serving: 24 | Prep: 15mins | Cook: 30mins | Ready in:

Ingredients

- 1 (15.25 ounce) package yellow cake mix (such as Betty Crocker®)
- 1/2 cup butter, melted
- 3 eggs
- 1/2 cup lime margarita mix (such as Jose Cuervo®)
- 1 egg yolk
- 3/4 cup lemon-lime soda
- 1 1/2 (1.5 fluid ounce) jiggers tequila (such as Jose Cuervo®)

Direction

- Preheat an oven to 165°C/325°F; line paper liners on muffin cups.
- Mix butter and cake mix in a big bowl. Add egg yolks, margarita mix and eggs; mix till combined. Put lemon-lime soda in batter; mix till foam melts. Mix tequila into batter; put batter in prepped muffin cups.
- In the preheated oven, bake for 30 minutes till inserted toothpick in middle exits clean.

Nutrition Information

- Calories: 136 calories;
- Total Carbohydrate: 16
- Cholesterol: 42
- Protein: 1.7
- Total Fat: 6.7
- Sodium: 159

154. PHILLY Blackforest Stuffed Cupcakes

Serving: 24 | Prep: 10mins | Cook: | Ready in:

Ingredients

- 1 (18.25 ounce) package chocolate cake mix
- 1 (250 g) package PHILADELPHIA Brick Cream Cheese, softened
- 1 egg
- 2 tablespoons sugar
- 1 (19 ounce) can cherry pie filling
- 1 1/2 cups thawed COOL WHIP Whipped Topping

Direction

- Set an oven to heat to 350°F. Prepare the cake batter as instructed on the package for the low-fat or light version, then put aside. Combine the sugar, egg and cream cheese, until well combined.
- For the garnish, take off 3/4 cup of the cherry pie filling, then put aside. Scoop 2 tbsp. of the cake batter on each of the 24 medium muffin cups lined with paper. Put 1 tbsp. of leftover cherry pie filling and 1 tbsp. of the cream cheese mixture on top of each, then use the leftover cake batter to evenly cover.
- Let it bake for 20-25 minutes or until an inserted toothpick in the middle exits clean. Allow to cool for 5 minutes, then take it out from the pan and transfer to wire racks. Let it fully cool. Just prior to serving, put the reserved cherry pie filling and whipped topping on top.

Nutrition Information

- Calories: 167 calories;
- Total Fat: 7.3
- Sodium: 227
- Total Carbohydrate: 24.6
- Cholesterol: 20
- Protein: 2.3

155. Pineapple Upside Down Cupcakes

Serving: 12 | Prep: 15mins | Cook: 15mins | Ready in:

Ingredients

- 1 (15.25 ounce) package yellow cake mix
- 1 cup water
- 1/2 cup vegetable oil
- 3 eggs
- 1 (12.5 ounce) can pineapple tidbits in juice, drained and juice reserved
- 1 cup brown sugar, or as needed
- 1/2 cup butter, melted
- 1 (16.5 ounce) can pitted cherries, drained (optional)

Direction

- First, preheat your oven to 350 degrees F (175 degrees C). Prepare lightly oiled cupcake cups or use a cupcake liners lined with parchment paper.
- In a mixing bowl, combine eggs, cake mix, oil and water. Beat altogether using an electric blender for 30 seconds set in low speed. Beat for another 2 minutes increasing to medium speed. Add in prepared pineapple juice into the cake mixture and beat well until combined.
- Drizzle some brown sugar in each cupcake cups and pour butter into it. Put pineapple tidbits and 1 cherry on top of the brown sugar mixture. Add the cake mixture into the pineapple tidbits.
- Cook the cupcake for about 15 to 20 minutes using the preheated oven until it reaches a yellow brown color or when surface bounces back when lightly touched.

Nutrition Information

- Calories: 430 calories;
- Cholesterol: 68
- Protein: 3.7
- Total Fat: 22.2
- Sodium: 316
- Total Carbohydrate: 56.2

156. Rainbow Cupcake Cones

Serving: 24 | Prep: 20mins | Cook: 20mins | Ready in:

Ingredients

- 1 (18.25 ounce) package white cake mix
- 1 cup water
- 3 eggs
- 1/3 cup vegetable oil
- 1 drop red food coloring, or desired amount
- 1 drop green food coloring, or desired amount
- 1 drop yellow food coloring, or desired amount
- 1 drop blue food coloring, or desired amount
- 24 flat-bottomed wafer ice cream cones in assorted colors
- 1 (16 ounce) container prepared vanilla frosting

Direction

- Preheat the oven to 175 ° C or 350 ° F.
- In bowl, mix vegetable oil, eggs, water and cake mix to moisten; use electric mixer to whip batter for 2 minutes on moderate speed.
- Equally distribute cake batter among 4 separate bowls. Tint every bowl a different hue, mixing in blue, yellow, green and red food coloring to attain preferred shade.
- Place ice cream cones in 2 dozen muffin cups, upright.
- Scoop into cones with approximately 1 1/2 tablespoons each of the colored batter, keeping approximately an-inch headspace.
- Cautiously turn the cones onto prepped oven and bake for 20 to 25 minutes, till an inserted toothpick in the center of one filled cone gets out clean.
- Let cupcakes cool well for an hour prior to decorating.

Nutrition Information

- Calories: 217 calories;
- Total Fat: 9.5
- Sodium: 190
- Total Carbohydrate: 31.6
- Cholesterol: 23
- Protein: 2.3

157. SPAM® A Licious Cupcakes With Salted Caramel Frosting

Serving: 24 | Prep: 15mins | Cook: 30mins | Ready in:

Ingredients

- Cupcakes:
- 4 ounces fully cooked luncheon meat (such as SPAM®), grated
- 1 (15.25 ounce) package devil's food cake mix
- 1 1/3 cups water
- 1 cup mayonnaise
- 2 large eggs
- Frosting:
- 1/2 cup butter
- 1 cup dark brown sugar
- 1/3 cup heavy whipping cream
- 1/4 teaspoon salt
- 2 cups confectioners' sugar, or as needed

Direction

- Set the oven to 175°C or 350°F and use paper muffin liners to line 24 muffin cups or grease them all.
- Heat a big skillet on medium-high heat. Cook and stir the grated luncheon meat into the hot skillet for 5-7 minutes, or until crisp and turning brown. Turn meat to a plate lined with paper towel and allow it to cool thoroughly.
- In a big bowl, use an electric mixer to beat together eggs, mayonnaise, water and cake mix on low speed until just turning moistened. Beat the batter for 2 minutes on medium speed, or until smooth. Fold two-thirds of fried luncheon meat into cake batter, then scoop into prepared muffin cups.

- In the preheated oven, bake for 20 minutes, or until a toothpick comes out clean after inserting into the center of cupcake. Allow to cool in the pans set on wire racks until cool thoroughly.
- In a small saucepan, melt butter on medium heat. Put in heavy cream and brown sugar, then stir until sugar is dissolved. Bring the mixture to a simmer and cook for one minute without stirring. Take away from the heat, then mix salt into sauce and allow it to cool thoroughly.
- Turn the sauce to a big bowl and beat in confectioners' sugar, one cup at a time, until getting wanted consistency of frosting. Spread the frosting over cooled cupcakes and put leftover fried luncheon meat on top.

Nutrition Information

- Calories: 285 calories;
- Protein: 2.8
- Total Fat: 16.5
- Sodium: 310
- Total Carbohydrate: 32.6
- Cholesterol: 41

158.   Sopapilla Cupcakes

Serving: 18 | Prep: 20mins | Cook: 15mins | Ready in:

Ingredients

- Cake:
- 1 (16.5 ounce) package white cake mix
- 1 cup water
- 3 large egg whites
- 1/4 cup oil
- 2 tablespoons ground cinnamon, divided
- 1 teaspoon vanilla extract
- 1/2 teaspoon lemon extract
- 1 tablespoon white sugar
- Frosting:
- 1/2 cup butter, room temperature
- 3 cups confectioners' sugar, or more as needed
- 3 tablespoons honey
- 1/2 teaspoon ground cinnamon
- 2 tablespoons milk, or as needed
- 1 tablespoon honey, for drizzling

Direction

- Start preheating the oven to 325°F (165°C). Use paper liners to line 18 muffin cups.
- In the bowl of a stand mixer, combine lemon extract, vanilla extract, 1 tablespoon cinnamon, oil, egg whites, water, and cake mix; combine for 30 seconds on low. Raise the speed to medium and blend the batter for 2 minutes. Put the batter in the muffin cups until 2/3-full.
- In a small bowl, mix together 1 tablespoon cinnamon and white sugar; drizzle over the batter.
- Put in the preheated oven and bake for 15 minutes until a toothpick will come out clean when you stick it in the middle of the cake. Let the cupcakes cool to room temperature.
- In a bowl, use an electric mixer to whisk butter for 1-2 minutes until fluffy and creamy. Add 1/2 teaspoon cinnamon, 3 tablespoons honey, and confectioners' sugar; whisk just until blended. Stir milk into the creamed butter mixture, 1 tablespoon each time, until reaching the frosting consistency. Put the frosting in a plastic bag or a piping bag with a cut corner, pipe onto each cupcake. Sprinkle over each frosted cupcake with honey.

Nutrition Information

- Calories: 286 calories;
- Total Carbohydrate: 46.2
- Cholesterol: 14
- Protein: 1.9
- Total Fat: 11
- Sodium: 218

159. Sushi Cupcakes

Serving: 12 | Prep: 25mins | Cook: 12mins | Ready in:

Ingredients

- 1 (15.25 ounce) package vanilla cake mix (such as Betty Crocker®)
- 1 cup water
- 3 eggs
- 1/2 cup vegetable oil
- 1 (16 ounce) package vanilla icing
- 1 (7 ounce) package long shredded coconut
- 5 multicolored gum drops (such as Jujubes®), or more to taste
- 4 pieces dried mango, roughly chopped, or more to taste
- 4 pieces dried ginger, roughly chopped, or more to taste
- 1 (1.75 ounce) package red and green sprinkles
- 2 (.75 ounce) packages blueberry-flavored fruit snack rolls (such as Betty Crocker Fruit by the Foot®)

Direction

- Preheat the oven to 175°C or 350°F. Oil one muffin tin.
- Use an electric mixer to whip oil, eggs, water and cake mix in big bowl till incorporated. Add batter to prepped tin.
- In prepped oven, bake for 12 to 17 minutes, till an inserted toothpick into the middle gets out clean. Cool cupcakes for 20 minutes in tin.
- Turn the cupcakes onto an even work counter. Cut every cupcake resembling shape of rectangular maki or round sushi roll. Use icing and shredded coconut to coat the cake rolls. Put sprinkles, dried ginger, dried mango and gum drops on top. Encase around cake rolls with fruit rolls.

Nutrition Information

- Calories: 523 calories;
- Cholesterol: 47
- Protein: 4.2
- Total Fat: 26.9
- Sodium: 381
- Total Carbohydrate: 70.4

Chapter 6: Holiday Cupcake Recipes

***

160. 4th Of July Cupcakes

Serving: 10 | Prep: 20mins | Cook: 20mins | Ready in:

Ingredients

- 1 (16.9 ounce) package blueberry muffin mix (such as Betty Crocker®)
- 3/4 cup water
- 1/4 cup vegetable oil
- 2 eggs
- 3/4 cup cream cheese frosting, or as needed
- 2 strawberry-flavored fruit roll (such as Fruit Roll-Ups®), cut into thin strips, or as needed
- 20 blueberries, halved crosswise

Direction

- Set the oven to 425°F or 220°C for preheating. Use paper liners to line the 10 muffin cups, or you can also grease the cups.
- Drain the blueberries from the muffin mix. In a bowl, mix the muffin mix with eggs, water, and oil until the batter is just blended. Fold the blueberries into the mixture. Distribute the batter among the prepared muffin cups, filling them up to the top of the cups.
- Bake them inside the preheated oven for 16-21 minutes until the inserted toothpick into the center will come out clean. Let them cool until they can be handled easily. Cut the tops from

each cupcake off and reserve them for another use.
- Spread onto the bottom of each cupcake with the cream cheese frosting, making sure to start from the middle, working it outwards. Form stripes by arranging the fruit roll strips onto each cupcake. For the stars, arrange two blueberry halves into the left corner of each cupcake.

Nutrition Information

- Calories: 361 calories;
- Sodium: 550
- Total Carbohydrate: 48.9
- Cholesterol: 45
- Protein: 4.3
- Total Fat: 16.8

161. Almond Cupcake With Salted Caramel Buttercream Frosting

Serving: 12 | Prep: 30mins | Cook: 25mins | Ready in:

Ingredients

- 1 1/2 cups all-purpose flour
- 1 3/4 teaspoons baking powder
- 1 cup white sugar
- 1/2 cup margarine, softened
- 2 eggs
- 1 teaspoon vanilla extract
- 1 teaspoon almond extract
- 3/4 cup whole milk
- 1/2 cup brown sugar
- 1/2 cup margarine
- 2 tablespoons light corn syrup
- 1 tablespoon vanilla extract
- 1/2 cup heavy cream, or as needed
- 1 pinch salt
- 3/4 cup salted butter, softened
- 2 cups confectioners' sugar, sifted

Direction

- Set oven to 350°F (175°C) to preheat. Put paper liners into 12 cupcake cups. Combine baking powder and flour in a bowl.
- Beat well 1/2 cup margarine with sugar in a mixing bowl until thoroughly incorporated. Beat in eggs, one by one, until well blended; whisk in almond extracts and vanilla. Working in batches, slowly beat flour mixture into batter alternately with milk. Fill batter into the prepared cupcake cups to approximately two-thirds full.
- Bake cupcakes for 20 to 25 minutes in the preheated oven until a toothpick comes out clean from the center.
- For caramel: put vanilla, corn syrup, 1/2 cup margarine, and brown sugar over medium heat in a large saucepan; bring to a boil. Lower heat, and simmer for 3 to 4 minutes or until mixture is thickened; turn off the heat and allow mixture to cool slightly until warmed (not hot). Pour in cream, little by little, until caramel reaches honey consistency. Stir in a pinch of salt; let mixture cool to room temperature.
- In a bowl, beat salted butter and confectioners' sugar using an electric mixer on medium speed until fluffy; gradually add and whip in caramel, 1 tablespoon at a time, beating well until no lumps remain in the frosting.

Nutrition Information

- Calories: 526 calories;
- Total Carbohydrate: 62.5
- Cholesterol: 70
- Protein: 3.6
- Total Fat: 29.8
- Sodium: 353

162. Aloha Cupcakes

Serving: 1 dozen. | Prep: 20mins | Cook: 15mins | Ready in:

Ingredients

- 1-1/4 cups cake flour
- 1-1/4 teaspoons baking powder
- 1/2 teaspoon baking soda
- 1/2 teaspoon salt
- 2 large eggs
- 3/4 cup granulated sugar
- 1/2 cup canola oil
- 1 teaspoon coconut extract
- 1/2 cup coconut milk
- 1/2 teaspoon white vinegar
- PINEAPPLE FROSTING:
- 1/2 cup shortening
- 1/2 cup butter
- 4 cups confectioners' sugar
- 1/2 cup finely chopped fresh pineapple
- 3 tablespoons unsweetened pineapple juice
- TOPPING:
- 1/2 cup sweetened shredded coconut, toasted
- 1/2 cup coarsely chopped macadamia nuts, optional

Direction

- Prepare the oven by preheating to 350°F. Use foil liners or paper to line the 12 muffin cups. Mix together the four ingredients; reserve. Whisk sugar and eggs for 1 minute on medium speed. Add in the coconut extract and oil; whisk for 1 minute more. Add in the half of flour mixture; then mix on low speed. Mix together the vinegar and coconut milk. Then add the half of it to batter; mix until well combined. Mix in the remaining flour mixture, then the remaining coconut milk mixture until it becomes smooth. Fill the prepared cups 2/3 full. Place inside the preheated oven for 15 to 18 minutes until cupcakes are golden brown in color and bounces back when lightly touched (prevent from over baking). Let it cool on wire rack. To make the frosting, cream butter and shortening until fluffy and light. A half a cup at a time, mix in confectioners' sugar, then after beating in 2 cups of sugar, add the pineapple juice and finely chopped pineapple. To achieve the consistency that you want, add more pineapple juice and additional confectioners' sugar. Scoop frosting onto cupcakes. Place toasted coconut on top and chopped macadamia nuts if you want.

Nutrition Information

- Calories: 533 calories
- Fiber: 1g fiber)
- Total Carbohydrate: 67g carbohydrate (55g sugars
- Cholesterol: 51mg cholesterol
- Protein: 3g protein.
- Total Fat: 29g fat (11g saturated fat)
- Sodium: 287mg sodium

163. Ann's Chocolate Chip Carrot Cake Pumpkins

Serving: 12 | Prep: 20mins | Cook: 20mins | Ready in:

Ingredients

- Cupcakes:
- 2 cups cake flour
- 2 teaspoons ground cinnamon
- 1 1/2 teaspoons baking soda
- 1 teaspoon baking powder
- 1 teaspoon salt
- 2 cups white sugar
- 1 1/2 cups vegetable oil
- 4 eggs
- 2 cups grated carrots
- 1 (8 ounce) can crushed pineapple, drained
- 1 tablespoon cake flour
- 1/2 cup chopped walnuts
- 1/2 cup semisweet chocolate chips
- Frosting:
- 1/2 cup butter

- 1 (8 ounce) package cream cheese, softened
- 1 tablespoon vanilla extract
- 2 cups confectioners' sugar, or more as needed
- 1 tablespoon lemon juice
- 3 drops orange food coloring
- 1 (1.5 ounce) tube black decorating gel

Direction

- Set oven temperature to 325 degrees F (165 degrees C) and preheat. (Set temperature to 325 degrees F if using a countertop induction oven.) Take 12 pumpkin-shaped cupcake baking moulds and grease (silicon moulds are fine too).
- Using a sieve, sift 2 cups of cake flour, baking powder, baking soda, cinnamon, and salt into a bowl. Combine in eggs, oil, and sugar until mixed evenly. Mix pineapple and carrots into the batter.
- In a bowl, spoon in 1 tablespoon of cake flour. Throw chocolate chips and walnuts into the flour until covered evenly and incorporate gently into the batter.
- Pour the batter into the moulds up to 2/3 height and give a gentle tap to the moulds to remove any air bubbles.
- Bake for 20-25 minutes in preheated oven, or 15-20 minutes in a countertop induction oven, until inserted toothpick comes out with no residue sticking on it. Allow to cool until it reaches room temperature for 15-20 minutes and separate the cupcakes from their moulds.
- Mix cream cheese, vanilla extract, and butter in a bowl, and use an electric mixer to beat until even for 4-6 minutes. Combine confectioners' sugar, at 1/2 cup intervals, and continue mixing at low speed setting until the frosting has a smooth consistency for spreading. Mix in orange food coloring and lemon juice while stirring until mixed evenly. Keep in refrigerator until set for 15-20 minutes.
- Use cream cheese frosting on cupcakes, and finish with decoration of black gel.

Nutrition Information

- Calories: 818 calories;
- Total Carbohydrate: 89.4
- Cholesterol: 103
- Protein: 7.3
- Total Fat: 49.4
- Sodium: 595

164. Arnold Palmer Cupcakes

Serving: about 2-1/2 dozen. | Prep: 20mins | Cook: 25mins | Ready in:

Ingredients

- 1 cup butter, softened
- 2 cups sugar
- 3 large eggs, room temperature
- 1 tablespoon grated lemon zest
- 2 teaspoons lemon juice
- 3-1/2 cups all-purpose flour
- 1 teaspoon baking soda
- 1/2 teaspoon baking powder
- 1/2 teaspoon salt
- 2 cups (16 ounces) sour cream
- ICED TEA FROSTING:
- 9 tablespoons butter, softened
- 6-3/4 cups confectioners' sugar
- 3/4 cup 2% milk
- 3/4 cup iced tea mix with lemon and sugar

Direction

- Cream the butter and sugar in a big bowl until fluffy and light. Add one egg at a time, beat it well before each addition. Beat in lemon zest and juice. Mix the salt, baking powder, baking soda and flour; add to the creamed mixture alternately with the sour cream, beating well before adding the next (take note that the batter will be thick).
- Prepare 30 lined muffin cups and fill each cup with a quarter cup of batter. Let the cupcakes bake for 25-30 minutes at 350°. Do a toothpick test, it should come out clean when poked in the middle. Allow to cool for 10 minutes

before taking off from pans and transfer to wire racks to cool thoroughly.
- To make the frosting, mix together the confectioners' sugar and butter in a small bowl, until fluffy and light. In another small bowl, mix together the iced tea mix and milk until dissolved completely; add the mixture to the butter mixture and beat until the consistency turns smooth. Ice the cupcakes.

Nutrition Information

- Calories: 355 calories
- Total Fat: 14g fat (8g saturated fat)
- Sodium: 182mg sodium
- Fiber: 0 fiber)
- Total Carbohydrate: 57g carbohydrate (45g sugars
- Cholesterol: 48mg cholesterol
- Protein: 3g protein.

165. Autumn Pumpkin Cupcakes

Serving: 2 dozen. | Prep: 30mins | Cook: 20mins | Ready in:

Ingredients

- 2 cups sugar
- 1 can (15 ounces) solid-pack pumpkin
- 4 large eggs
- 3/4 cup canola oil
- 1 teaspoon vanilla extract
- 2 cups all-purpose flour
- 2 teaspoons baking soda
- 2 teaspoons pumpkin pie spice
- 1 teaspoon salt
- 1 teaspoon baking powder
- SAUCE:
- 1/2 cup packed brown sugar
- 6 tablespoons heavy whipping cream
- 1/4 cup butter, cubed
- 1/8 teaspoon salt
- 1/2 teaspoon vanilla extract
- FROSTING:
- 1 package (8 ounces) cream cheese, softened
- 1 cup butter, softened
- 1 teaspoon vanilla extract
- 3 cups confectioners' sugar

Direction

- Set the oven to 350° and start preheating. Using paper liners, line 24 muffin cups. Whisk vanilla, oil, eggs, pumpkin and sugar in a large bowl until well blended. Beat baking powder, salt, pie spice, baking soda and flour in another bowl; beat into pumpkin mixture gradually.
- Fill 2/3 of prepared cups. Bake until the inserted toothpick in the center is clean when coming out or for 20-22 minutes. Cool 10 minutes in pans; transfer to wire racks to completely cool.
- To prepare sauce: Mix salt, butter, cream and brown sugar in a small heavy saucepan; bring to boiling. Lower the heat; cook while stirring until thickened or for 2-3 minutes. Take out of the heat; stir in vanilla. Cool to room temperature.
- At the meantime, whisk vanilla, butter and cream cheese until blended in a large bowl. Whisk in confectioners' sugar gradually until smooth. Frost cupcakes; drizzle with sauce.

Nutrition Information

- Calories: 391 calories
- Fiber: 1g fiber)
- Total Carbohydrate: 47g carbohydrate (37g sugars
- Cholesterol: 70mg cholesterol
- Protein: 3g protein.
- Total Fat: 22g fat (10g saturated fat)
- Sodium: 357mg sodium

166. Black Cat Cupcakes

Serving: 2 dozen. | Prep: 15mins | Cook: 20mins | Ready in:

Ingredients

- 1 package chocolate cake mix (regular size)
- 1 can (16 ounces) dark chocolate frosting
- 12 Oreo cookies, quartered
- Assorted candies: M&M's, black licorice, Runts and Starburst

Direction

- Follow the package instructions to prepare and bake the cake mix for the cupcakes, filling the paper-lined muffin cups with 2/3 full of the mixture. Let them cool for 10 minutes. Remove them from the pans and place them on wire racks. Let them cool completely.
- Frost the cupcakes' tops using the star tip. For the ears, insert 2 pieces of cookie, breaking the Oreos if necessary to expose its filling. Use assorted candies to style the faces.

Nutrition Information

- Calories: 259 calories
- Sodium: 234mg sodium
- Fiber: 1g fiber)
- Total Carbohydrate: 49g carbohydrate (32g sugars
- Cholesterol: 0 cholesterol
- Protein: 2g protein.
- Total Fat: 6g fat (2g saturated fat)

167. Boston Creme Mini Cupcakes

Serving: 24 | Prep: 30mins | Cook: 15mins | Ready in:

Ingredients

- cooking spray
- 1 (18.25 ounce) box yellow cake mix
- 1 cup water
- 3 eggs
- 1/3 cup vegetable oil
- 1 (3.5 ounce) package instant French vanilla pudding
- 2 cups cold milk
- 1 (16 ounce) can prepared chocolate frosting
- 1 cup whipped cream (optional)
- 6 maraschino cherries, quartered (optional)

Direction

- Heat oven to 175°C (350°F) beforehand.
- Use cooking spray to spray 24 mini muffin cups.
- In a bowl, stirring vegetable oil, eggs, water and yellow cake mix till moistened. Using an electric mixer to beat for 2 minutes on medium speed.
- In the prepared mini muffin cups, spooning cake batter till each is about 2/3 full.
- In the preheated oven, allow to bake for 15-19 minutes till cupcakes turn golden brown lightly and risen. After 10 minutes, checking for doneness. Cooking is finished when insert a toothpick into the center of a cupcake, it comes out clean. Let cupcakes cool down for approximately 20 minutes.
- In a bowl, whisking together milk and instant French vanilla pudding mix for 2 minutes. Let pudding rest for another 5 minutes to thicken.
- Piping into each cupcake with approximately one and a quarter teaspoon of vanilla pudding.
- Let filled cupcakes freeze for no less than an hour for easier frosting.
- On each cupcake, spreading a very thin coating of chocolate frosting; let cupcakes sit for 15 minutes in the refrigerator.
- Spreading over the first layer with second, thicker layer of frosting. In the center of each frosted cupcake, lay small dollop of whipped cream and place 1/4 of a maraschino cherry on top. Let mini cupcakes sit in the refrigerator till serving.

Nutrition Information

- Calories: 248 calories;
- Total Fat: 11.7
- Sodium: 253
- Total Carbohydrate: 34.2
- Cholesterol: 32
- Protein: 2.7

168. Candied Holly Cupcakes

Serving: 1-1/2 dozen. | Prep: 10mins | Cook: 20mins | Ready in:

Ingredients

- 1/2 cup shortening
- 1 cup sugar
- 2 eggs
- 1-1/2 cups all-purpose flour
- 1/2 teaspoon baking soda
- 1/2 teaspoon each ground cinnamon, allspice, nutmeg and cloves
- 1/2 cup buttermilk
- 1/2 cup cherry jam or flavor of your choice
- 1/2 cup chopped pecans
- 1/4 cup finely chopped candied cherries
- 1/4 cup finely chopped candied orange peel
- 2 cups prepared vanilla frosting
- 9 candied cherries, halved
- 18 green citron pieces or green candied pineapple pieces, cut into strips

Direction

- Cream sugar and shortening in a large bowl until fluffy and light. Then beat in the eggs. Combine spices, flour and baking soda. Put alternately with buttermilk into the creamed mixture; beat well after each addition. Mix in orange peel, cherries, pecans and jam.
- Fill 3/4 full the paper-lined muffin cups. Bake for 20-25 mins at 350°, until a toothpick inserted in comes out clean. Let cool for 10 mins, then discard from pans to cool completely on wire racks.
- Frost the cooled cupcakes. Garnish with the citron for leaves and the cherries for holly berries.

Nutrition Information

- Calories:
- Total Carbohydrate:
- Cholesterol:
- Protein:
- Total Fat:
- Sodium:
- Fiber:

169. Candied Yam Cupcakes

Serving: 24 | Prep: 20mins | Cook: 35mins | Ready in:

Ingredients

- 1 pound yams, peeled and cubed
- 4 eggs
- 1 cup canola oil
- 1 cup white sugar
- 1 teaspoon vanilla extract
- 2 cups all-purpose flour
- 2 teaspoons baking powder
- 1 teaspoon baking soda
- 2 teaspoons ground cinnamon
- 1 teaspoon salt
- 3 ounces cream cheese
- 1/2 cup butter, softened
- 1 teaspoon vanilla extract
- 2 cups confectioners' sugar

Direction

- Put a steamer insert into a big saucepan; fill with water to right under the bottom of the steamer. Cover; boil on high heat. Add yams; recover. Steam for 15 minutes till very tender. Take yams from the steamer; slightly cool.

- Preheat an oven to 175°C/350°F; line paper liners on 2 12 cup cupcake tins.
- Use an electric mixer to beat cooked yams, vanilla extract, sugar, oil and eggs till fluffy and light in a big bowl. Sift salt, cinnamon, baking soda, baking powder and flour. Mix dry ingredients into the yam mixture; stir till just combined. Put batter, filling 2/3 full, to paper liners.
- In a preheated oven, bake for 17-20 minutes till inserted toothpick in the middle of a cupcake exits clean; cool for 5 minutes in pans. Put on a wire rack; fully cool.
- Beat butter and cream cheese together till fluffy; beat confectioners' sugar and vanilla extract in till smooth. Use cream cheese frosting to frost cool cupcakes.

Nutrition Information

- Calories: 276 calories;
- Cholesterol: 45
- Protein: 2.7
- Total Fat: 15.4
- Sodium: 241
- Total Carbohydrate: 32.4

170. Candy Corn Cupcakes

Serving: 24 | Prep: 15mins | Cook: 20mins | Ready in:

Ingredients

- 1 (18.25 ounce) package white cake mix
- 1 cup water
- 1/3 cup vegetable oil
- 3 eggs
- 14 drops red food coloring, or as needed - divided
- 22 drops yellow food coloring, or as needed - divided
- 6 drops green food coloring, or as needed
- 2 cups prepared white frosting
- 12 pieces of yellow, orange, and white candy corn
- 12 pieces of brown, orange, and white candy corn

Direction

- Preheat an oven to 175°C/350°F; line paper liners on 24 cupcake cups.
- Put cake mix, water, vegetable oil then 3 eggs in a bowl; beat them with electric mixer at low speed for 2 minutes till thoroughly combined. Put 1/2 cake mix into 2nd bowl; divide leftover cake mix in half. Put into 2 different small bowls.
- Mix in 4 red food coloring drops with 6 yellow food coloring drops in biggest cake mix portion to make it orange. Mix in 6 green food coloring drops, 12 yellow food coloring drops and 10 red food coloring drops in 2nd smaller cake mix bowl to make it brown. Mix in 5 yellow food coloring drops into leftover small cake mix bowl to make it yellow.
- Put yellow cake batter on bottoms of 12 prepped cupcake cups; fill to 1/3 full. Put brown batter on bottoms of leftover 12 prepped cupcake cups; fill to 1/3 full. Put orange cupcake mix on brown and yellow layers, filling cupcakes to 2/3 full. Don't shake/jar filling cupcakes to not mix the layers.
- In preheated oven, put cupcakes carefully; bake for 18-22 minutes till inserted toothpick in middle of cupcake exits clean. Cool.
- Use white frosting to frost each cooled cupcake; put piece of white, orange and yellow candy corn over each orange and yellow cupcake. Put white, orange and brown candy corn piece over each orange and brown cupcake.

Nutrition Information

- Calories: 238 calories;
- Protein: 2
- Total Fat: 10.6
- Sodium: 199

- Total Carbohydrate: 35
- Cholesterol: 23

171. Candy'D Sweet Potato Cupcakes With Brown Sugar Icing

Serving: 48 | Prep: 30mins | Cook: 25mins | Ready in:

Ingredients

- 2 pounds sweet potatoes, peeled and cubed
- 1/2 cup orange juice, or as needed
- 1 cup butter at room temperature
- 1 cup light brown sugar
- 1 cup white sugar
- 4 eggs at room temperature
- 2 teaspoons vanilla extract
- 1 large orange, zested
- 3 cups all-purpose flour
- 2 teaspoons baking powder
- 2 teaspoons ground cinnamon
- 1 1/2 teaspoons ground ginger
- 1 teaspoon baking soda
- 1/4 teaspoon salt
- 1 cup confectioners' sugar, sifted
- 3/4 cup packed dark brown sugar
- 1/2 cup heavy cream
- 1/4 cup unsalted butter
- 1/4 teaspoon vanilla extract

Direction

- Arrange a steamer insert in a saucepan then fill with water to just below the base of the steamer; cover then boil on high heat. Put in sweet potato cubes then cover; steam for 15-20 minutes according on thickness until tender. Take the sweet potatoes out of the steamer then cool; move to a blender then add orange juice. Cover then puree until the mixture is smooth. Pour in a tablespoon of orange juice at a time if the mixture is too thick until blended.
- Preheat oven to 175°C or 350°Fahrenheit. Line paper muffin liners on 48 muffin cups.
- In a big bowl, mix white sugar, light brown sugar, and a cup of butter and beat using an electric mixer until fluffy and light. Mix in one egg at a time, blend each egg well before adding another. Whisk in 2 tsp. of vanilla extract with the final egg; mix in the orange zest and sweet potato puree.
- In a bowl, sift salt, flour, baking soda, baking powder, ginger, and cinnamon together; stir into the sweet potato mixture a cup at a time, mixing until just combined. The result will be a thick batter. Scoop batter in the lined-muffin tins.
- Bake for 18 minutes in the preheated oven until an inserted toothpick in the middle of a cupcake comes out without residue. Cool for 10 minutes in the pans then transfer on a wire rack to completely cool.
- Prepare the frosting. In a big bowl, strain the confectioners' sugar; set aside. In a saucepan set on low heat, heat a quarter cup butter, heavy cream, and brown sugar until the sugar dissolves, mix from time to time. Turn to medium-high heat, then boil the mixture for 3 minutes while constantly mixing until thick. Take off heat then mix in a quarter teaspoon of vanilla extract. Stir the brown sugar mixture with the confectioners' sugar for 1-2 minutes until smooth. Cool the sugar mixture then thicken prior to icing the cupcakes.

Nutrition Information

- Calories: 161 calories;
- Total Carbohydrate: 25
- Cholesterol: 32
- Protein: 1.8
- Total Fat: 6.2
- Sodium: 106

172. Cannoli Cupcakes

Serving: 8 cupcakes. | Prep: 50mins | Cook: 25mins | Ready in:

Ingredients

- 1 package white cake mix (regular size)
- 3/4 cup heavy whipping cream, divided
- 1 cup ricotta cheese
- 1 cup confectioners' sugar
- 1/2 cup Mascarpone cheese
- 1/4 teaspoon almond extract
- 1/2 cup chopped pistachios
- 4 ounces white baking chocolate, chopped
- White chocolate curls

Direction

- Prepare cake mix batter following the package instructions. Pour the batter in jumbo muffin cups lined with paper to fill 3/4 full. Let it bake for 24 to 28 minutes following the package instructions or until an inserted toothpick in the middle exits clean. Allow to cool for 10 minutes prior to taking it out of the pans and transferring to wire racks to fully cool.
- Beat half a cup of cream in small bowl until it forms stiff peaks, then put aside. Mix together the extract, Mascarpone cheese, confectioners' sugar and ricotta cheese in a big bowl until it becomes smooth, then fold in whipped cream and pistachios.
- Trim off the top of every cupcake. Pipe or spread the cheese mixture on the cupcakes, then place back the tops. Melt the leftover cream with white baking chocolate in a small saucepan on low heat, then mix until it becomes smooth. Take it out of the heat and allow to cool to room temperature. Scoop on top of the cupcakes and sprinkle chocolate curls on top. Put the leftovers in the fridge.

Nutrition Information

- Calories: 786 calories
- Cholesterol: 81mg cholesterol
- Protein: 13g protein.
- Total Fat: 48g fat (21g saturated fat)
- Sodium: 565mg sodium
- Fiber: 1g fiber)
- Total Carbohydrate: 78g carbohydrate (53g sugars

173. Carrot Cake Cupcakes With Cream Cheese Icing

Serving: 12 | Prep: 20mins | Cook: 30mins | Ready in:

Ingredients

- 2 cups all-purpose flour
- 2 cups white sugar
- 2 teaspoons baking soda
- 2 teaspoons ground cinnamon
- 1/2 teaspoon ground ginger
- 2 tablespoons canola oil
- 4 large eggs
- 4 large carrots, grated
- 1 cup unsalted butter, softened
- 2 (8 ounce) packages cream cheese, softened
- 1 tablespoon vanilla extract
- 2 cups confectioners' sugar

Direction

- Set the oven for preheating to 350°F (175°C).
- Grease 12 muffin cups using the butter, or you can just line them using the paper liners.
- Combine ginger, cinnamon, baking soda, white sugar and flour; sift together in a big bowl.
- Beat the eggs and canola oil into the flour mixture using an electric mixer. Make sure to beat each egg well before each addition.
- Add the carrots to the mixture and stir until well incorporated.
- Pour the carrot mixture in the prepared muffin cups, filling them about 2/3 full.

- Let it bake inside the preheated oven for 30 to 40 minutes, until the cupcakes turn lightly browned and a toothpick poked into the middle comes out clean. Allow them to cool through.
- Set an electric mixer on high speed and beat the cream cheese and the unsalted butter together in a bowl until the mixture becomes fluffy. Adjust the speed to low and add in confectioners' sugar and vanilla extract; beat until incorporated. Adjust the speed to high, and continue to beat until the frosting is fluffy, about 3 minutes more.
- Put the cream cheese frosting in a pastry bag and pipe onto the cupcakes.

Nutrition Information

- Calories: 611 calories;
- Sodium: 363
- Total Carbohydrate: 74
- Cholesterol: 144
- Protein: 7.5
- Total Fat: 32.6

174. Carrot Cake Cupcakes With Lemon Cream Cheese Frosting

Serving: 24 | Prep: 30mins | Cook: 20mins | Ready in:

Ingredients

- Carrot Cake Cupcakes:
- 2 cups flour
- 2 cups granulated sugar
- 2 teaspoons baking powder
- 2 teaspoons McCormick® Cinnamon, Ground
- 1/2 teaspoon McCormick® Nutmeg, Ground
- 1/2 teaspoon salt
- 1 1/4 cups vegetable oil
- 4 eggs, lightly beaten
- 1 tablespoon McCormick® Pure Vanilla Extract
- 3 cups finely grated carrots
- Lemon Cream Cheese Frosting:
- 1 (8 ounce) package cream cheese, softened
- 1/2 cup butter, softened
- 1/2 teaspoon McCormick® Pure Lemon Extract
- 1 (16 ounce) box confectioners' sugar
- 1 tablespoon milk, or as needed

Direction

- Preheat an oven to 350 °F. For Cupcakes, in big bowl, stir salt, nutmeg, cinnamon, baking powder, granulated sugar and flour. Put vanilla, eggs and oil; stir thoroughly. Put the carrots; stir till well incorporated. Scoop batter into 2 dozen muffin cups lined with paper, filling every cup two thirds full.
- Bake till toothpick pricked into the cupcake gets out clean, for 20 minutes. Cool for 5 minutes in pans on a wire rack. Take out of pans; cool fully.
- For icing, in big bowl, whip lemon extract, butter and cream cheese, till fluffy and light. Slowly whip in confectioners' sugar till smooth. Incase icing is very thick to scatter, slowly whip in milk. With icing, ice cooled cupcakes.

Nutrition Information

- Calories: 362 calories;
- Sodium: 166
- Total Carbohydrate: 45.2
- Cholesterol: 51
- Protein: 3
- Total Fat: 19.5

175. Carrot Pineapple Cupcakes

Serving: 12 | Prep: 20mins | Cook: 20mins | Ready in:

Ingredients

- 1 cup white sugar
- 2/3 cup vegetable oil
- 2 eggs, beaten
- 1 1/2 cups all-purpose flour
- 2 teaspoons baking powder
- 1 teaspoon baking soda
- 1 teaspoon ground cinnamon
- 1/2 teaspoon salt
- 1 cup finely grated carrot
- 1 cup crushed pineapple, drained
- 1 teaspoon vanilla extract
- 1/2 cup butter, softened
- 1 (8 ounce) package cream cheese, softened
- 3 cups confectioners' sugar
- 1 teaspoon vanilla extract
- 1 tablespoon milk

Direction

- Preheat the oven to 375°F (190°C).
- Prepare 12 muffin cups by either lining them with paper or greasing them.
- Mix eggs, vegetable oil and white sugar together in a big mixing bowl and stir thoroughly.
- In a different bowl, beat baking soda, flour, salt, cinnamon and baking powder together.
- Blend flour mixture into liquid mixture; stir in 1 teaspoon vanilla extract, pineapple and carrot.
- Fill the muffin cups to the brim with batter.
- Place cupcakes in the oven and bake for 20 minutes. When an inserted toothpick comes out spotless, the cupcakes can be placed aside to cool off entirely.
- Using an electric hand mixer, blend cream cheese and butter in a bowl until smooth.
- For a spreadable frosting, beat milk, vanilla extract and confectioners' sugar into the mixture then apply it across the cupcakes once they're cooled.

Nutrition Information

- Calories: 515 calories;
- Total Fat: 27.4
- Sodium: 412
- Total Carbohydrate: 64.9
- Cholesterol: 72
- Protein: 4.4

176. Carrot Topped Cupcakes

Serving: 2 dozen. | Prep: 25mins | Cook: 20mins | Ready in:

Ingredients

- 1 package spice cake mix (regular size)
- 1-1/2 cups shredded carrots
- 1/2 cup chopped walnuts
- 1 teaspoon ground cinnamon
- 1 can (16 ounces) cream cheese frosting
- Orange paste food coloring
- Fresh parsley sprigs

Direction

- Prepare cake batter according to the direction on the package. Fold in cinnamon, walnuts and carrots.
- Fill batter to half of the paper-lined muffin cups. Bake at 350° until the inserted toothpick in the center comes out clean or for 18-23 minutes. Take out of the pans, transfer to wire racks to completely cool.
- Frost cupcakes with 1-1/4 cups frosting. Transfer the rest of frosting to a small resealable bag; use orange fruit coloring to tint. Create a small hole in the bag's corner; pipe a carrot on each cupcake. For greens, add a parsley sprig.

Nutrition Information

- Calories:
- Protein:
- Total Fat:
- Sodium:

- Fiber:
- Total Carbohydrate:
- Cholesterol:

177. Champagne Cupcakes

Serving: 24 | Prep: 15mins | Cook: 20mins | Ready in:

Ingredients

- cooking spray
- 1 (18.25 ounce) package white cake mix
- 1 1/4 cups Champagne or other sparkling white wine at room temperature
- 1/3 cup vegetable oil
- 3 eggs
- 1/2 cup butter, softened
- 4 cups confectioners' sugar
- 1/4 cup Champagne or other sparkling white wine at room temperature
- 1 teaspoon vanilla extract

Direction

- Preheat the oven to 175°C or 350°Fahrenheit.
- Use cooking spray to grease 24 muffin cups.
- In a big mixing bowl, combine 1 1/4 cup champagne and cake mix; mix in eggs and vegetable oil. Beat for 2 minutes on medium speed using an electric mixer.
- Transfer in greased muffin cups until 3/4 full.
- Bake for 20 minutes in the preheated oven until an inserted toothpick in the center comes out without residue.
- Cool for 10 minutes in the pan then remove. Completely cool for another half hour.
- In a bowl, combine vanilla extract, butter, quarter cup champagne and a cup of confectioners' sugar. Mix in the rest of the confectioners' sugar, a cup at one time, until creamy and smooth; slather over cooled cupcakes.

Nutrition Information

- Calories: 255 calories;
- Protein: 1.8
- Total Fat: 9.9
- Sodium: 178
- Total Carbohydrate: 37.9
- Cholesterol: 33

178. Cherry Amish Friendship Bread Cupcakes With Buttercream Frosting

Serving: 24 | Prep: 20mins | Cook: 20mins | Ready in:

Ingredients

- 1 cup Amish Friendship Bread Starter (see footnote for recipe link)
- 3 eggs
- 1 cup vegetable oil
- 1/2 cup milk
- 1 cup white sugar
- 1/2 teaspoon vanilla extract
- 1 1/2 teaspoons baking powder
- 1/2 teaspoon baking soda
- 1/2 teaspoon salt
- 2 cups all-purpose flour
- 1 (3 ounce) package cherry Jell-O®
- 1/2 cup vegetable shortening
- 1/2 cup butter, softened
- 1 teaspoon vanilla extract
- 4 cups sifted confectioners' sugar
- 2 tablespoons milk
- 1/2 cup white chocolate chips, or as needed (optional)

Direction

- Preheat the oven to 165 degrees C (325 degrees F). Line paper liners onto 24 cupcake cups.
- Combine together the Amish friendship bread starter, baking powder, eggs, sugar, vegetable oil, salt, 1/2 cup of milk, baking soda, and 1/2 teaspoon of vanilla extract in a mixing bowl until mixed well. Stir in the cherry gelatin

powder and flour. Scoop batter into the cupcake cups prepared.
- Bake for about 20 to 25 minutes until a toothpick comes out clean when inserted in the middle of a cupcake. Allow to cool.
- Use an electric mixer on medium speed to beat vegetable shortening together with butter in a large bowl until fluffy. Then pour in vanilla extract. Beat in the confectioners' sugar, one cup at a time and stop frequently to scrape down the bowl's sides. Stir in milk and then beat until frosting becomes fluffy and light. Pour over cooled cupcakes. If desired, drizzle some white chocolate chips onto each cupcake.

Nutrition Information

- Calories: 366 calories;
- Total Fat: 19.5
- Sodium: 166
- Total Carbohydrate: 45.6
- Cholesterol: 35
- Protein: 3.3

179. Cherry Cheese Cupcakes

Serving: about 2 dozen. | Prep: 20mins | Cook: 35mins | Ready in:

Ingredients

- 3 packages (8 ounces each) cream cheese, softened
- 1-1/2 cups sugar, divided
- 1-1/2 teaspoons vanilla extract, divided
- 5 large eggs
- 1 cup sour cream
- 1-1/2 cups cherry pie filling
- Mint leaves, optional

Direction

- Beat 1 teaspoon of vanilla, 1 cup of sugar and cream cheese until smooth in a large bowl. Put in eggs, one by one, beating thoroughly between additions.
- Scoop to muffin cups lined with foil. Bake at 300 degrees until a toothpick pricked into the middle comes out clean, or for 25 to 30 minutes. Allow to cool for 5 minutes.
- Mix vanilla, the rest of the sugar and sour cream together until smooth in a small bowl. Scoop over cupcakes. Bring back into the oven for 6 to 8 minutes or until set. Allow to cool for 10 minutes in pans, then transfer onto wire racks until cooled thoroughly.
- Add pie filling on top; if preferred, add mint to decorate. Keep in the fridge.

Nutrition Information

- Calories: 202 calories
- Total Carbohydrate: 18g carbohydrate (17g sugars
- Cholesterol: 82mg cholesterol
- Protein: 4g protein.
- Total Fat: 13g fat (8g saturated fat)
- Sodium: 105mg sodium
- Fiber: 0 fiber)

180. Chesscakes

Serving: 24 | Prep: 20mins | Cook: 30mins | Ready in:

Ingredients

- 1 (18.25 ounce) package white cake mix
- 2 (9 inch) unbaked pie crusts
- 1 (10 ounce) jar raspberry preserves

Direction

- Preheat an oven to 175°C/350°F; for this recipe, you'll need 2 12-cup ungreased muffin tins. So cake doesn't stick, you can spray nonstick cooking spray on tops of muffin pans.
- Follow package directions to prep cake mix; put aside. Roll pastry dough out to 18-in. thick; cut 24 dough circles out using round,

floured cookie cutter slightly bigger than muffin cups. In each muffin cup, put 1 dough circle, gently pressing dough into sides and bottom. Dough should reach halfway up each muffin cup's sides.
- In each pastry-lined cup, put rounded 1 tbsp. raspberry jam; put prepped cake batter in every cup on pastry and jam, filling to just top of every cup.
- In preheated oven, bake till inserted toothpick in cake exits clean for 25-30 minutes; briefly cool in pans. Loosen with knife. Transfer cakes onto wire rack; fully cool.

Nutrition Information

- Calories: 196 calories;
- Protein: 1.9
- Total Fat: 7.3
- Sodium: 219
- Total Carbohydrate: 31
- Cholesterol: 0

181. Chocolate Chai Cupcakes

Serving: 6 | Prep: 25mins | Cook: 15mins | Ready in:

Ingredients

- 6 tablespoons nonfat dry milk powder
- 3/4 cup hot black tea, or as needed
- nonstick cooking spray with flour
- 2 teaspoons ground cinnamon
- 1 teaspoon ground nutmeg
- 1 teaspoon ground allspice
- 1/2 teaspoon ground cloves
- 1/4 teaspoon ground black pepper
- 1 cup all-purpose flour
- 1 cup lightly packed brown sugar
- 6 tablespoons unsweetened cocoa powder
- 1 teaspoon baking soda
- 1/2 teaspoon baking powder
- 1/2 teaspoon salt
- 1/4 cup sunflower seed oil
- 1 egg, lightly beaten
- 1 teaspoon grated fresh ginger

Direction

- Pour the nonfat milk powder into the measuring cup. Mix in enough amount of black tea until you have a total of 1 cup. Whisk the mixture until the milk has dissolved; put aside until cool.
- Set the oven to 375°F or 190°C for preheating. Use the nonstick cooking spray to coat the muffin pan.
- In a small bowl, whisk the nutmeg, black pepper, cloves, cinnamon, and allspice.
- Sift the cocoa powder, baking powder, salt, baking soda, flour, spice mixture, and brown sugar into the large bowl. Whisk the egg, cooled tea mixture, and oil into the flour mixture until the batter is just incorporated. Fold in the ginger. Pour the batter into the prepared muffin cups, filling each cup to 3/4 full.
- Let them bake inside the preheated oven for 12-15 minutes until the inserted toothpick in its center comes out clean. Allow the cupcakes to cool on wire racks.

Nutrition Information

- Calories: 305 calories;
- Cholesterol: 29
- Protein: 6.9
- Total Fat: 11.1
- Sodium: 504
- Total Carbohydrate: 47.9

182. Chocolate Gingerbread Cupcakes

Serving: 1 dozen. | Prep: 40mins | Cook: 15mins | Ready in:

Ingredients

- 1 package (8 ounces) cream cheese, softened
- 1/2 cup white baking chips, melted and cooled
- 1/2 teaspoon vanilla extract
- 1/4 teaspoon salt
- 1-1/2 cups confectioners' sugar
- 1/2 cup marshmallow creme
- CUPCAKES:
- 1 package (14-1/2 ounces) gingerbread cake/cookie mix
- 2 teaspoons pumpkin pie spice
- 1/2 teaspoon ground ginger
- 2 ounces semisweet chocolate, melted
- Grated semisweet chocolate

Direction

- Set oven to 375 degrees and start preheating. Whip the first 4 ingredients until combined; slowly whisk in confectioners' sugar. Fold marshmallow crème into the mixture. Cover and refrigerate, then prepare cupcakes.
- Line paper liners on 12 muffin cups. Follow instructions on the package to prepare cake mix batter, putting in ginger and pie spice before mixing. Whisk in melted chocolate.
- Pour mixture into lined cups until it reaches 3/4 of each cup. Bake for 15 to 18 minutes until a toothpick slid into the middle comes out with no batter streaks. Allow to cool for 10 minutes in pan, then transfer to a wire rack to cool through.
- Cut a 1 1/2-inch circle with 1-inch depth in the top of each cupcake with a sharp knife. Gently take out cut part and save. Pour 2 tablespoons of filling into cut-out hole; sprinkle grated chocolate on top. Return the cut tops, while gently pressing down. Sprinkle more confectioners' sugar on top. Leave the rest in the fridge.

Nutrition Information

- Calories: 356 calories
- Fiber: 1g fiber)
- Total Carbohydrate: 52g carbohydrate (41g sugars
- Cholesterol: 38mg cholesterol
- Protein: 4g protein.
- Total Fat: 15g fat (7g saturated fat)
- Sodium: 359mg sodium

183. Chocolate And Red Wine Cupcakes

Serving: 2 dozen. | Prep: 15mins | Cook: 20mins | Ready in:

Ingredients

- 1-1/2 cups dry red wine
- 2 eggs
- 3 tablespoons canola oil
- 1 teaspoon vanilla extract
- 1-1/2 cups all-purpose flour
- 1-1/2 cups sugar
- 3/4 cup baking cocoa
- 1-1/2 teaspoons baking soda
- 3/4 teaspoon salt
- 3/4 teaspoon baking powder
- 16 ounces bittersweet chocolate, chopped
- 2 cups heavy whipping cream

Direction

- Beat vanilla, oil, eggs, and wine in a large bowl until well blended. Mix flour, baking powder, salt, baking soda, cocoa, and sugar; beat into the wine mixture gradually until blended.
- Fill half full into the paper-lined muffin cups. Next, bake for around 18-20 minutes at 350°, or until a toothpick comes out clean. Then let it cool for around 10 minutes before transferring from pans to wire racks in order to completely cool.
- Put the chocolate in a small bowl. Bring cream just to a boil in a small saucepan. Pour over the chocolate, then whisk until smooth. Freeze until chilled. Next, beat for about 15 seconds, until it forms soft peaks. Pipe over the cupcakes.

Nutrition Information

- Calories: 274 calories
- Sodium: 179mg sodium
- Fiber: 2g fiber)
- Total Carbohydrate: 29g carbohydrate (20g sugars
- Cholesterol: 45mg cholesterol
- Protein: 3g protein.
- Total Fat: 18g fat (9g saturated fat)

184. Christmas Reindeer Cupcakes

Serving: 12 | Prep: 1hours | Cook: 18mins | Ready in:

Ingredients

- Cupcakes:
- 9 tablespoons unsalted butter, room temperature
- 3/4 cup white sugar
- 1 teaspoon vanilla extract
- 2 eggs
- 1 1/2 cups sifted self-rising flour
- 1/2 cup milk
- Frosting:
- 1 cup confectioners' sugar
- 1 tablespoon unsalted butter, room temperature
- 1 tablespoon milk
- 1 drop brown food coloring
- Decoration:
- 6 vanilla wafer cookies (such as Nilla®)
- 12 red jelly beans
- 24 candy eyeballs
- 24 chewy chocolate-flavored candy (such as Tootsie Roll®)
- 24 pretzels

Direction

- Set the oven to 375°F or 190°C for preheating. Grease the 12-cup muffin tin or use the paper liners to line the cups.
- In a large bowl, mix the white sugar, vanilla extract, and 9 tbsp. of butter using the electric mixer until creamy and smooth. Add the eggs, one at a time. Whisk the mixture until well-blended. Fold in 1/4 cup of milk and 1/2 of the flour. Whisk the mixture until combined. Do the same with the remaining milk and flour. Pour the batter into the prepared muffin cups, filling them to 3/4 full.
- Bake them inside the preheated oven for 18 minutes until the inserted toothpick into the center comes out clean.
- Get the tin from the oven and let it cool on a wire rack for about 5 minutes. Remove the cupcakes from the tin. Place the cupcakes on a wire rack and let them cool fully for 1 hour before decorating them.
- In a large bowl, combine 1 tbsp. of milk, confectioners' sugar, and 1 tbsp. of butter. Whisk the mixture using an electric mixer until it turns creamy and smooth. If necessary, thin the frosting with more water or milk. Add the food coloring. Whisk the mixture until the frosting is brown uniformly. You can add more food coloring, 1 drop at a time until the desired color was reached.
- Top each cupcake with a thin layer of frosting. Divide the vanilla cookies in half and place each half on each cupcake for its mouth. Glue a jelly bean onto the cookie using a little bit of frosting for Rudolph's red nose. Insert each cupcake with 2 candy eyeballs. Crack a piece of pretzel until it looks like antlers, and then insert 2 antlers on top of each cupcake. For the ears, shape the chewy candies and insert 2 of them into each cupcake's sides.

Nutrition Information

- Calories: 427 calories;
- Total Fat: 13.9
- Sodium: 815
- Total Carbohydrate: 77.1
- Cholesterol: 57
- Protein: 6.3

185. Christmas Tree Cupcakes

Serving: 12 | Prep: 30mins | Cook: |Ready in:

Ingredients

- 2 1/2 cups vanilla frosting, divided
- 12 unfrosted cupcakes
- 2 drops green food coloring, or as needed
- 1/4 cup sprinkles, colored sugar, or candies
- 12 unfrosted cupcakes, cooled

Direction

- Pour 1/2 cup of vanilla frosting into the bowl. Spread the top of each cupcake with a thin layer of frosting using a knife. To make the decorating part easier, refrigerate the cupcakes for half an hour.
- In a bowl, combine the greed food coloring and leftover 2 cups of vanilla frosting. Whisk the mixture until the frosting turns uniformly green. Drop in additional green food coloring, 1 drop at a time, until your desired color was reached.
- Pour the frosting into a piping bag. Pipe the edge of each cupcake around with the green frosting, working this perpendicular to the top of the cupcake. Make sure you work this in a circular motion to come up with the shape of a tree. Do the same with the remaining cupcakes.
- Style the Christmas trees with colored sugar, candies, or sprinkles as tree ornaments.

Nutrition Information

- Calories: 461 calories;
- Protein: 3.7
- Total Fat: 18.4
- Sodium: 320
- Total Carbohydrate: 70.8
- Cholesterol: 37

186. Cinnabon® Cupcakes

Serving: 24 | Prep: 1hours | Cook: 20mins |Ready in:

Ingredients

- Cinnamon syrup:
- 1/2 cup unsalted butter
- 1/2 cup brown sugar
- 2 tablespoons ground cinnamon
- Cake batter:
- 2 1/2 cups sifted cake flour
- 1 tablespoon baking powder
- 1/2 teaspoon salt
- 1 cup whole milk at room temperature
- 2 large egg whites at room temperature
- 1 egg at room temperature
- 1/4 teaspoon vanilla extract
- 1/4 teaspoon almond extract
- 1/2 cup unsalted butter at room temperature
- 1 1/2 cups white sugar
- 1/2 cup cold heavy whipping cream
- 1 cup chopped pecans
- Cream cheese frosting:
- 1/4 cup unsalted butter at room temperature
- 1 (8 ounce) package cream cheese at room temperature
- 1 1/2 cups confectioners' sugar
- 1 drop vanilla extract
- 1 teaspoon ground cinnamon for sprinkling, or to taste

Direction

- Set the oven to 350°F (175°C) for preheating. Grease or line the 24 cupcake cups with the paper liners.
- In a saucepan, melt a half cup of the unsalted butter over low heat. Mix in 2 tbsp. of the cinnamon and brown sugar for 2 minutes until the cinnamon syrup is hot and the brown sugar is already dissolved. Put the mixture aside.
- Sift the baking powder, salt, and cake flour into the bowl. In a separate bowl, mix the egg

whites, almond extract, milk, egg, and 1/4 tsp. of the vanilla extract. In a large bowl, mix 1/2 cup of the room temperature butter and white sugar using the electric mixer for 5 minutes until creamy and pale yellow. Whisk the flour mixture into the creamed butter mixture gradually, adding it alternately with the milk mixture until the batter is well-combined. Beat the mixture for 2 more minutes.

- Use an electric mixer and clean batters to beat the cold cream into the chilled metal or glass bowl for 4 minutes until the cream holds soft peaks and fluffy. Fold the whipped cream into the batter. Distribute the batter among the prepared cups, filling each cup up to 2/3 full.
- Add 1 tsp. of cinnamon syrup into each batter in each cupcake cup. Put the rest of the cinnamon syrup aside.
- Let the cupcakes bake inside the preheated oven for 16 minutes until browned lightly and the inserted toothpick into the center of the cupcake will come out with some moist crumbs. Get the cupcakes from the pans and let them cool on racks, arranging them upside down.
- In a saucepan, heat the remaining cinnamon syrup over medium heat. Mix in the pecans and allow the mixture to boil at a low point. Remove it from the heat immediately. Spread the pecan mixture onto the wooden cutting board. Allow the pecan mixture to cool completely. Finely chop the pecan candy.
- In a bowl, whisk 1/4 cup of the butter that is in room temperature using the electric mixer until creamy and soft. Whisk in the cream cheese until blended. Add a drop of vanilla extract and confectioners' sugar to the mixture. Whisk it on high speed for at least 5 minutes until the frosting turns fluffy.
- Use the frosting to frost the cooled cupcakes. Style each cupcake with a sprinkle of cinnamon and a pinch of chopped pecan candy.

Nutrition Information

- Calories: 329 calories;
- Total Fat: 18.6
- Sodium: 154
- Total Carbohydrate: 38.7
- Cholesterol: 51
- Protein: 3.5

187. Creepy Halloween Skull Cupcakes

Serving: 24 | Prep: 30mins | Cook: 18mins | Ready in:

Ingredients

- 1 (18.25 ounce) package devil's food cake mix (such as Duncan Hines®)
- 1 cup water
- 3 eggs
- 1/3 cup vegetable oil
- 1 1/2 (16 ounce) packages prepared vanilla frosting
- 1 (7 ounce) pouch prepared chocolate frosting

Direction

- Preheat an oven to 175°C/350°F. Line paper liners (Halloween-themed/dark-colored ones are best) on 2 12-cup muffin tins.
- Beat oil, eggs, water and cake mix with an electric mixer at low speed for 30 seconds in a big bowl; beat for 2 minutes at medium speed till batter is creamy and smooth. Put batter in prepped muffin cups; fill each to 3/4 full.
- In preheated oven, bake for 18-21 minutes till inserted toothpick in middle exits clean; remove from oven. Cool tins for 15 minutes on wire rack. Remove cupcakes from tins; fully cool on wire rack for 1 hour before decorating.
- Use thin white vanilla frosting layer to frost each cupcake; to easily decorate, refrigerate for 30 minutes.
- Take cupcakes from fridge; apply 2nd white frosting layer. Use chocolate frosting to fill pipping bag with small round tip; draw skull face onto cupcakes. For eyes, pipe big ovals, 2

dots for nostrils then big stitched smile for its mouth.

Nutrition Information

- Calories: 276 calories;
- Sodium: 234
- Total Carbohydrate: 38.6
- Cholesterol: 25
- Protein: 2.8
- Total Fat: 13.1

188. Cupcake Princess' Vanilla Cupcakes

Serving: 12 | Prep: 15mins | Cook: 20mins | Ready in:

Ingredients

- 1 1/4 cups all-purpose flour
- 3/4 teaspoon baking soda
- 1 pinch salt
- 5 tablespoons butter, cut into pieces
- 2/3 cup milk
- 1 cup white sugar
- 2 eggs
- 1 egg yolk
- 1 teaspoon vanilla extract

Direction

- Set oven temperature to 350 degrees F (175 degrees C) and preheat. Use 12 paper cupcake liners to line a conventional muffin tin. Mix salt, flour and baking soda in a bowl leave to one side.
- Put milk and butter in a small saucepan and heat on low heat setting until the butter complete melts. Mix eggs, vanilla, egg yolk, and sugar in a big bowl by beating with an electric mixer, until the consistency is thicker and it has a lighter color. At low speed setting, introduce the flour mix while beating until evenly mixed. Gradually pour in the heated milk and continue beating until mixed evenly.
- Separate the batter equally between the cupcake liners. Bake for 20 minutes until an inserted toothpick can be removed without any residue. Allow to cool for 10 minutes on the cupcake pan. Shift cupcakes onto a cooling rack to allow cooling to occur completely.

Nutrition Information

- Calories: 178 calories;
- Cholesterol: 62
- Protein: 3.1
- Total Fat: 6.4
- Sodium: 131
- Total Carbohydrate: 27.4

189. Cute Bunny Cupcakes

Serving: 24 | Prep: 1hours | Cook: 30mins | Ready in:

Ingredients

- 2 1/2 cups all-purpose flour
- 2 cups white sugar
- 1 teaspoon baking powder
- 1/2 teaspoon baking soda
- 1 1/3 cups buttermilk
- 1/2 cup vegetable shortening
- 1 teaspoon vanilla extract
- 1/8 teaspoon salt
- 4 egg whites
- 2 (16 ounce) packages vanilla frosting, divided
- sweetened flake coconut, or as needed
- 1 drop red food coloring, or as needed
- 12 whole graham cracker squares (4 cookies each)
- 48 miniature semisweet chocolate chips

Direction

- Set oven temperature to 350 degrees F (175 degrees C) and leave aside to preheat. Prepare

24 cupcake cups by lining the insides with paper.
- Add sugar, flour, baking soda, and baking powder into a bowl and whisk together. Add vegetable shortening, buttermilk, salt, and vanilla extract into dry ingredients, and beat together until evenly mixed. Add egg whites to batter and continue beating. Fill prepared cupcake cups with batter up to 2/3 full.
- Bake for around 30 minutes in the preheated oven until cupcakes have light-browned appearance. Set aside to cool.
- Separate the first container of frosting into half and add red food coloring to give a pink hue. Leave the remaining half of vanilla frosting aside. Frost cupcakes using the second container of frosting. Scatter coconut over the cupcakes.
- Form individual cookies by breaking graham crackers and carefully cutting out leaf shapes that is pointed at both ends, forming 48 ears. Apply white frosting on the outside of each ear and pink frosting on the insides. Push 2 ears into each cupcake. Stick 2 mini chocolate chips into the cupcake to make eyes and make a nose using a dot of pink frosting.

Nutrition Information

- Calories: 401 calories;
- Total Fat: 16.5
- Sodium: 199
- Total Carbohydrate: 60.8
- Cholesterol: < 1
- Protein: 3.4

190. Easter Bunny Cupcakes

Serving: 30 | Prep: 30mins | Cook: 20mins | Ready in:

Ingredients

- 1 cup unsalted butter, softened
- 2 tablespoons unsalted butter, softened
- 1 3/4 cups white sugar
- 3 eggs
- 2 teaspoons grated lemon zest
- 1 teaspoon vanilla extract
- 3 1/2 cups all-purpose flour
- 1 teaspoon baking soda
- 1/2 teaspoon baking powder
- 1/2 teaspoon salt
- 1 (16 ounce) container sour cream
- Buttercream Frosting:
- 1 cup unsalted butter, softened
- 2 tablespoons unsalted butter, softened
- 1 teaspoon vanilla extract
- 5 cups confectioners' sugar
- 2 tablespoons milk
- Decoration:
- 30 large marshmallows, cut in half lengthwise
- 1 cup pink sugar sprinkles
- 30 candy-coated milk chocolate pieces (such as M&M's®)
- 1 (1.5 ounce) tube black decorating gel

Direction

- Preheat an oven to 175 degrees C (350 degrees F). Line cups with paper liners or coat 30 individual muffin cups with grease.
- Beat white sugar and one cup plus two tablespoons of butter in a large bowl using an electric blender until the mixture is creamy. Place in the eggs, one at a time, and beat thoroughly after every addition. Beat in vanilla extract and lemon zest.
- In a separate bowl, mix salt, baking powder, baking soda and flour. Pour into the butter mixture and alternate with sour cream. Combine thoroughly to form a thick batter. Scoop 1/4 cup batter into every muffin cup.
- Bake for 20 to 25 minutes in the preheated oven until the tops spring back when pressed lightly. Let it cool for ten minutes in tins. Place onto a wire rack and cool for about 20 minutes.
- Make frosting as the cupcakes cool. Use an electric blender to cream together vanilla extract and 1 cup plus 2 tablespoons of butter. Slowly beat in the confectioners' sugar, one

cup at a time, and mix thoroughly after every addition. Beat in milk and continue to beat until the frosting is fluffy and light.
- Spread the marshmallow halves with the cut-side down onto a clean surface. Spread a small amount of frosting in the middle of every marshmallow half. Sprinkle with the pink decorating sugar to form bunny ears.
- Spread the frosting in an even layer atop every cooled cupcake. For the ears, put two of prepared marshmallow halves onto every cupcake. For the nose, put a piece of chocolate in the center of every cupcake and then draw the eyes and whiskers using black decorating gel.

Nutrition Information

- Calories: 401 calories;
- Sodium: 137
- Total Carbohydrate: 55.7
- Cholesterol: 62
- Protein: 3.1
- Total Fat: 19.2

191. Easter Nests

Serving: 24 | Prep: 30mins | Cook: 25mins | Ready in:

Ingredients

- 1 (15.25 ounce) package chocolate cake mix
- 1 1/4 cups water
- 1/2 cup vegetable oil
- 3 eggs
- 1 (10 ounce) package sweetened flaked coconut
- 1 (16 ounce) can prepared chocolate frosting
- 1 cup egg-shaped chocolate candies (such as peanut M&Ms®), or as needed

Direction

- Preheat the oven to 175°C or 350°F. Line paper liners on 2 dozen cupcake cups.
- In mixing bowl, whip eggs, vegetable oil, water and cake mix on low speed in an electric mixer, to moisten the mixture, for half a minute. Raise the speed to moderate and whip for additional of 2 minutes, till batter becomes smooth. Pour batter into prepped cupcake cups, filling them 2/3 full.
- Let cupcakes bake for 18 to 23 minutes in prepped oven till an inserted toothpick in one cupcake gets out clean. Take cupcakes out of oven and raise oven temperature to 205°C or 400°F. Cool the cupcakes.
- Scatter coconut to a shallow, big baking pan or on one baking sheet; in hot oven, toast for 7 minutes, till coconut turn golden brown. Cool down.
- Cut out a portion form top of every cupcake, leaving a hollow indentation approximately 1 1/2-inch across and half-inch deep. Throw cut-out parts. Use chocolate frosting to frost the cupcakes and put toasted coconut on frosting to cover. Put 3 candies with shape of egg, in small indentation on top of every cupcake.

Nutrition Information

- Calories: 291 calories;
- Total Carbohydrate: 35.5
- Cholesterol: 24
- Protein: 3.1
- Total Fat: 16.4
- Sodium: 229

192. Easter Surprise Cupcakes

Serving: 24 | Prep: 15mins | Cook: 20mins | Ready in:

Ingredients

- 2 1/4 cups all-purpose flour
- 2 1/2 teaspoons baking powder
- 1 teaspoon salt

- 2/3 cup margarine, softened
- 1 cup brown sugar
- 3/4 cup white sugar
- 2 eggs
- 1 teaspoon vanilla extract
- 1 1/4 cups milk
- 24 small chocolate eggs, unwrapped

Direction

- Set the oven to 350°F or 175°C for preheating. Grease the 24 muffin cups or line them with paper liners. Sift the salt, flour, and baking powder, and then put the mixture aside.
- In a large bowl, cream the brown sugar, white sugar, and margarine together until fluffy and light. Whisk in the eggs, one at a time. Mix in the vanilla. Whisk in the flour mixture, adding it alternately with milk and whisking well until just incorporated.
- Fill each muffin cup with 1/3 full of the mixture. Stuff each center with a chocolate egg. Pour the remaining batter among the cups until they are 2/3 full.
- Bake them inside the preheated oven for 18-20 minutes or until the cupcakes are golden brown and their tops spring back when tapped lightly.

Nutrition Information

- Calories: 196 calories;
- Sodium: 212
- Total Carbohydrate: 29
- Cholesterol: 18
- Protein: 2.6
- Total Fat: 8

193. Easy Eggnog Cupcakes

Serving: 24 | Prep: 15mins | Cook: 20mins | Ready in:

Ingredients

- Cupcakes:
- 1 (15.25 ounce) package yellow cake mix
- 1 1/2 cups eggnog
- 4 eggs
- 1/4 cup butter, melted
- 1 teaspoon nutmeg
- Frosting:
- 1 cup eggnog
- 2 tablespoons all-purpose flour
- 1/4 cup butter
- 1/4 cup shortening
- 1 cup white sugar

Direction

- Preheat an oven to 175°C/350°F; line paper muffin liners/grease 24 muffin cups.
- Mix nutmeg, 1/4 cup melted butter, eggs, 1 1/2 cups eggnog and yellow cake mix till batter is smooth in a bowl. Put cupcake batter in prepped muffin cups so they are 2/3 full.
- In preheated oven, bake for 12-14 minutes till top springs back when pressed lightly and golden. Put cupcakes onto wire rack; fully cool.
- Mix flour and 1 cup eggnog in a saucepan on medium high heat for 5-7 minutes till it thickens. Take off heat; fully cool.
- Beat sugar, shortening and butter using an electric mixer for 2-3 minutes till fluffy and light; beat in the cooled eggnog mixture slowly. Beat till you get desired frosting consistency; spread frosting on cooled cupcakes.

Nutrition Information

- Calories: 213 calories;
- Cholesterol: 57
- Protein: 3
- Total Fat: 10.9
- Sodium: 171
- Total Carbohydrate: 26.6

194. Easy Halloween Mummy Cupcakes

Serving: 24 | Prep: 30mins | Cook: 18mins | Ready in:

Ingredients

- 1 (18.25 ounce) package devil's food cake mix (such as Duncan Hines®)
- 1 cup water
- 3 eggs
- 1/3 cup vegetable oil
- 1 (16 ounce) can vanilla frosting
- 48 chocolate chips

Direction

- Preheat an oven to 175°C/350°F. Line paper liners, Halloween-themed/dark-colored ones are best, on 2 12-cup muffin tins.
- Beat oil, eggs, water and cake mix with an electric mixer at low speed for 30 seconds till moist in a big bowl; beat for 2 minutes at medium speed till batter is creamy and smooth. Put batter in prepped muffin cups; fill each to 3/4 full.
- In the preheated oven, bake for 18-21 minutes till inserted toothpick in middle exits clean. Remove from oven; cool tins for 15 minutes on wire rack. Remove cupcakes from tins; fully cool for 1 hour on wire rack prior to decorating.
- Put frosting into plastic/pastry bag with corner cut off; onto bottom and top of cupcakes, pipe frosting strands, leaving oval eye-shape exposed in center. In exposed middle, pipe 2 dots for mummy's eyes. Put 2 chocolate chips in middle of every dot, flat-side up, for pupils.

Nutrition Information

- Calories: 361 calories;
- Sodium: 205
- Total Carbohydrate: 48
- Cholesterol: 28
- Protein: 3.8
- Total Fat: 19.3

195. Eggnog Cupcakes

Serving: 24 | Prep: 20mins | Cook: 20mins | Ready in:

Ingredients

- Cupcakes:
- 1 (16 ounce) package pound cake mix
- 1 1/4 cups eggnog
- 2 large eggs
- 1/2 teaspoon freshly grated nutmeg
- 1/2 teaspoon vanilla extract
- Icing:
- 1/2 cup softened butter
- 1 (3 ounce) package cream cheese, softened
- 1 (16 ounce) package confectioners' sugar
- 1/4 cup eggnog
- 1/2 teaspoon vanilla extract
- 1/2 teaspoon freshly grated nutmeg

Direction

- Preheat an oven to 175°C/350°F; line paper liners on 24 muffin cups.
- Beat 1/2 tsp. vanilla extract, 1/2 tsp. nutmeg, eggs, 1 1/4 cups eggnog and cake mix using an electric mixer at low till batter is blended in a bowl. Put speed on medium; beat for 2 minutes. Put batter in prepped muffin cups.
- In preheated oven, bake for 18-20 minutes till inserted toothpick in middle of cupcake exits clean. Put cupcakes onto wire rack; fully cool.
- Beat cream cheese and butter using an electric mixer till creamy and smooth in a bowl. Beat alternately small quantity of 1/4 cup eggnog and confectioners' sugar, finishing with confectioners' sugar, into butter mixture with an electric mixer at low speed till icing is fluffy and smooth. Beat 1/2 tsp. nutmeg and 1/2 tsp. vanilla extract into icing till incorporated; spread on cooled cupcakes.

Nutrition Information

- Calories: 239 calories;
- Total Carbohydrate: 33.5
- Cholesterol: 50
- Protein: 2.6
- Total Fat: 11
- Sodium: 124

196. Eggnog Chai Cupcakes

Serving: 12 | Prep: 20mins | Cook: 22mins | Ready in:

Ingredients

- Cupcakes:
- 1 (15.25 ounce) package spiced cake mix (such as Betty Crocker®)
- 1 cup brewed chai tea
- 1/2 cup vegetable oil
- 3 eggs
- Frosting:
- 1/2 cup butter, softened
- 1 (8 ounce) package cream cheese, softened
- 2 cups confectioners' sugar
- 1 teaspoon vanilla extract
- 1/2 teaspoon ground nutmeg
- 2 tablespoons eggnog
- 1 teaspoon rum extract

Direction

- Set the oven to 350°F (175°C) for preheating. Use paper liners to line the muffin cups.
- In a bowl, whisk the chai tea, vegetable oil, eggs and cake mix using the electric mixer at low speed for 30 seconds. Adjust the speed of the mixer to medium. Whisk the mixture for 2 more minutes until the batter is smooth. Pour the batter into the prepared muffin cups, filling them up to 2/3 full.
- Bake them inside the preheated oven for 22-24 minutes until the inserted toothpick into the center comes out clean. Let the cupcakes cool in the tin, about 5 minutes. Transfer them onto a wire rack; cool completely.
- In a bowl, whisk the cream cheese and butter using the electric mixer at medium speed for 20-30 seconds until smooth. Add the vanilla extract, nutmeg, and confectioners' sugar. Whisk the mixture at medium-high speed for 1 minute until smooth. If necessary, scrape the sides of the bowl. Add the eggnog. Whisk the mixture until well-incorporated. Whisk in rum extract at medium-low speed.
- Pour the frosting mixture into the plastic or pastry bag with a corner snipped. Use it to pipe the frosting onto the cooled cupcakes.

Nutrition Information

- Calories: 472 calories;
- Total Fat: 29.2
- Sodium: 372
- Total Carbohydrate: 48.3
- Cholesterol: 89
- Protein: 5.3

197. Firecracker Cupcakes

Serving: 24 | Prep: 35mins | Cook: 16mins | Ready in:

Ingredients

- 1 (15.25 ounce) package white cake mix (such as Duncan Hines®)
- 1 cup water
- 3 eggs
- 1/3 cup vegetable oil
- 1 (14 ounce) package sweetened flaked coconut (such as Bakers® Angel Flake®)
- 8 drops blue food coloring
- 8 drops red food coloring
- 1 (16 ounce) package vanilla frosting
- 1 (.68 oz. tube) red decorating gel
- 1 toothpick
- 24 (4 inch) pieces red licorice strings

Direction

- Set the oven to 350°F or 175°C for preheating. Use paper liners to line the two 12-cup muffin tins or grease the cups.
- In a bowl, combine the eggs, oil, cake mix, and water. Whisk the mixture until moistened. Whisk the mixture using the electric mixer with low speed for 2 minutes. Pour the mixture into the prepared muffin cups.
- Bake the cupcakes inside the preheated oven for 16-20 minutes until lightly golden.
- Divide the coconut into 3 even portions. Pour 2 portions of coconut into separate resealable plastic bags. Put the remaining portion of coconut on a plate. Add the red food coloring to one of the plastic bags and blue food coloring to the other bag. Seal and shake the bags until the coconuts are perfectly colored. Transfer the colored coconuts onto separate plates.
- Get the paper liners from the cupcakes. Frost the sides and tops of the cupcakes. Dip each of the cupcakes into the 3 plates filled with coconut, making sure that all sides are well coated. Use the decorating gel to make a star shape on top of the cupcake. Use a toothpick to form a hole in the center of the star. Insert the licorice "fuse" piece into the hole.

Nutrition Information

- Calories: 339 calories;
- Protein: 2.6
- Total Fat: 13.3
- Sodium: 233
- Total Carbohydrate: 53.2
- Cholesterol: 23

---

198. Flower Garden Cupcakes

Serving: 24 servings | Prep: 15mins | Cook: | Ready in:

Ingredients

- 1 pkg. (2-layer size) white cake mix
- 1 cup boiling water
- 1 pkg. (3 oz.) JELL-O Strawberry Flavor Gelatin
- 1 tub (8 oz.) COOL WHIP Whipped Topping, thawed
- food colorings (assorted colors)
- suggested decorations: JET-PUFFED Marshmallows, colored sugar, small hard candies, BAKER'S ANGEL FLAKE Coconut, JET-PUFFED BUNNY MALLOWS Marshmallows, vanilla wafers, JET-PUFFED Miniature Marshmallows

Direction

- 1. Follow the directions on the package to prepare the cake batter and bake 24 cakes. Let the cakes cool in pans for 10 minutes. Then use a fork to piece the tops.
- 2. Stir the gelatin with boiling water in a small bowl for 2 minutes until completely dissolved. Scoop the mixture over the cupcakes. Put into a refrigerator for half an hour. You can tint the cool whip with food coloring if you want then spread over the cakes.
- 3. You can decorate the cupcakes your ways.

Nutrition Information

- Calories: 180
- Saturated Fat: 2 g
- Fiber: 0 g
- Protein: 2 g
- Total Fat: 4 g
- Sodium: 180 mg
- Sugar: 23 g
- Total Carbohydrate: 33 g
- Cholesterol: 0 mg

---

199. Fluffy Pumpkin Spiced Cupcakes

Serving: 24 | Prep: 15mins | Cook: 30mins | Ready in:

Ingredients

- 1 (15 ounce) can pumpkin puree
- 1 1/2 cups white sugar
- 1 cup packed brown sugar
- 1/2 cup butter-flavored shortening
- 1/2 cup butter, softened
- 1/4 cup whole milk
- 1/4 cup vegetable oil
- 4 eggs
- 2 cups cake flour
- 1/4 cup dry buttermilk powder
- 1/4 cup cornstarch
- 2 teaspoons pumpkin pie spice
- 2 teaspoons baking powder
- 1 teaspoon baking soda
- 3/4 teaspoon salt

Direction

- Set the oven to 350°F or 175°C for preheating. Use paper muffin liners to line the 24 muffin cups.
- In a large bowl, whisk the white sugar, butter, vegetable oil, eggs, milk, pumpkin puree, brown sugar, and shortening until smooth. In a separate bowl, whisk the dry buttermilk powder, pumpkin pie spice, salt, cake flour, baking soda, cornstarch and baking powder. Add the dry ingredients to the pumpkin mixture, whisking the mixture well until combined. Pour the mixture into the prepared muffin cups, filling them up to 2/3 full.
- Bake them inside the preheated oven for 30 minutes until the middle of the cupcakes springs back once touched. Let them cool in the pans for 10 minutes. Transfer them onto a wire rack and let them cool completely.

Nutrition Information

- Calories: 250 calories;
- Protein: 2.8
- Total Fat: 11.7
- Sodium: 258
- Total Carbohydrate: 34.5
- Cholesterol: 42

200. Fruity Mini Cupcakes

Serving: 48 | Prep: 15mins | Cook: 15mins | Ready in:

Ingredients

- 1 (18.25 ounce) package white cake mix
- 1 cup water
- 1/3 cup vegetable oil
- 3 eggs
- 4 (0.13 ounce) packages unsweetened fruit-flavored drink mix (such as Kool-Aid®)

Direction

- Set the oven to 350°F (175°C), and start preheating.
- Line mini paper liners on 48 mini muffin cups.
- Beat unsweetened drink mix powder, eggs, vegetable oil, water and cake mix till the batter is evenly colored and smooth.
- Fill batter into the mini muffin cups till about 2/3 full.
- Bake in the prepped oven for about 15 minutes, till the cupcakes are set in the center. A toothpick put into the middle of a cupcake should go out clean.
- Cool the mini cupcakes before decorating.

Nutrition Information

- Calories: 63 calories;
- Total Fat: 3
- Sodium: 80
- Total Carbohydrate: 8.3
- Cholesterol: 12
- Protein: 0.9

201. Gingerbread Cupcakes

Serving: 24 | Prep: 15mins | Cook: 15mins | Ready in:

Ingredients

- 1 (18.25 ounce) box vanilla cake mix
- 1/2 cup buttermilk
- 1/2 cup molasses
- 1/3 cup vegetable oil
- 4 large eggs
- 1 1/2 teaspoons ground ginger
- 1/2 teaspoon ground cinnamon
- 1/4 teaspoon ground nutmeg

Direction

- Preheat the oven to 175°C or 350°F. Line paper muffin liners on 2 dozen muffin cups.
- In big bowl, combine nutmeg, cinnamon, ginger, eggs, vegetable oil, molasses, buttermilk and cake mix till barely incorporated. Scoop batter to a big sealable plastic bag, release excess air, and enclose the top of bag. Snip one corner of bag approximately quarter-inch from bottom. Pipe batter to prepped muffin cups, approximately 2/3 full.
- Bake for 15 to 20 minutes in prepped oven till an inserted toothpick in the middle gets out clean. Cool for 10 minutes in pans prior to transferring on wire rack to fully cool.

Nutrition Information

- Calories: 155 calories;
- Cholesterol: 32
- Protein: 2.2
- Total Fat: 6.5
- Sodium: 161
- Total Carbohydrate: 22.4

202. Gluten Free Lovely Lemon Cupcakes

Serving: 14 | Prep: 30mins | Cook: 25mins | Ready in:

Ingredients

- 2 cups almond flour
- 3/4 cup gluten-free all-purpose baking flour
- 1/4 teaspoon baking powder
- 1 cup butter, softened
- 2 cups sucanat (crystallized sugar cane juice)
- 1 (15 ounce) container ricotta cheese
- 4 eggs
- 1 teaspoon vanilla extract
- 1/2 teaspoon pure lemon oil
- 1/2 cup prepared lemon curd
- 14 ounces cream cheese, softened
- 1 cup butter, softened
- 1 1/3 cups confectioners' sugar
- 1 1/2 teaspoons vanilla extract
- 1 1/2 teaspoons pure lemon oil

Direction

- Set the oven for preheating to 350°F (175°C).
- Prepare 14 muffin cups lined with paper liners.
- Sift together the baking powder, gluten-free all-purpose baking flour and almond flour in a bowl.
- Cream 1 cup butter with sucanat in a mixing bowl of the stand mixer until fluffy and light, 1 to 2 minutes; stir in ricotta cheese.
- Beat in eggs, one at a time, beating each egg well before each addition. Beat in almond flour mixture little by little, about a quarter cup at a time, and scrape down the sides of the bowl frequently. Mix half a teaspoon of lemon oil and a teaspoon of vanilla extract into the batter until evenly incorporated.
- Pour the batter in the prepared muffin cups about 2/3 full.
- Let it bake inside the preheated oven for 25 minutes to half an hour, until cupcakes turn very lightly golden brown and have risen. Avoid opening the oven doors until 25 minutes of the baking time have passed.
- Let the cupcakes cool completely.
- Cut plugs out of the cores of each cupcakes and fill the hole with about 1 1/2 teaspoon lemon curd.
- Beat a cup of butter and cream cheese in a mixing bowl of the stand mixer until the

mixture turns creamy and smooth. Mix in 1 1/2 teaspoon lemon oil, 1 1/2 teaspoon vanilla extract and confectioners' sugar to make a smooth and spreadable frosting. Ice the filled cupcakes.

Nutrition Information

- Calories: 643 calories;
- Total Fat: 43.5
- Sodium: 346
- Total Carbohydrate: 53.8
- Cholesterol: 171
- Protein: 14.1

203. Grownup Chai Chocolate Cupcakes

Serving: 10 | Prep: 15mins | Cook: 30mins | Ready in:

Ingredients

- 1/2 cup unsalted butter
- 2 (1 ounce) squares unsweetened chocolate, chopped
- 4 chai tea bags
- 1/2 cup all-purpose flour, sifted
- 3/4 cup white sugar
- 2 eggs
- 1 teaspoon vanilla extract

Direction

- Set the oven to 325°F or 165°C for preheating. Use 10 paper liners to line the muffin tin.
- In the double boiler's top, melt the chocolate and butter over simmering water for 5-10 minutes, stirring often and scraping the sides down using the rubber spatula to prevent it from scorching until smooth.
- Open the tea bags and pour the chai mixture into the spice grinder and grind for 5-10 seconds until it is grounded into a fine powder.

- In a large bowl, mix the chai powder, sugar, and flour. Add the eggs, one at a time and beat well every after addition until the batter is smooth. Mix in the vanilla extract. Drizzle the batter with the chocolate mixture, mixing well until just blended. Distribute the batter among the prepared muffin cups.
- Bake them inside the preheated oven for 25 minutes until the tops are cracked slightly and glossy and the inserted toothpick into the muffin's center comes out clean. Transfer the muffins from the tin onto the wire rack immediately; cool.

Nutrition Information

- Calories: 207 calories;
- Protein: 2.7
- Total Fat: 13.2
- Sodium: 17
- Total Carbohydrate: 21.8
- Cholesterol: 62

204. Halloween Chocolate Cupcakes With Monster Peanut Butter Eyes

Serving: 12 | Prep: 50mins | Cook: 15mins | Ready in:

Ingredients

- Chocolate Cupcakes:
- 9 tablespoons unsweetened cocoa powder
- 5 tablespoons boiling water, or more if needed
- 3/4 cup unsalted butter
- 3/4 cup white sugar
- 2 tablespoons white sugar
- 1 cup all-purpose flour
- 2 teaspoons baking powder
- 3 eggs
- 1 teaspoon vanilla extract
- Peanut Butter Eyes:
- 4 cups confectioners' sugar

- 1 3/4 cups peanut butter
- 1 cup white chocolate chips
- 1/4 cup butter
- 1 (1.5 ounce) tube red decorating gel
- 1 (16 ounce) package prepared chocolate frosting
- 1 (1.5 ounce) tube white decorating gel

Direction

- Preheat an oven to 95°C/200°F; grease/line cups with paper liners on 12-cup muffin tin.
- Sift cocoa powder in big bowl; add 5 tbsp. boiling water. Mix into thick paste; if needed, 1 tbsp. at a time, add extra water. Add 3/4 cup and 2 tbsp. sugar and 3/4 cup butter; use electric mixer to beat till creamy and smooth. One by one, beat eggs in; beat well with every addition till batter is smooth.
- Mix baking powder and flour in bowl; mix into batter till combined well. Put batter in prepped muffin cups; fill each to 2/3 to top using ice cream scoop.
- In preheated oven, bake for 10-15 minutes till toothpick exits clean and lightly pressing tops makes them spring back. Cool for few minutes in muffin tin; put on wire rack. Completely cool for 1 hour.
- Beat vanilla extract, 1/4 cup butter, peanut butter and confectioners' sugar till thick dough forms in bowl; refrigerate for half an hour.
- Line baking parchment on baking sheet.
- Take peanut butter mixture from fridge; roll to small balls for monster eyes. Moisten hands/chill mixture if it begins to stick. Put balls on prepped baking sheet; freeze for half an hour.
- In top of double boiler above simmering water, put white chocolate on top; continuously mix, scraping sides down with rubber spatula to prevent scorching, for 5 minutes till chocolate melts.
- Take eyes from freeze; pick them up individually with toothpick. In melted chocolate, dip balls; leave small circle on 1 side blank. Remove extra chocolate by twirling toothpick; put on parchment lined baking sheet.
- Dig out little peanut butter mixture from every ball that isn't covered in chocolate to create room for red decorating gel; use red decorating gel to fill holes.
- Use chocolate frosting to frost cupcakes; put 2 peanut butter eyes over. Use white decorating gel to draw on a mouth.

Nutrition Information

- Calories: 890 calories;
- Sodium: 500
- Total Carbohydrate: 109.8
- Cholesterol: 85
- Protein: 14.3
- Total Fat: 48.2

205. Halloween Fondant Ghost Cupcakes

Serving: 12 | Prep: 40mins | Cook: 16mins | Ready in:

Ingredients

- 1 cup all-purpose flour
- 2 tablespoons all-purpose flour
- 1/2 cup unsweetened cocoa powder
- 1 teaspoon baking soda
- 1 teaspoon salt
- 1 cup white sugar
- 1/2 cup butter
- 1 egg
- 1 teaspoon vanilla extract
- 1 cup milk
- Decorating:
- 1 (16 ounce) package vanilla frosting
- 6 large marshmallows, cut in half crosswise
- 2 tablespoons confectioners' sugar, or as needed
- 8 ounces ready-to-use white fondant
- 12 raisins, halved

Direction

- Set the oven to 350°F or 175°C for preheating. Grease the 12-cup muffin tin or use the paper liners to line the cups.
- Sift the baking soda, salt, 1 cup plus 2 tbsp. of flour, and cocoa powder into the bowl.
- In a large bowl, combine the butter and sugar, and then whisk the mixture using the electric mixer until fluffy and light. Whisk in the vanilla extract and egg. Stir in the flour mixture, adding it alternately with the milk. Whisk the batter until just combined.
- Let them bake inside the preheated oven for 16-20 minutes until their tops will spring back when pressed lightly and the inserted toothpick into the center will come out clean. Remove them from the oven and place them on a wire rack. Let them cool for 15 minutes. Get the cupcakes from the tin and let them cool completely for 2 hours.
- Use a thin layer of white vanilla frosting to frost each of the cupcakes. Arrange one marshmallow half into the center of the cupcake, cut-side up.
- Sprinkle the confectioners' sugar all over the work surface. Pinch some walnut-sized pieces of the white fondant off. Roll the pieces into thin circles until they look a little bigger than the cupcakes. For it to look like ghosts, drape the marshmallows over them. Make two holes near the top by poking them for the eyes. Fill each hole with one raisin half.

Nutrition Information

- Calories: 454 calories;
- Sodium: 441
- Total Carbohydrate: 75.6
- Cholesterol: 36
- Protein: 3.2
- Total Fat: 16.4

206. Halloween Gingerbread Cupcakes

Serving: 12 | Prep: 40mins | Cook: 20mins | Ready in:

Ingredients

- Reynolds® StayBrite® Baking Cups
- 6 tablespoons butter, softened
- 1/2 cup granulated sugar
- 1 1/2 teaspoons baking powder
- 1 teaspoon ground cinnamon
- 1/4 teaspoon ground ginger
- 1/4 teaspoon baking soda
- 1/4 teaspoon salt
- 2 eggs
- 1 cup milk
- 1/2 cup molasses
- 1 3/4 cups all-purpose flour
- Orange and black decorating sugar
- Cinnamon Vanilla Frosting:
- 1/3 cup butter, softened
- 1/3 cup sour cream
- 1 teaspoon vanilla
- 4 cups powdered sugar
- 1 teaspoon ground cinnamon

Direction

- Set the oven to 350°F for preheating. Use 12-18 Reynolds® StayBrite® Baking Cups that have a black swirl design to line the muffin pans.
- In a large bowl, beat the sugar and butter using the electric mixer at medium speed for 30 seconds. Add the salt, ginger, cinnamon, baking powder, and baking soda. Beat the mixture, scraping the sides of the bowl if needed until well-combined. Whisk in eggs, one at a time.
- In a medium bowl, whisk the molasses and milk. Add the flour and milk mixture alternately to the butter mixture, whisking it at low speed after every addition until just blended. Distribute the batter among the prepared muffin cups and fill them to 3/4 full.
- Bake them for 18-20 minutes until the inserted wooden toothpick near their centers comes out

clean. Let them cool in pans that are set on a wire rack for 5 minutes. Remove the cupcakes from the pans carefully and let them cool on a wire rack completely.
- Frost the cupcakes using the Cinnamon Vanilla Frosting. Sprinkle the cupcakes with the colored decorating sugars.
- For the Cinnamon Vanilla Frosting, combine the vanilla, butter, and sour cream in a large mixing bowl. Use an electric mixer to beat the mixture at medium speed for 30 seconds. Beat in the ground cinnamon and powdered sugar gradually. Thin the mixture with 1-2 tbsp. of milk until the desired consistency is reached.

Nutrition Information

- Calories: 437 calories;
- Total Carbohydrate: 76.2
- Cholesterol: 64
- Protein: 3.9
- Total Fat: 13.8
- Sodium: 242

207. Harvest Pumpkin Cupcakes

Serving: 32 | Prep: 20mins | Cook: 30mins | Ready in:

Ingredients

- Cupcakes:
- 4 eggs, slightly beaten
- 3/4 cup Mazola® Vegetable Plus! Oil
- 2 cups sugar
- 1 (15 ounce) can pumpkin
- 1 3/4 cups all-purpose flour
- 1/4 cup Argo® OR Kingsford's® Corn Starch
- 4 teaspoons Spice Islands® Pumpkin Pie Spice
- 2 teaspoons Argo® Baking Powder
- 1 teaspoon baking soda
- 3/4 teaspoon salt
- Frosting:
- 1 (8 ounce) package cream cheese, softened
- 3 tablespoons butter OR margarine, softened
- 1 tablespoon orange juice
- 2 teaspoons Spice Islands® 100% Pure Bourbon Vanilla Extract
- 1 1/2 teaspoons freshly grated orange peel
- 4 cups powdered sugar

Direction

- For the cupcakes: In a large mixing bowl, blend pumpkin, sugar, oil and eggs together; set aside. In a separate bowl, mix dry ingredients together. Put the dry ingredients into the pumpkin mixture; beat till well blended. Transfer into lined muffin tins. Fill around two-thirds full. Bake for 30 minutes in the preheated 350° oven, or till the center springs back when touched. Allow to cool for 30 minutes. Spread the frosting over.
- For the frosting: Beat butter and cream cheese till fluffy. Put in the remaining ingredients; beat till smooth. Spread on top of the cooled cupcakes.

Nutrition Information

- Calories: 233 calories;
- Sodium: 194
- Total Carbohydrate: 35.9
- Cholesterol: 34
- Protein: 2.2
- Total Fat: 9.6

208. Hummingbird Cupcakes

Serving: about 2 dozen. | Prep: 40mins | Cook: 20mins | Ready in:

Ingredients

- 1 cup butter, softened
- 2 cups sugar
- 3 eggs
- 2 teaspoons vanilla extract
- 2 cups mashed ripe bananas

- 1/2 cup drained canned crushed pineapple
- 3 cups all-purpose flour
- 1 teaspoon baking soda
- 1 teaspoon ground cinnamon
- 1/2 teaspoon salt
- 1 cup sweetened shredded coconut
- 1 cup chopped walnuts
- CREAM CHEESE FROSTING:
- 1 package (8 ounces) cream cheese, softened
- 1/2 cup butter, softened
- 3-3/4 cups confectioners' sugar
- 1 teaspoon vanilla extract

Direction

- Cream sugar and butter in a big bowl till fluffy and light. Put in eggs, one by one, whipping thoroughly after every increment. Whip vanilla in. Mix pineapple and bananas in small bowl.
- Mix salt, cinnamon, baking soda and flour; put to creamed mixture alternating with mixture of banana, whipping thoroughly after every increment. Fold in walnuts and coconut.
- Fill muffin cups lined with paper 2/3 full. Bake for 20 to 25 minutes at 350° or till an inserted toothpick in the middle gets out clean. Let cool for 10 minutes prior to transferring from pans onto wire racks to fully cool.
- Whip butter and cream cheese in small bowl till fluffy. Put in vanilla and confectioners' sugar; whip till smooth. Frost the cupcakes.

Nutrition Information

- Calories: 410 calories
- Total Fat: 20g fat (11g saturated fat)
- Sodium: 230mg sodium
- Fiber: 2g fiber)
- Total Carbohydrate: 56g carbohydrate (39g sugars
- Cholesterol: 67mg cholesterol
- Protein: 4g protein.

209. Independence Day Cupcakes

Serving: 24 | Prep: 45mins | Cook: 25mins | Ready in:

Ingredients

- 2 1/4 cups all-purpose flour
- 1 1/2 cups white sugar
- 1 1/2 teaspoons baking powder
- 1/2 teaspoon salt
- 1/2 cup vegetable shortening
- 3 egg whites
- 2 teaspoons vanilla extract
- 1 cup milk
- 1 (1 ounce) package instant sugar-free vanilla pudding mix
- 2 cups skim milk
- 1 (7 ounce) container light whipped cream
- 12 thinly sliced strawberries, or as needed
- 24 fresh blueberries

Direction

- Set the oven to 350°F (175°C) for preheating. Use paper liners to line the 24 cupcake cups. In a large mixing bowl, mix the baking powder, flour, salt, and sugar.
- Cut in the shortening using the pastry cutter until the mixture turns crumbly. Mix in the vanilla extract, a cup of milk, and egg whites until the batter is smooth. Fill the paper-lined cupcake cups with the batter, about 2/3 full.
- Bake them inside the preheated oven for 22-26 minutes until the inserted toothpick into the cupcake's center comes out clean. Let the cupcakes cool completely.
- Beat 2 cups of skim milk and pudding mix in a bowl for 2 minutes until the pudding turns thick. Let the mixture stand for 5 minutes to finish thickening. Fill the pastry bag fitted with a medium tip with the pudding.
- To fill and style the cupcakes, cut a small hole into the top of the cupcake using the thin paring knife, making sure it has a diameter of 1/2-inch. Remove its core by inserting the knife 3/4 down into the cupcake. Fill the hole

of the cupcake with the pudding in a pastry bag, enough to fill the hole up to the top of the cupcake. Use the light whipped cream to frost the tops of the cupcakes, spreading the cream well in a smooth layer.
- Garnish the center of the cupcake with the blueberry. Arrange five slices of strawberry all around the blueberry, positioning their pointed ends outward until you form a star shape. Store the cupcakes inside the fridge.

Nutrition Information

- Calories: 172 calories;
- Protein: 2.8
- Total Fat: 6.7
- Sodium: 147
- Total Carbohydrate: 25.9
- Cholesterol: 6

210.   Jelly Doughnut Cupcakes

Serving: 24 | Prep: 30mins | Cook: 20mins | Ready in:

Ingredients

- cooking spray
- 1 (18.5 ounce) package yellow cake mix
- 1 (3.5 ounce) package instant French vanilla pudding mix
- 1 cup whole milk
- 1 cup vegetable oil
- 4 eggs
- 1 (12 ounce) jar seedless raspberry jam
- 2 tablespoons confectioners' sugar for dusting

Direction

- Preheat the oven to 175 ° C or 350 ° F.
- Use cooking spray to coat 2 dozen muffin cups; line paper liners on cups.
- In big bowl, whip eggs, vegetable oil, milk, instant French vanilla pudding mix and yellow cake mix using electric hand mixer till no dry patches in batter remain and cake mix is moistened completely. Scrape bowl and mix once more.
- Fill prepped muffin cups with batter, approximately 1/2 full of.
- Let cupcakes bake in prepped oven for 18 to 20 minutes, till slightly golden brown. An inserted toothpick or cake tester in the center of cupcake must get out clean.
- Cool cupcakes.
- Cut plug approximately 1 1/2-inch long and 3/4-inch diameter out of the middle of every cupcake.
- Put raspberry jam to opening, filling it.
- Lightly dust confectioners' sugar on cupcakes.

Nutrition Information

- Calories: 246 calories;
- Sodium: 216
- Total Carbohydrate: 31
- Cholesterol: 32
- Protein: 2.3
- Total Fat: 12.9

211.   Key Lime Cupcakes

Serving: 24 | Prep: 20mins | Cook: 20mins | Ready in:

Ingredients

- Cake:
- 1 (15.25 ounce) package white cake mix (such as Pillsbury® Classic White)
- 1 cup water
- 3 eggs
- 1/3 cup vegetable oil
- 2 tablespoons lime zest
- 1 tablespoon fresh lime juice
- 3 drops green food coloring (optional)
- Frosting:
- 1/2 cup butter, softened
- 1 (8 ounce) package cream cheese, softened
- 2 tablespoons lime zest

- 1/2 teaspoon vanilla extract
- 1 1/2 cups confectioners' sugar, sifted
- 2 tablespoons pearlized sprinkles, or as needed (optional)

Direction

- Preheat the oven to 175°C or 350°F. Line 2 dozen muffin cups with paper liners or use cooking spray to coat them.
- Use an electric mixer to combine vegetable oil, eggs, water and cake mix in bowl for 2 minutes to make a smooth batter. Put lime juice, food coloring and 2 tablespoons of lime zest; combine thoroughly. Put the batter to prepped muffin cups.
- Bake for 18 minutes in prepped oven till golden in color and an inserted toothpick into the middle of one cupcake gets out clean. Let cupcakes cool on wire rack.
- Use an electric mixer to whip cream cheese and butter in bowl till creamy and smooth. Put vanilla extract and 2 tablespoons of lime zest into mixture of creamed butter; combine thoroughly. Combine into creamed butter mixture with confectioners' sugar, half cup at one time, until achieves a smooth frosting; refrigerate to chill till frosting thickens, approximately half an hour.
- Smear frosting on every cupcake and put sprinkles on top.

Nutrition Information

- Calories: 215 calories;
- Total Carbohydrate: 23.1
- Cholesterol: 44
- Protein: 2.4
- Total Fat: 12.9
- Sodium: 184

212. Lemon Frosted Carrot Cake Cupcakes

Serving: 24 | Prep: 30mins | Cook: 18mins | Ready in:

Ingredients

- Reynolds® StayBrite® Baking Cups
- 2 cups all-purpose flour
- 1 cup granulated sugar
- 2 teaspoons ground cinnamon
- 1 teaspoon baking powder
- 1 teaspoon baking soda
- 1/4 teaspoon ground nutmeg
- 1/8 teaspoon salt
- 2 cups shredded carrots
- 1/2 cup canola oil
- 1/2 cup unsweetened applesauce
- 1 egg, lightly beaten
- 1 teaspoon vanilla
- 1 cup flaked coconut, toasted
- 1 cup mini jelly beans or chocolate egg candies
- Lemon Cream Cheese Frosting:
- 3 ounces cream cheese, softened
- 3 tablespoons butter, softened
- 2 tablespoons lemon curd
- 3 cups powdered sugar, divided
- 2 teaspoons milk, or more as needed

Direction

- Set the oven to 350°F for preheating. Use 24 Reynolds® StayBrite® Baking Cups to line the muffin pans.
- In a large bowl, mix the baking soda, flour, cinnamon, baking powder, nutmeg, salt, and sugar.
- In a medium bowl, combine the applesauce, vanilla, egg, oil, and carrots. Pour the carrot mixture into the flour mixture and whisk until well-combined. Distribute the batter into the prepared muffin cups.
- Let them bake for 16-18 minutes until the inserted toothpick into the centers will come out very clean. Let them cool in the muffin pan for 5 minutes. Place them onto a cooling rack and let them cool completely.

- Top the cupcakes with the Lemon Cream Cheese Frosting, making sure to reserve a small amount. Form a nest using the coconut. Dip the candy eggs or jelly beans into the reserved frosting lightly and arrange them into the nests, keeping them in place.
- For the Lemon Cream Cheese Frosting, combine the softened butter, cream cheese, and lemon curd in a big mixing bowl. Use an electric mixer to whisk the mixture at medium to high speed until smooth. Add 1 1/2 cups of powdered sugar gradually to the mixture and whisk well. Mix in 2 tsp. of milk. Beat in 1 1/2 cups of powdered sugar gradually. Add more milk if necessary, 1 tsp. at a time until the desired consistency is reached.

Nutrition Information

- Calories: 262 calories;
- Sodium: 130
- Total Carbohydrate: 45.3
- Cholesterol: 17
- Protein: 1.8
- Total Fat: 8.6

213. Lemon Filled Cupcakes

Serving: 24 | Prep: 30mins | Cook: 20mins | Ready in:

Ingredients

- 1 (18.25 ounce) package lemon cake mix
- 1 cup water
- 1/3 cup vegetable oil
- 3 eggs
- 1/4 cup vegetable shortening
- 1/4 cup butter
- 1/4 cup fresh lemon juice, or to taste
- 2 cups confectioners' sugar
- 4 ounces white chocolate, chopped
- 1 (8 ounce) package cream cheese, softened
- 1/2 cup butter, softened
- 1 teaspoon vanilla extract
- 4 cups confectioners' sugar
- 3 tablespoons orange juice
- 1 tablespoon grated lemon zest, or as needed (optional)

Direction

- Set the oven to 350°F or 175°C for preheating.
- Use paper liners to line the 24 muffin cups.
- In a large bowl, whisk the vegetable oil, lemon cake mix, eggs, and water for 2 minutes.
- Fill the prepared muffin cups with the batter, filling them to 2/3 full.
- Bake the cupcakes inside the preheated oven for 18-22 minutes until browned lightly and the inserted toothpick into the center will come out clean. Let the cupcakes cool completely.
- Use a pastry cutter to cut 1/4 cup of butter and vegetable shortening into a bowl until well-blended. Beat in lemon juice until creamy.
- Stir in 2 cups of confectioners' sugar, adding it 1/2 cup at a time until the filling is already smooth. Put the filling aside.
- Heat the white chocolate in a microwave-safe bowl inside the microwave with high heat for 15 seconds. Stir the chocolate, and heat it again with 15-second intervals, whisking well between heating until the white chocolate has melted and smooth.
- For the frosting, beat 1/2 cup of butter and cream cheese in a bowl until creamy and smooth. Mix in the vanilla extract and melted white chocolate.
- Whisk in 4 cups of confectioners' sugar gradually, adding it alternately with drizzles of orange juice until the frosting turns creamy and smooth.
- Make holes through the top of each of the cupcakes. Take note that the holes must be deep enough since the filling will be filled inside.
- Fill the holes with the lemon filling.
- Pipe the top of the cupcakes with the cream cheese frosting. Sprinkle the cupcakes with lemon zest.

Nutrition Information

- Calories: 379 calories;
- Total Fat: 19
- Sodium: 237
- Total Carbohydrate: 50.4
- Cholesterol: 55
- Protein: 3.2

214. Lemon Yogurt Tea Cakes

Serving: about 1 dozen. | Prep: 20mins | Cook: 20mins | Ready in:

Ingredients

- 2-1/4 cups all-purpose flour
- 1 cup sugar
- 3/4 teaspoon baking powder
- 1/2 teaspoon baking soda
- 1/2 teaspoon salt
- 1/2 cup cold butter
- 1 cup (8 ounces) fat-free plain yogurt
- 3 large egg whites
- 2 tablespoons lemon juice
- 4 teaspoons grated lemon peel
- 1 teaspoon lemon extract

Direction

- Mix salt, baking soda, baking powder, sugar and flour in a big bowl; cut in the butter until the mixture looks like coarse crumbs. Whip together the extract, peel, lemon juice, egg whites and yogurt; mix into the crumb mixture just until it is moistened.
- Pour into muffin cups coated with cooking spray or lined with papers, filling three-fourths full. Bake for 18-22 minutes at 350° until a toothpick comes out clean after inserting in the middle of the cake. Let it cool for 10 minutes before you transfer it from pan to a wire rack to cool completely.

Nutrition Information

- Calories: 232 calories
- Total Fat: 8g fat (5g saturated fat)
- Sodium: 255mg sodium
- Fiber: 1g fiber)
- Total Carbohydrate: 37g carbohydrate (18g sugars
- Cholesterol: 20mg cholesterol
- Protein: 4g protein.

215. Light And Airy Strawberry Cupcakes

Serving: 12 | Prep: 10mins | Cook: 20mins | Ready in:

Ingredients

- 2 cups all-purpose flour
- 1 cup white sugar
- 2 teaspoons baking soda
- 1 cup water
- 1 cup mayonnaise
- 2 1/2 tablespoons strawberry preserves
- 1 teaspoon vanilla extract
- 12 large fresh strawberries (optional)

Direction

- Set oven to preheat at 175°C (350°F). Line 12 muffin cups with paper liners or grease them.
- In a large bowl, combine baking soda, sugar, and flour; create a well in the middle. Add vanilla extract, strawberry preserves, mayonnaise, and water to the well and mix until the batter is just blended. Scoop the batter into the prepared muffin cups. Press 1 strawberry into each one.
- In the preheated oven, bake for 20 to 25 minutes until tops spring back when pressed.

Nutrition Information

- Calories: 289 calories;
- Cholesterol: 7
- Protein: 2.4
- Total Fat: 14.8
- Sodium: 315
- Total Carbohydrate: 37.3

216. Mascarpone Strawberry Cupcakes

Serving: 12 | Prep: 15mins | Cook: 20mins | Ready in:

Ingredients

- 1 (18.25 ounce) package moist white cake mix
- 1 cup water
- 1 (8 ounce) container mascarpone cheese
- 1/4 cup vegetable oil
- 2 egg whites
- 1/2 cup frozen strawberries, thawed
- 2 1/2 cups confectioners' sugar

Direction

- Set the oven to 350°F (175°C) for preheating.
- Use liners to line the 12 muffin cups.
- In a bowl, mix the mascarpone cheese, egg whites, vegetable oil, cake mix, and water until well-blended.
- Distribute the cake mixture among the prepared muffin cups.
- Bake them inside the preheated oven for 20 minutes until browned lightly.
- In a blender or food processor, puree the strawberries until smooth.
- In a bowl, mix the pureed strawberries with confectioners' sugar.
- Top the cupcakes with the strawberry mixture.

Nutrition Information

- Calories: 409 calories;
- Total Fat: 17.9
- Sodium: 303
- Total Carbohydrate: 60.1
- Cholesterol: 23
- Protein: 3.9

217. Mini Christmas Cakes

Serving: 24 | Prep: 1hours | Cook: 1hours30mins | Ready in:

Ingredients

- Cake:
- 3 cups dried currants
- 1 1/4 cups raisins
- 1 cup sultana raisins
- 1/2 cup candied red cherries, chopped
- 8 fluid ounces brandy
- grated zest of 1 large orange
- grated zest of 1 large lemon
- 1 cup unsalted butter, softened
- 2 tablespoons unsalted butter, softened
- 1 cup brown sugar
- 2 tablespoons brown sugar
- 3 large eggs, beaten
- 1 tablespoon molasses, or more to taste
- 1 cup all-purpose flour
- 1/2 cup self-rising flour
- 1/4 cup ground almonds
- 2 teaspoons mixed spice
- 1/2 cup ground almonds
- Decoration:
- 6 tablespoons apricot jam
- 2 1/2 (4 ounce) packages marzipan
- 1/2 (1 lb 8 oz) box white fondant
- 1 teaspoon blue food coloring

Direction

- In a plastic container with a lid, combine candied cherries, sultana raisins, raisins and currants. Pouring over dried fruit with brandy; stirring in lemon and orange zest. Cover container and put aside for 2-3 days for soaking. Shaking or stirring container each few hours when you remember.

- Heat oven to 135°C (275°F) beforehand. Use 24 cupcake cases to line a baking sheet or grease 24 ramekins lightly.
- In a bowl, combine a cup and 2 tablespoons of brown sugar together with a cup and two tablespoons of butter; using an electric mixer to beat till combined well. Adding molasses and eggs and beating well. Stirring in mixed spice, almonds, self-rising flour, and all-purpose flour till combined well. Folding in soaked fruit and almonds; mix well. In the prepared ramekins or cases, spooning mixture.
- In the preheated oven, allow to bake for approximately 90 minutes on the center rack till when insert a toothpick in the center of a cake, it comes out clean. Let it sit in the cases for cooling down.
- Before decorating, tightly wrap them in aluminum foil and greaseproof paper or storing in airtight tins for no less than 10 days.
- In the microwave, heating jam till warmed for 10 seconds and brushing onto every cake.
- Between two sheets of plastic wrap, rolling out marzipan. Using a glass or a round cookie cutter with the same size as the cake to cut out circles. On every mini fruitcake, place marzipan circles on top of the jam. Before completing the final decoration, storing fruitcakes for 8 hours to overnight in an airtight container.
- Between 2 sheets of plastic wrap, rolling white fondant out and cutting out circles with the same size in diameter as the cakes. Using a snowflake pattern to press a cookie stencil onto the fondant circles. Using a small brush to brush blue food coloring onto the snowflake pattern and lay on top of the marzipan layer. Continue with remaining cakes.

Nutrition Information

- Calories: 422 calories;
- Total Fat: 14.2
- Sodium: 58
- Total Carbohydrate: 66.5
- Cholesterol: 46
- Protein: 4.8

218. Monster Chocolate Cupcakes For Halloween

Serving: 12 | Prep: 45mins | Cook: 14mins | Ready in:

Ingredients

- Chocolate Cupcakes:
- 1/2 cup milk
- 1 tablespoon white vinegar
- 1/2 cup unsalted butter, at room temperature
- 10 tablespoons white sugar
- 2 teaspoons vanilla sugar
- 2 large eggs
- 3/4 cup all-purpose flour
- 1 tablespoon all-purpose flour
- 1/2 cup unsweetened cocoa powder
- 1/2 teaspoon baking powder
- 1/4 teaspoon baking soda
- 1 pinch salt
- Cream Cheese Frosting:
- 1 (8 ounce) package cream cheese, softened
- 1/4 cup unsalted butter, at room temperature
- 1 teaspoon vanilla extract
- 1 cup confectioners' sugar, sifted
- 2 drops green food coloring
- 24 candy eyeballs

Direction

- In a bowl, mix vinegar and milk. Allow to stand for 5 minutes until milk curdles.
- Set the oven to 350°F (175°C) and start preheating. Grease a 12-cup muffin tin or use paper liners to line cups.
- In a large bowl, mix vanilla sugar, white sugar and half cup butter; use an electric mixer to whisk until creamy and smooth. Add eggs, one per time; after each addition, whisk well.
- In a bowl, salt, mix baking powder, cocoa powder, baking soda and 3/4 cup plus 1 tablespoon flour. Add curdled milk and flour

mixture alternately to the creamed butter mixture; combine until batter is blended well. Scoop batter into prepared muffin cups, filling each 3/4 full.
- Bake in the prepared oven for about 14 minutes until the tops spring back when pressed lightly and the inserted toothpick in the center of a cupcake is clean when coming out. Cool for a few minutes in the muffin tin; place on wire rack for about an hour to cool completely.
- In a bowl, mix 1/4 cup butter and cream cheese; use an electric mixer to whisk until combined well. Combine in vanilla extract. Gradually stir in confectioners' sugar. Drop some food coloring to color frosting green.
- In a pastry bag fitted with a grass tip, place green frosting. Hold the pastry bag 1/8 inch above the surface of a cupcake at a 90-degree angle. Squeeze bag to create green 'fur' by pulling tip up and away when the icing strand is about half inch high. Do the same to cover cupcake with fur evenly. Attach 2 eyes to each cupcake.

Nutrition Information

- Calories: 316 calories;
- Total Fat: 20
- Sodium: 133
- Total Carbohydrate: 32.1
- Cholesterol: 83
- Protein: 4.5

219. Moon Rocks

Serving: 24 | Prep: 20mins | Cook: 20mins | Ready in:

Ingredients

- 1 cup semisweet chocolate chips
- 2 cups all-purpose flour
- 1 1/2 teaspoons baking soda
- 1/2 teaspoon salt
- 1/2 cup butter, softened
- 1 1/2 cups packed light brown sugar
- 3 eggs
- 1 teaspoon vanilla extract
- 1 cup water
- 2 cups miniature marshmallows

Direction

- Set the oven to 350°F or 175°C for preheating.
- On top of a double boiler, melt the chocolate and let it cool.
- Combine the salt, baking soda, and flour in a mixing bowl. In a separate bowl, cream the sugar and butter. Whisk eggs into the butter mixture, adding them one at a time. Whisk the flour mixture, vanilla, chocolate, and water into the butter and egg mixture thoroughly. Mix in the marshmallows. Fill the paper-lined cupcake pans with the mixture, about half-full.
- Let them bake inside the preheated oven for 20 minutes. Let them cool on a wire rack. Serve.

Nutrition Information

- Calories: 181 calories;
- Sodium: 170
- Total Carbohydrate: 29.3
- Cholesterol: 37
- Protein: 2.3
- Total Fat: 6.7

220. Nana's Chocolate Cupcakes With Mint Frosting

Serving: 1 dozen. | Prep: 25mins | Cook: 15mins | Ready in:

Ingredients

- 1/2 cup baking cocoa
- 1 cup boiling water
- 1/4 cup butter, softened
- 1 cup sugar

- 2 large eggs
- 1-1/3 cups all-purpose flour
- 2 teaspoons baking powder
- 1/4 teaspoon salt
- 1/4 cup unsweetened applesauce
- FROSTING:
- 1 cup confectioners' sugar
- 3 tablespoons butter, softened
- 4 teaspoons heavy whipping cream
- Dash peppermint extract
- 1 drop green food coloring, optional
- 2 tablespoons miniature semisweet chocolate chips
- Mint Andes candies, optional

Direction

- Set the oven at 375° to preheat. Use foil or paper liners to line 12 muffin cups. Mix boiling water and cocoa until smooth; let it cool completely.
- Beat sugar and butter until blended. Beat in eggs, 1 egg at a time. Whip together salt, baking powder and flour in another bowl; pour into butter mixture alternately with applesauce, beat well after each addition. Beat in cocoa mixture.
- Pour into prepared muffin cups, filling each three-fourths full. Bake until a toothpick inserted in the center of the cupcakes comes out clean, about 15-18 minutes. Allow the cakes to cool for 10 minutes, then transfer them to a wire rack to cool completely.
- Beat the extract, cream, butter and confectioners' sugar until smooth. Use food coloring to tint the frosting green if desired. Put in chocolate chips and stir. Spread on top of the cupcakes. If desired, sprinkle with candies.

Nutrition Information

- Calories: 253 calories
- Total Carbohydrate: 41g carbohydrate (28g sugars
- Cholesterol: 51mg cholesterol
- Protein: 3g protein.
- Total Fat: 9g fat (5g saturated fat)
- Sodium: 196mg sodium
- Fiber: 1g fiber)

221. Neapolitan Cupcakes

Serving: 48 | Prep: 30mins | Cook: 20mins | Ready in:

Ingredients

- 2 (19.8 ounce) packages brownie mix
- 1 cup vegetable oil
- 4 eggs
- 1/2 cup water
- 1 (18.25 ounce) package strawberry cake mix
- 1 cup water
- 3 eggs
- 1/3 cup vegetable oil
- 1 1/2 cups unsalted butter at room temperature
- 1 (16 ounce) package confectioners' sugar, sifted
- 1/2 teaspoon vanilla extract

Direction

- Preheat an oven to 175°C/350°F.
- Use paper liners to line 48 muffin cups.
- Mix 1/2 cup water, 4 eggs, 1 cup vegetable oil and both brownie mix packages till smooth and evenly combined in a big bowl.
- Mix 1/3 cup vegetable oil, 3 eggs, 1 cup water and strawberry cake mix till moist in another bowl; beat with electric mixer for 2 minutes on medium speed.
- Put 2 tbsp. brownie batter into bottom of every prepped muffin cup.
- Put strawberry cake batter over brownie batter; fill each cup to 2/3 full.
- In preheated oven, bake for 20 minutes till inserted toothpick in middle exits clean and cupcake springs back when pressed lightly.
- Cool for 10 minutes in pans. Transfer onto racks; fully cool.

- Beat unsalted butter using electric mixer at medium high speed for 2 minutes till butter is creamy and pale in a bowl.
- 1/2 cup at 1 time, beat confectioners' sugar into butter, beating well after every addition, scraping bowl's sides down as needed. Put mixer speed on high to beat as much as air as you can into frosting after every confectioners' sugar addition; lower speed to low then beat till frosting is smooth. Repeat for around 5 minutes for beating time till you incorporate all confectioners' sugar; beat in vanilla extract.
- Spread buttercream frosting on cooled cupcakes.

Nutrition Information

- Calories: 294 calories;
- Cholesterol: 42
- Protein: 2.1
- Total Fat: 16.7
- Sodium: 148
- Total Carbohydrate: 35.7

222. Pecan Pie Cupcakes

Serving: 9 | Prep: 15mins | Cook: 20mins | Ready in:

Ingredients

- cooking spray
- 1 cup brown sugar
- 1 cup chopped pecans
- 1/2 cup all-purpose flour
- 2 eggs
- 1/2 cup butter, melted
- 1 teaspoon vanilla extract, or to taste

Direction

- Set the oven to 350°F or 175°C for preheating. Use paper liners to line the muffin tin, and then coat the liners using the cooking spray.
- In a large bowl, mix the pecans, flour, and brown sugar. Create a well into the center of the mixture.
- Use an electric mixer to whisk the eggs in a large bowl for 3-5 minutes until foamy. Fold in vanilla and butter. Pour the mixture into the middle of the brown sugar mixture. Whisk the butter until well-blended.
- Fill the cups of the muffin tin with the batter, filling them 2/3 full.
- Bake them inside the preheated oven for 20-25 minutes until the inserted toothpick into the center will come out clean.

Nutrition Information

- Calories: 310 calories;
- Total Carbohydrate: 31.1
- Cholesterol: 68
- Protein: 3.4
- Total Fat: 20.1
- Sodium: 95

223. Pineapple Upside Down Cupcakes

Serving: 24 | Prep: 20mins | Cook: 20mins | Ready in:

Ingredients

- cooking spray
- 1/2 cup butter, melted
- 1 1/2 cups brown sugar
- 24 maraschino cherries
- 1 (20 ounce) can crushed pineapple
- 1 (18.25 ounce) package pineapple cake mix (such as Duncan Hines® Pineapple Supreme)
- 3 eggs
- 1 1/3 cups pineapple juice
- 1/3 cup vegetable oil
- 1 tablespoon confectioners' sugar for dusting, or as needed

Direction

- Place one rack of oven to the center of oven. Preheat the oven to 175°C to 350 °F.
- Use cooking spray to coat 2 dozen muffin cups.
- Line waxed paper on a work counter.
- Scoop a teaspoon of liquified butter to the base of every prepped muffin cup.
- In every muffin cup, scoop a tablespoon of brown sugar.
- Force one maraschino cherry in the middle of brown sugar in every muffin cup.
- Top cherry with one heaping tablespoon of crushed pineapple and use the back of spoon to compact into a smooth layer.
- In big bowl, combine vegetable oil, pineapple juice, eggs and pineapple cake mix on low speed using an electric mixer to moisten, for half a minute. Raise speed of mixer to moderate and whip for two minutes.
- Fill muffin cups to top with pineapple cake batter; avoid excessive filling.
- In prepped oven, bake for 20 minutes, till an inserted toothpick into the middle of one cupcake gets out clean.
- Cool cupcakes for not less than 5 minutes prior to flipping muffin cups over to waxed paper to loosen. Serve with cherry and pineapple sides facing up. Lightly dust confectioners' sugar on cupcakes.

Nutrition Information

- Calories: 236 calories;
- Sodium: 174
- Total Carbohydrate: 38.6
- Cholesterol: 33
- Protein: 1.5
- Total Fat: 9

224. Pink Lemonade Cupcakes With Pink Buttercream Frosting

Serving: 12 | Prep: 20mins | Cook: 20mins | Ready in:

Ingredients

- Cupcakes:
- 1/2 cup white sugar
- 1/4 cup vegetable oil
- 1/4 cup cold water
- 2 eggs
- 3 tablespoons pink lemonade powder
- 1/3 cup buttermilk
- 1 cup all-purpose flour
- 1/2 teaspoon baking soda
- 1/2 teaspoon baking powder
- 1 dash red food coloring, or as desired
- Buttercream Frosting:
- 4 1/2 cups confectioners' sugar
- 1/2 cup unsalted butter, at room temperature
- 1/4 cup half-and-half
- 2 tablespoons pink lemonade powder
- 1 dash red food coloring, or as desired

Direction

- Set oven to 350°F (175°C) to preheat. Line 12 muffin cups using paper liners.
- In a mixing bowl, mix together 3 tablespoons pink lemonade powder, eggs, water, oil, and white sugar; whisk in buttermilk until no lumps remain. In another mixing bowl, combine baking powder, baking soda, and flour; whisk into sugar mixture until just incorporated. Create pink batter with just enough food coloring added. Fill batter into prepared muffin cups.
- Bake for 20 to 25 minutes in the preheated oven until cupcake becomes elastic.
- In a mixing bowl, beat 2 tablespoons pink lemonade powder, half-and-half, butter, and confectioners' sugar together with an electric mixer until frosting is creamy and smooth. Tint the pink frosting with enough food coloring; frost cupcakes with pink frosting.

Nutrition Information

- Calories: 404 calories;
- Total Carbohydrate: 69.4
- Cholesterol: 53
- Protein: 2.6
- Total Fat: 13.8
- Sodium: 97

225. Pink Peppermint Cupcake

Serving: 24 | Prep: 10mins | Cook: 20mins | Ready in:

Ingredients

- 1 (18.25 ounce) package white cake mix
- 1 1/3 cups water
- 3 egg whites
- 2 tablespoons butter, melted
- 1/2 teaspoon peppermint extract
- 1 dash red food coloring, or as desired (optional)
- 1 (16 ounce) package vanilla frosting
- 1/2 cup crushed peppermint candies

Direction

- Set the oven to 350°F (175°C) to preheat. Use aluminum foil liners or paper liners to line muffin cups.
- In a bowl, use an electric mixer to whisk together food coloring, peppermint extract, butter, egg whites, water, and cake mix for 30 seconds on low speed. Raise the speed to medium and keep whisking for 2 minutes until smooth, scraping down sides when necessary. Fill the batter into the muffin cups to approximately 3/4 full.
- Put in the preheated oven and bake for 20-22 minutes until a toothpick comes out clean when you insert it into the middle. Once the cupcakes have baked for 1/2 of the baking time, rotate the tins to aid even baking. Remove the cupcakes to a wire rack to fully cool.
- Frost vanilla frosting onto the cupcakes and put crushed candies on top.

Nutrition Information

- Calories: 202 calories;
- Sodium: 193
- Total Carbohydrate: 34.6
- Cholesterol: 3
- Protein: 1.4
- Total Fat: 6.4

226. Pull Apart Spider Web Cupcakes

Serving: 24 | Prep: 20mins | Cook: 20mins | Ready in:

Ingredients

- 1 (18.25 ounce) package white cake mix
- 1 cup water
- 1/3 cup vegetable oil
- 3 eggs
- 2 (16 ounce) containers prepared fluffy white frosting
- 3 drops orange gel food coloring, or as needed
- 1 (.68 oz. tube) black decorating gel

Direction

- Set the oven to 350°F (175°C) for preheating. Use the paper muffin liners to line 24 muffin cups.
- In a large bowl, mix the eggs, water, cake mix, and oil using the electric mixer with medium speed for 2 minutes until the batter is smooth. Distribute the batter among the prepared muffin cups, filling them up to 2/3 full.
- Let them bake inside the preheated oven for 19-23 minutes until their tops will spring back once pressed. Allow them to cool in the pans

- for 10 minutes. Transfer them on a wire rack and let them cool completely.
- In a bowl, whisk the orange food coloring and frosting until you reach your desired consistency and shade.
- Place the cooled cupcakes close together onto the large platter, arranging them in solid circular shape. Make a large and round frosted surface by spreading the frosting onto each cupcake. Squeeze in the center of the frosting with one large dot of a black decorating gel. Make some concentric circles around the dot, making sure the circles are 2-inches apart. Use the toothpick to trace the center dot to the outermost circle. Repeat the same step 12 times until it resembles a spider's web.

Nutrition Information

- Calories: 285 calories;
- Total Fat: 12
- Sodium: 232
- Total Carbohydrate: 42.5
- Cholesterol: 23
- Protein: 1.7

227. Pumpkin Cupcakes With Cream Cheese Frosting

Serving: 36 | Prep: 20mins | Cook: 20mins | Ready in:

Ingredients

- Cupcakes:
- 3 cups baking mix (such as Bisquick ®)
- 1 (15 ounce) can pumpkin puree
- 1 cup white sugar
- 1 cup brown sugar
- 4 eggs
- 1/4 cup butter, softened
- 1/4 cup milk
- 2 teaspoons pumpkin pie spice
- Cream Cheese Frosting:
- 1/2 (8 ounce) package cream cheese, softened
- 1/2 cup butter, softened
- 4 1/2 cups confectioners' sugar, divided
- 2 teaspoons vanilla extract

Direction

- Set the oven at 175°C (350°F) to preheat. Grease or use paper liners to line 36 muffin cups.
- In a bowl, use an electric mixer to beat pumpkin pie spice, milk, 1/4 cup butter, brown sugar, eggs, white sugar, pumpkin puree, and baking mix on low speed until well mixed; scoop into the prepared muffin cups.
- In the preheated oven, bake for 20-30 minutes, until inserting a toothpick in the center and it comes out clean. Allow the cupcakes to cool for 5 minutes in the pan before transferring to cool completely on a wire rack.
- On low speed, use an electric mixer to beat 1/2 cup butter and cream cheese in a bowl until creamy and smooth. Next, beat vanilla extract and 2 cups confectioners' sugar on low speed into the creamed butter mixture until well mixed; then increase to high speed and continue to beat until fluffy. Pour 2 1/2 cups confectioners' sugar gradually into the frosting; on medium speed, keep beating until the frosting is thickened.
- Scoop the frosting into a resealable plastic bag and cut 1 corner. Pipe the frosting onto the cooled cupcakes.

Nutrition Information

- Calories: 197 calories;
- Sodium: 201
- Total Carbohydrate: 32.5
- Cholesterol: 34
- Protein: 1.9
- Total Fat: 7.1

228. Pumpkin Ginger Cupcakes

Serving: 24 | Prep: 20mins | Cook: 20mins | Ready in:

Ingredients

- 2 cups all-purpose flour
- 1 (3.4 ounce) package instant butterscotch pudding mix
- 2 teaspoons baking soda
- 1/4 teaspoon salt
- 1 tablespoon ground cinnamon
- 1/2 teaspoon ground ginger
- 1/2 teaspoon ground allspice
- 1/4 teaspoon ground cloves
- 1/3 cup finely chopped crystallized ginger
- 1 cup butter, room temperature
- 1 cup white sugar
- 1 cup packed brown sugar
- 4 eggs, room temperature
- 1 teaspoon vanilla extract
- 1 (15 ounce) can pumpkin puree

Direction

- Set the oven to 350°F or 175°C for preheating. Grease or line 24 muffin cups using the paper muffin liners. In a bowl, mix the cinnamon, pudding mix, flour, ground ginger, crystallized ginger, allspice, salt, baking soda, and cloves; put aside.
- Use an electric mixer to whisk the brown sugar, white sugar, and butter in a large bowl until fluffy and light. Once the mixture has a noticeable light color, add the eggs, one at a time and let each egg incorporate into the mixture before adding the next one. Whisk in the pumpkin puree and vanilla together with the last egg. Mix in the flour mixture until just incorporated. Spread the batter into the prepared cups.
- Bake them inside the preheated oven for 20 minutes until they are golden and their tops spring back when pressed lightly. Let them cool in the pans for 10 minutes, and then remove them from the pans onto the wire rack to cool completely.

Nutrition Information

- Calories: 211 calories;
- Total Fat: 8.7
- Sodium: 303
- Total Carbohydrate: 31.8
- Cholesterol: 51
- Protein: 2.4

229. Pumpkin Pie Cupcakes

Serving: 12 | Prep: 10mins | Cook: 20mins | Ready in:

Ingredients

- Cupcakes:
- 1 (18.25 ounce) box yellow cake mix
- 1 3/4 cups canned pumpkin pie mix
- 2 eggs
- 2 teaspoons pumpkin pie spice
- Frosting:
- 1 (8 ounce) package cream cheese, softened
- 1/4 cup confectioners' sugar
- 1 teaspoon pumpkin pie spice

Direction

- Start preheating the oven at 350°F (175°C). Oil or line paper liners on muffin cups.
- Combine 2 teaspoons of pumpkin pie spice, eggs, pumpkin pie mix, and yellow cake mix in a bowl until well-combined. Pour batter in muffin cups, about 1/4 cup per cupcake.
- Bake in the prepared oven for about 18 minutes until a toothpick comes out clean when inserted in the center. Let cupcakes cool in the tin for 5 minutes before removing to a wire rack to cool fully.
- Whisk 1 teaspoon of pumpkin pie spice, confectioners' sugar, and cream cheese in a

bowl, with an electric mixer, until frosting is puffy; scoop onto each cupcake.

Nutrition Information

- Calories: 316 calories;
- Total Fat: 12.4
- Sodium: 432
- Total Carbohydrate: 47.5
- Cholesterol: 52
- Protein: 4.8

230. Pumpkin Spice Cupcakes With Cream Cheese Frosting

Serving: 24 | Prep: 20mins | Cook: 20mins | Ready in:

Ingredients

- Cupcakes:
- 2 1/2 cups white sugar
- 3/4 cup butter, softened
- 3 eggs
- 1 (15 ounce) can solid-pack pumpkin puree
- 2 1/3 cups all-purpose flour
- 1 tablespoon pumpkin pie spice
- 1 tablespoon ground cinnamon
- 3/4 teaspoon baking powder
- 1/2 teaspoon ground ginger
- 1 cup buttermilk
- Frosting:
- 1 (8 ounce) package cream cheese, softened
- 1/2 cup butter, softened
- 4 cups confectioners' sugar
- 2 teaspoons ground cinnamon
- 1 teaspoon vanilla extract

Direction

- Set the oven at 350°F (175°C) and start preheating. Use paper liners to line 24 muffin cups.
- In a bowl, beat 3/4 cup of butter and white sugar with an electric mixer till creamy and smooth; put in eggs; one at a time, beating well after each addition. Beat pumpkin into the creamed butter mixture.
- In a bowl, combine ginger, baking powder, 1 tablespoon of cinnamon, pumpkin pie spice and flour; mix alternately with buttermilk into the creamed butter mixture, till the batter becomes smooth. Fill the batter into each muffin cup by 3/4 full.
- Bake in the preheated oven for 20-25 minutes, till a toothpick comes out clean when inserted into the center of a cupcake. Allow to cool for 10 minutes in the muffin tin; remove onto a wire rack.
- In a bowl, beat 1/2 cup of butter and cream cheese with an electric mixer till fluffy. Beat together vanilla extract, 2 teaspoons of cinnamon and confectioners' sugar till the frosting is smooth. Evenly spread on each cupcake.

Nutrition Information

- Calories: 345 calories;
- Total Fat: 13.8
- Sodium: 174
- Total Carbohydrate: 53.8
- Cholesterol: 59
- Protein: 3.4

231. Pumpkin Streusel Cupcakes

Serving: 2 dozen. | Prep: 25mins | Cook: 20mins | Ready in:

Ingredients

- 1 package spice cake mix (regular size)
- 1-1/4 cups water
- 3 large eggs
- 1/2 cup canned pumpkin
- STREUSEL:
- 1/2 cup packed brown sugar

- 1/2 teaspoon ground cinnamon
- 1 tablespoon butter
- FROSTING:
- 1 package (8 ounces) cream cheese, softened
- 2 tablespoons butter
- 2 cups confectioners' sugar
- 1/2 teaspoon vanilla extract

Direction

- Mix pumpkin, eggs, water and cake mix in a big bowl. Beat the mixture on low speed just until it is moistened. Switch to medium speed and beat for 2 more minutes.
- Mix cinnamon and brown sugar together in a small bowl; cut in butter until the mixture is crumbly. Pour the batter into muffin cups lined with papers, filling one-fourth full. Put heaping teaspoonfuls of streusel into the center of each cupcake. Pour in remaining batter t cover.
- Bake for 18-20 minutes at 350° until a toothpick comes out clean after inserting into the middle of the cake. Let it cool for 10 minutes, then transfer from pans to wire racks to fully cool.
- Beat butter and cream cheese in a small bowl until the mixture is fluffy. Put in vanilla and confectioners' sugar; beat until the mixture becomes smooth. Pipe the frosting on top of the cupcakes. Keep them in the fridge.

Nutrition Information

- Calories: 204 calories
- Fiber: 0 fiber)
- Total Carbohydrate: 31g carbohydrate (23g sugars
- Cholesterol: 46mg cholesterol
- Protein: 3g protein.
- Total Fat: 8g fat (4g saturated fat)
- Sodium: 213mg sodium

232. REALLY Real Strawberry Cupcakes

Serving: 20 | Prep: 30mins | Cook: 17mins | Ready in:

Ingredients

- 1 1/4 ounces freeze-dried strawberries
- 3/4 cup all-purpose flour
- 3/4 cup cake flour
- 1 1/2 teaspoons baking powder
- 1/4 teaspoon baking soda
- 1/2 teaspoon salt
- 1/2 cup unsalted butter, room temperature
- 1 1/3 cups white sugar
- 3 eggs, room temperature
- 1 teaspoon vanilla extract
- 2/3 cup whole milk, room temperature

Direction

- Set oven to preheat at 175°C (350°F). Line muffin tins with 20 cupcake liners (line 72 mini muffin tins to make mini cupcakes).
- Use a food processor or a coffee grinder to grind strawberries into a fine powder. In a bowl, whisk together salt, baking soda, baking powder, strawberry powder, all-purpose flour, and cake flour.
- In a bowl, beat sugar and butter with an electric mixer until light and fluffy. Mixture should have a noticeably lighter color. Add room-temperature eggs one by one, letting each egg blend into butter mixture before adding the next one. Mix in vanilla extract.
- Mix in alternately the flour mixture with the milk, into butter mixture until just combined. Fill cupcake batter in lined tins.
- In preheated oven, bake until cupcakes spring back when touched gently with a fingertip or a toothpick inserted in the middle comes out clean, from 16 to 18 minutes for regular cupcakes, and 8 to 10 minutes for mini cupcakes.

Nutrition Information

- Calories: 145 calories;
- Total Fat: 5.7
- Sodium: 125
- Total Carbohydrate: 21.6
- Cholesterol: 41
- Protein: 2.2

233. Raspberry Iced Tea Cupcakes

Serving: 36 | Prep: 45mins | Cook: 30mins | Ready in:

Ingredients

- 3 cups all-purpose flour
- 4 1/2 teaspoons baking powder
- 1 1/2 teaspoons salt
- 1 cup unsalted butter, softened
- 2 cups white sugar
- 1 (3.4 ounce) package instant lemon pudding mix
- 4 eggs
- 1 cup milk
- 1/2 teaspoon vanilla extract
- 1 lemon, juiced and zested
- 2 egg whites
- 2/3 cup white sugar
- 1 cup unsalted butter at room temperature
- 8 drops oil-based creme de menthe candy flavoring
- 8 ounces cream cheese, softened
- 1/2 cup frozen unsweetened raspberries, thawed
- 1/4 cup unsweetened instant tea powder
- 4 teaspoons unsweetened instant tea powder
- 1 teaspoon vanilla extract
- 1/2 cup white sugar
- 2 cups heavy cream

Direction

- Start preheating the oven at 350°F (175°C). Line paper liners on 36 cupcake cups.
- In a bowl, sift salt, baking powder, and flour until well-combined and sifted. Beat 1 cup of unsalted butter in a large mixing bowl with an electric mixer on medium speed until fluffy. Stir in lemon pudding mix and 2 cups of sugar, then beat on high speed for about 8 minutes until fluffy and well-mixed. Whisk in eggs, one at a time. Mix in milk, in 1/3 cup increments, alternately with the flour mixture while the electric mixer is running; stir in lemon zest, lemon juice, and vanilla extract until well-blended. Stuff the prepared cupcake cups with batter, about 2/3 full.
- Bake in the prepared oven for 18 to 23 minutes until the cupcakes look lightly browned and a toothpick comes out clean when inserted into the center. Let the cupcakes cool.
- In the meantime, prepare the filling; pour about 2 inches of water into the base of a double boiler, place on medium heat, and heat the water to a boil. Lower the heat to a simmer and put 2/3 cup of sugar and egg whites into the top of the double boiler. Do not let the water reach the upper part of the double boiler. Stir until the sugar is dissolved; combine using electric mixer set on high speed for about 5 to 10 minutes until the meringue forms soft peaks. Lower the mixer speed to medium and whisk in the butter, about 2 or 3 tablespoons each time. When butter is thoroughly beaten, blend in the creme de menthe candy flavoring oil for an extra 1 to 2 minutes until well-incorporated and the filling is fluffy. Take filling off from the heat and put aside. Once cooled, put the filling into a piping bag with a medium-sized round tip.
- Preparing the frosting: In a bowl, put 1/2 cup of sugar, 1 teaspoon f vanilla extract, both amounts of tea powder, raspberries, and cream cheese, then beat with an electric mixer on high speed until smooth. While beating, slowly add the cream into the bowl and beat for about 3 minutes until it forms stiff peaks. Scrape down the side of the bowl frequently.
- Place the piping tip into the top of each cupcake and squeeze about 1/2 tablespoon of filling into each cupcake. Spread a generous

dollop of frosting on top of each cupcake, then enjoy.

Nutrition Information

- Calories: 289 calories;
- Protein: 3.2
- Total Fat: 18.1
- Sodium: 232
- Total Carbohydrate: 29.8
- Cholesterol: 73

234. Real Strawberry Cupcakes

Serving: 12 | Prep: 40mins | Cook: 25mins | Ready in:

Ingredients

- 8 large fresh strawberries, or as needed
- 2 eggs
- 1 cup white sugar
- 1/3 cup vegetable oil
- 1/2 teaspoon vanilla extract
- 1/2 teaspoon lemon zest
- 1 1/2 cups all-purpose flour
- 2 teaspoons baking powder
- 1/4 teaspoon salt
- 3 tablespoons instant vanilla pudding mix (optional)
- 1 drop red food coloring, or as needed (optional)
- 3/4 cup cream cheese, softened
- 2 tablespoons butter, softened
- 1/2 cup confectioners' sugar
- 1/2 teaspoon vanilla extract
- 3 large fresh strawberries, sliced

Direction

- Set oven to preheat at 165°C (325°F). Into the cupcake cups, line cupcake liners or spray cooking spray.
- Into a blender, add 8 strawberries and blend smoothly. Run the puree through a strainer to eliminate seeds. The resulting puree should equal about 3/4 cup. Put it aside.
- Beat lemon zest, strawberry puree, eggs, white sugar, vegetable oil and 1/2 teaspoon vanilla extract together in a large bowl until well mixed. Stir in the vanilla pudding mix (for a moister cupcake), salt, baking powder, flour, and red food coloring to create a shade of pink you like. Into the prepared cupcake cups, scoop the batter to about 2/3 full each.
- In the preheated oven, bake until the cupcakes have risen and a toothpick comes out clean when inserted into the center of the cupcake for about 23 minutes. Let them cool down for at least 10 minutes before frosting.
- For the frosting, use an electric mixer to beat together butter and cream cheese in a mixing bowl until smooth; mix in 1/2 teaspoon vanilla extract and confectioners' sugar to achieve a no lump-icing. Use about 2 tablespoons of icing to frost each cupcake, and top a strawberry slice on each.

Nutrition Information

- Calories: 295 calories;
- Protein: 3.9
- Total Fat: 14.1
- Sodium: 249
- Total Carbohydrate: 39
- Cholesterol: 52

235. Santa Hat Cupcakes

Serving: 12 | Prep: 45mins | Cook: | Ready in:

Ingredients

- 1 (16 ounce) package vanilla frosting, divided
- 12 unfrosted cupcakes, cooled
- 1/4 cup red colored sugar or sprinkles
- 4 fresh strawberries, hulled

- 3 ounces ready-to-use white fondant
- 2 drops red food coloring, or as needed
- 2 tablespoons confectioners' sugar, or as needed

Direction

- For the Santa hat cupcakes with sprinkles: Place some of the frosting into a piping bag with a large round tip. Pipe frosting at a 90° angle to the center of the cupcake in the shape of a Santa hat, slowly reduce the pressure to make a cone. Top cone with red sprinkles or red colored sugar. Scoop a little frosting into a piping bag fitted with a small star-shaped tip. Create the rim by piping the frosting around the hat's base and pipe a small pom-pom on top. Repeat the process with 3 more cupcakes.
- To make the strawberries Santa hat cupcakes: Frost a thin vanilla frosting layer on 4 cupcakes. Put a strawberry in the middle, placing the tip facing up. Use the small star-shaped tip to pipe a small pom-pom atop the strawberry. Make the hat's rim by using the large round tip to pipe frosting around the cupcake's base. Use a finger to make swirls in the rim. Repeat the process with the other 3 frosted cupcakes.
- To make the fondant Santa hat cupcakes: Use red food coloring to color white fondant. Sprinkle confectioners' sugar over a work surface and roll 1/4 the fondant out into a really thin circle of 2 1/2-inch diameter. Cut a wedge from the circle and leave a Pac-Man shape. Pipe a frosting cone in the middle of each cupcake using the large round tip. Create a cone by folding the cut edges of the fondant together. Put red fondant hat surrounding the frosting cone. Make the rim of the hat by using a star-shaped tip to pipe frosting around the base and put a small pom-pom on top. Repeat with the other 3 cupcakes.

Nutrition Information

- Calories: 335 calories;
- Total Fat: 11.6
- Sodium: 188
- Total Carbohydrate: 56.1
- Cholesterol: 18
- Protein: 1.8

236. Spiced Spider Cupcakes

Serving: 24 | Prep: 1hours | Cook: 25mins | Ready in:

Ingredients

- Spice Cake:
- 3 cups all-purpose flour
- 2 cups white sugar
- 2 teaspoons baking soda
- 1 teaspoon salt
- 1 teaspoon ground cinnamon
- 1/2 teaspoon ground cloves
- 1/2 teaspoon ground nutmeg
- 2 cups water
- 2/3 cup canola oil
- 2 tablespoons distilled white vinegar
- 2 teaspoons vanilla extract
- Cream Cheese Frosting:
- 2 (3 ounce) packages cream cheese, softened
- 1/2 cup butter, softened
- 2 teaspoons vanilla extract
- 1/4 teaspoon salt
- 1/8 teaspoon ground cinnamon
- 5 cups sifted confectioners' sugar, or more as needed
- Decorations:
- 1 (.68 oz. tube) black decorating gel
- 24 large spiced gumdrops
- black shoestring licorice

Direction

- Set the oven to 350°F or 175°C for preheating. Use the paper liners to line the cupcake pans.
- In a bowl, mix the white sugar, 1 tsp. of cinnamon, nutmeg, cloves, baking soda, flour, and 1 tsp. of salt until well-mixed. In a separate bowl, combine the vinegar, 2 tsp. of vanilla extract, water, and canola oil. Add the

liquid mixture into the dry mixture. Whisk it until the batter is smooth and very thin.
- Pour the batter into the pitcher or measuring cup. Distribute the batter among the prepared cupcake pans.
- Let them bake inside the preheated oven for 25 minutes until their tops will spring back when pressed gently using your fingertip and the inserted toothpick into the center will come out clean. Let the cupcakes cool on a wire rack completely.
- Use an electric mixer to whisk 2 tsp. of vanilla extract, 1/8 tsp. of cinnamon, 1/4 tsp. of salt, cream cheese, and butter until smooth. Gradually whisk in the confectioners' sugar until the frosting reaches the spreading consistency and creamy. Once the cupcakes are cool, use this mixture to frost them.
- To style the cupcakes, make a small circle into the center of each cupcake using the black decorating gel. Create a larger circle around the first circle. Continue drawing larger circles until the last circle is already near the edge, about 1/4-inch. Each cupcake must have a total of 5 rings. Create 8 lines that radiate from the center of each cupcake to its edge using the toothpick for the webs. Make sure it resembles spokes on a wheel.
- For the legs, cut the licorice strings into 1 1/4-inch long pieces. Place 4 licorice legs into the two sides of the gumdrop. Draw the eyes using the decorating gel and draw a smiley mouth onto each gumdrop. Put in the center of the webs on each cup cake with a gumdrop spider.

Nutrition Information

- Calories: 402 calories;
- Total Fat: 12.7
- Sodium: 302
- Total Carbohydrate: 70.7
- Cholesterol: 18
- Protein: 2.3

237.   Strawberry Cupcakes

Serving: 12 | Prep: 15mins | Cook: 20mins | Ready in:

Ingredients

- 10 tablespoons butter, room temperature
- 3/4 cup white sugar
- 3 eggs
- 1 teaspoon strawberry extract
- 1 3/4 cups self-rising flour
- 1/4 teaspoon salt
- 1/4 cup finely chopped fresh strawberries, drained

Direction

- Preheat the oven to 165 o C (325 o F). Line 12 cupcake pan cups with paper liners or grease them.
- Beat together the sugar and butter in a large bowl until fluffy and light. Beat in the eggs, one by one, then mix in strawberry extract. Combine the salt and self-rising flour; mix into the batter until just incorporated. Lastly, fold in strawberries. Scoop the batter into the lined or greased cups, split the batter evenly.
- In the preheated oven, bake until the tops bounce back when pressed lightly, about 20 to 25 minutes. Let cool in the pan over a wire rack. Arrange the cooled cupcakes onto a serving platter. Frost with frosting of your choice.

Nutrition Information

- Calories: 218 calories;
- Total Fat: 11
- Sodium: 366
- Total Carbohydrate: 26.4
- Cholesterol: 72
- Protein: 3.5

238. Strawberry Cupcakes With Lemon Zest Cream Cheese Icing

Serving: 14 | Prep: 25mins | Cook: 20mins | Ready in:

Ingredients

- Strawberry Puree:
- 1 cup frozen strawberries
- 2 tablespoons water
- 1 teaspoon honey
- 1/2 teaspoon fresh lemon zest
- 1 tablespoon white sugar
- Cupcake Batter:
- 1 box strawberry cake mix (such as Betty Crocker®)
- 1 cup water
- 3 eggs
- 1/2 cup vegetable oil
- 1/2 teaspoon lemon zest
- Lemon Zest Cream Cheese Icing:
- 1 (8 ounce) package cream cheese, softened
- 1/4 cup unsalted butter at room temperature
- 2 cups sifted confectioners' sugar
- 1/2 teaspoon vanilla extract
- 1/2 teaspoon fresh lemon juice
- 1/2 teaspoon lemon zest

Direction

- Prepare the oven by preheating to 325°F (165°C). Use paper liners to line 14 cupcake cups. For creating the strawberry purée, in a blender or food processor, place frozen strawberries and blend until chopped evenly. Add in the sugar, 1/2 teaspoon lemon zest, honey and 2 tablespoons water. Mix until it becomes smooth.
- In a large bowl, beat vegetable oil, eggs, 1 cup water, cake mix, using an electric mixer on low speed until become moist; raise the mixer speed to medium and mix for 2 minutes. Mix lemon zest into batter. Fill prepared cupcake cups about 2/3 full. In the middle of each piece of cupcake batter, drop a spoonful of strawberry purée. Place the cupcakes in preheated oven for 18 to 22 minutes until golden in color and the tops bounce back when pressed lightly. The inserted toothpick near the middle should come out neat as well. Let the cupcakes cool for at least 30 minutes.
- Making the icing, in a bowl, put butter and cream cheese then beat using an electric mixer until it becomes Smooth. Add in confectioners' sugar; mix in Lemon zest, lemon juice and vanilla extract. Place inside the refrigerator until cupcakes are cool enough to frost. Then Frost cooled cupcakes with icing.

Nutrition Information

- Calories: 392 calories;
- Total Fat: 20.2
- Sodium: 291
- Total Carbohydrate: 50.9
- Cholesterol: 61
- Protein: 3.4

239. Strawberry Chocolate Mini Cupcakes With White Chocolate Ganache

Serving: 48 | Prep: 30mins | Cook: 20mins | Ready in:

Ingredients

- 2 cups all-purpose flour
- 1/4 teaspoon baking soda
- 1 tablespoon baking powder
- 1 cup unsweetened cocoa powder
- 5 tablespoons unsweetened cocoa powder
- 1 (0.13 ounce) package unsweetened strawberry-flavored drink mix
- 1/4 teaspoon salt
- 5 tablespoons butter
- 2 1/2 cups white sugar
- 4 eggs
- 2 1/2 teaspoons vanilla extract, or to taste
- 1 3/4 cups milk

- 1/4 cup heavy cream
- 2 cups heavy cream
- 2 (0.13 ounce) packages unsweetened strawberry-flavored drink mix
- 36 ounces white chocolate, chopped

Direction

- Preheat an oven to 150°C/300°F; line paper liners on cups of 4 24-cup mini cupcake pans. Sift salt, 1 strawberry drink mix package, all cocoa powder, baking powder, baking soda and flour in mixing bowl.
- Use electric mixer to beat white sugar and butter on medium speed till fluffy and light in another bowl; one by one, beat eggs in, adding each egg after last one is incorporated fully. Beta vanilla extract in; in 4 additions, mix flour-cocoa mixture, alternating each time using milk. Lower mixer speed to low; beat cream in. Fill cupcake cups to 1/2-3/4 full.
- In preheated oven, bake for 10-15 minutes till an inserted toothpick in cupcake's middle exits clean. Transfer to racks; cool cupcakes.
- Put 2 cups cream to almost boiling in saucepan on medium high heat; melt 2 strawberry drink mix packets in cream. Mix white chocolate in till chunks melt and mixture is shiny, smooth and melted. Put aside; cool ganache to warm temperature, about 35°C/95°F; use ganache to frost each cupcake.

Nutrition Information

- Calories: 238 calories;
- Sodium: 85
- Total Carbohydrate: 29
- Cholesterol: 39
- Protein: 3.3
- Total Fat: 13

240. Sweet Potato Cupcakes With Toasted Marshmallow Frosting

Serving: 12 | Prep: 25mins | Cook: 20mins | Ready in:

Ingredients

- Sweet Potato Cupcakes:
- 1/2 cup butter, room temperature
- 1 1/2 cups brown sugar
- 2 eggs, room temperature
- 1 teaspoon vanilla extract
- 1 cup cooked, mashed sweet potatoes
- 2 cups unbleached all-purpose flour
- 2 teaspoons baking powder
- 1/2 teaspoon baking soda
- 1/2 teaspoon salt
- 1 teaspoon ground cinnamon
- 1 teaspoon ground ginger
- 1/2 teaspoon ground nutmeg
- 1/4 teaspoon ground cloves
- 1/2 cup milk, room temperature
- Marshmallow Frosting:
- 1/3 cup white sugar
- 1/4 teaspoon cream of tartar
- 1 pinch salt
- 2 egg whites
- 3 tablespoons cold water
- 1 teaspoon vanilla extract
- 1/2 cup marshmallow creme

Direction

- Preheat an oven to 175°C/350°F; line cupcake liners on 12 muffin cups.
- Use an electric mixer to beat brown sugar and butter till fluffy and light in a big bowl. One by one, add room-temperature eggs; blend each egg into butter mixture prior to adding next one. Blend in sweet potatoes and vanilla extract.
- Whisk cloves, nutmeg, ginger, cinnamon, 1/2 tsp. salt, baking soda, baking powder and flour in a bowl; put 1/2 of flour into the sweet potato mixture, mixing just till incorporated. Blend in the leftover flour mixture and milk.

- Scoop batter into prepped cupcake pan; in preheated oven, bake for 18-22 minutes till lightly touch with a finger make the cupcake tops spring back and an inserted toothpick in the middle of cupcake exits clean. On rack, cool.
- Frosting: Mix together cold water, egg whites, a pinch of salt, cream of tartar and white sugar in a heatproof mixing bowl; set mixing bowl above a pan with simmering water. Beat with an electric mixer for 5-7 minutes till stiff peaks form and very hot to touch. Take off the heat; beat for another 1 minute. Add marshmallow crème and 1 tsp. vanilla extract; beat till combined.
- Frost cupcake: fill a pastry bag with a big plain tip with frosting; all over cupcakes, pipe mini marshmallow-shaped dots. Alternately, generously frost with lots of swirls and swoops using a knife.
- Put oven rack about 6-in. from heat source; preheat oven broiler.
- Put 3 or 4 cupcakes on a baking sheet; put in the oven under broiler. Toast for approximately 90 seconds till frosting begins to brown, checking every 20 seconds then rearranging baking sheet if needed. Repeat with the leftover cupcakes till all are toasted.

Nutrition Information

- Calories: 292 calories;
- Total Fat: 8.9
- Sodium: 347
- Total Carbohydrate: 48.8
- Cholesterol: 48
- Protein: 4.6

241. Sweet Pumpkin Cupcakes With Cream Cheese Frosting

Serving: 24 | Prep: 15mins | Cook: 20mins | Ready in:

Ingredients

- Cupcakes:
- 1 (18.25 ounce) package yellow cake mix
- 3 eggs
- 3/4 cup water
- 1/3 cup canola oil
- 1 (16 ounce) can pumpkin puree
- Cream Cheese Frosting:
- 1 (8 ounce) package cream cheese, softened
- 1/4 cup butter, softened
- 1 1/2 teaspoons vanilla extract
- 1 1/4 cups confectioners' sugar

Direction

- Set the oven at 350°F (175°C) and start preheating. Use grease to coat 24 muffin cups or line them with paper liners.
- In a bowl, using a hand mixer, beat canola oil, water, eggs and cake mix together on medium speed for around 2 minutes, till smooth. Put in pumpkin; beat till the batter becomes smooth; transfer into the prepared muffin cups.
- Bake in the preheated oven for 18-20 minutes, till a toothpick comes out clean when inserted into the center of a cupcake. Allow the cupcakes to cool completely on a wire rack.
- In a bowl, using an electric mixer, beat butter and cream cheese together till smooth; put in vanilla extract; beat till smooth. Beat into the cream cheese mixture with confectioners' sugar, 1/4 cup at a time, till the frosting turns creamy and smooth. Refrigerate for at least 30 minutes, till the frosting is chilled.
- Spread the frosting onto the cupcakes; refrigerate for at least 1 hour, till the frosted cupcakes are chilled.

Nutrition Information

- Calories: 212 calories;
- Sodium: 237
- Total Carbohydrate: 25.2
- Cholesterol: 39
- Protein: 2.7
- Total Fat: 11.5

- Protein: 1.4
- Total Fat: 5.3
- Sodium: 149

242. Sweetheart Cupcakes

Serving: 24 | Prep: 20mins | Cook: 20mins | Ready in:

Ingredients

- 1 (18.25 ounce) package white cake mix
- 1 1/4 cups water
- 1/3 cup vegetable oil
- 3 egg whites
- 8 drops red food coloring
- 2 drops raspberry candy oil

Direction

- Preheat oven to 175°C/350°F; line paper cupcake liners on a standard muffin tin.
- Beat egg whites, vegetable oil, water and cake mix for 30 seconds on low speed; beat till smooth on medium for 2 minutes. Use white batter to fill cupcake liners to 1/3 full; put aside.
- Mix 4 red food coloring drops into leftover bowl of batter so batter gets pink; mix in raspberry oil. Put 1/3 pink batter into resealable plastic bag; put aside.
- Mix extra food coloring into leftover bowl of pink batter till it is a red/orange color; put batter in resealable plastic bag. Cut corner off bag; stick open tip into middle of every cup with white batter. Squeeze in 2 tbsp. red batter.
- Cut corner off bag with pink batter; stick open tip into middle of red batter. Squeeze 1 tbsp. pink batter in every cup.
- In preheated oven, bake layered cupcakes for 15-20 minutes till inserted toothpick in middle exits clean. Fully cool then frost.

Nutrition Information

- Calories: 119 calories;
- Total Carbohydrate: 16.6
- Cholesterol: 0

243. White Chocolate Chip Pumpkin Cupcakes

Serving: 24 | Prep: 10mins | Cook: 20mins | Ready in:

Ingredients

- 1 (16.25 ounce) package moist white cake mix (such as Betty Crocker® SuperMoist®)
- 1 1/4 cups water
- 1/3 cup vegetable oil
- 3 egg whites
- 1 (15 ounce) can pumpkin puree
- 1 teaspoon pumpkin pie spice
- 1 (8 ounce) package miniature white chocolate chips (such as Nestle® Toll House®)
- 1 (16 ounce) container cream cheese frosting

Direction

- Preheat the oven to 175°C or 350°F. Grease 2 dozen muffin cups or line using paper liners.
- In bowl, whip egg whites, oil, water and cake mix on low with electric mixer for 30 seconds. Raise the speed to moderate and whip till batter becomes smooth, for an additional of 2 minutes. Mix pumpkin pie spice and pumpkin puree in batter; fold white chocolate chips in. Scoop the batter to prepped muffin cups, keeping roughly half-inch headspace. Cupcakes rise quite a bit.
- In prepped oven, bake for 20 to 25 minutes, till an inserted toothpick in the middle of one cupcake gets out clean. Turn cupcakes onto wire rack to fully cool. Use cream cheese frosting to frost the cupcakes.

Nutrition Information

- Calories: 255 calories;

- Total Fat: 13
- Sodium: 233
- Total Carbohydrate: 33.1
- Cholesterol: 2
- Protein: 2.2

244.   Zucchini Cupcakes

Serving: about 1-1/2 dozen. | Prep: 20mins | Cook: 20mins | Ready in:

Ingredients

- 3 large eggs
- 1-1/3 cups sugar
- 1/2 cup canola oil
- 1/2 cup orange juice
- 1 teaspoon almond extract
- 2-1/2 cups all-purpose flour
- 2 teaspoons ground cinnamon
- 2 teaspoons baking powder
- 1 teaspoon baking soda
- 1 teaspoon salt
- 1/2 teaspoon ground cloves
- 1-1/2 cups shredded zucchini
- FROSTING:
- 1 cup packed brown sugar
- 1/2 cup butter, cubed
- 1/4 cup 2% milk
- 1 teaspoon vanilla extract
- 1-1/2 to 2 cups confectioners' sugar

Direction

- Set the oven at 350° and start preheating. Whisk together the first five ingredients. Mix dry ingredients together; slowly put into the egg mixture and blend properly. Mix in zucchini.
- Fill 2/3 of each of paper-line muffin cups with the batter. Bake for 20-25 minutes, or till a toothpick comes out clean when inserted into the center. Allow to cool for 10 minutes. Take away and place on a wire rack.
- Mix milk with butter and brown sugar in a large saucepan for frosting. Boil over medium heat; cook while stirring for 1-2 minutes, or till thickened. Take away from the heat; mix in vanilla. Allow to cool to lukewarm.
- Slowly whisk in confectioner' sugar till the frosting achieves spreading consistency. Frost the cupcakes.

Nutrition Information

- Calories: 327 calories
- Total Carbohydrate: 52g carbohydrate (38g sugars
- Cholesterol: 45mg cholesterol
- Protein: 3g protein.
- Total Fat: 12g fat (4g saturated fat)
- Sodium: 305mg sodium
- Fiber: 1g fiber)

Chapter 7: Cupcake Recipes For Kids

***

245.   Baby Rattles

Serving: 3 dozen mini cupcakes. | Prep: 20mins | Cook: 15mins | Ready in:

Ingredients

- 1-1/2 cups all-purpose flour
- 2/3 cup sugar
- 1 teaspoon baking powder
- 1/2 teaspoon baking soda
- 1/4 teaspoon salt
- 1 cup sour cream
- 2 large eggs
- 1 teaspoon almond extract

- 1/2 teaspoon vanilla extract
- 1/3 cup butter, softened
- 1/2 cup milk chocolate or pastel chocolate chips
- ICING:
- 1-1/2 cups confectioners' sugar
- 2 tablespoons milk
- 4 teaspoons butter, softened
- 1/2 teaspoon vanilla extract
- Pastel sprinkles
- 36 pieces of red shoestring licorice (5 inches each)
- 36 pieces of ribbon (8 inches each)

Direction

- Combine the salt, baking soda, sugar, flour, and baking powder in a bowl. Mix the eggs with the extract and sour cream, and then add the mixture to the dry ingredients together with butter; whisk well. Fill the paper-lined miniature muffin cups with 1 heaping teaspoonful of the mixture. Stuff each cup with 3 chocolate chips. Top the chips with the batter, filling the cups 2/3 full.
- Bake them at 350° until golden brown, for about 15 minutes. Remove them from the tins immediately, and then let them cool on a wire rack completely.
- For the icing, mix the milk, vanilla, sugar, and butter. Spread the mixture all over the cupcakes and top each with sprinkles. For the handles, make a small hole in the cupcake's side using the sharp knife. Insert both ends of the licorice piece into the hole. Tie the bowl with a ribbon around the licorice.

Nutrition Information

- Calories:
- Fiber:
- Total Carbohydrate:
- Cholesterol:
- Protein:
- Total Fat:
- Sodium:

246. Banana Chip Mini Cupcakes

Serving: 3-1/2 dozen. | Prep: 30mins | Cook: 15mins | Ready in:

Ingredients

- 1 package (14 ounces) banana quick bread and muffin mix
- 3/4 cup water
- 1/3 cup sour cream
- 1 egg
- 1 cup miniature semisweet chocolate chips, divided
- 1 tablespoon shortening

Direction

- Set the oven to 375° for preheating. Combine the egg, muffin mix, sour cream, and water in a large bowl and whisk the mixture until just moistened. Fold 1/2 cup of chocolate chips into the mixture.
- Pour the mixture into the paper-lined or greased miniature muffin cups, filling them to 2/3 full. Bake them for 12 to 15 minutes until the inserted toothpick into the center comes out clean. Let them cool for 5 minutes. Remove them from the pans and transfer them onto wire racks. Let them cool completely.
- Melt the remaining chocolate chips and shortening inside the microwave for the frosting. Whisk the mixture until smooth. Use this to frost the cupcakes.

Nutrition Information

- Calories: 65 calories
- Sodium: 57mg sodium
- Fiber: 0 fiber)
- Total Carbohydrate: 10g carbohydrate (6g sugars

- Cholesterol: 6mg cholesterol
- Protein: 1g protein.
- Total Fat: 2g fat (1g saturated fat)

247. Berry Surprise Cupcakes

Serving: 2 dozen. | Prep: 20mins | Cook: 15mins | Ready in:

Ingredients

- 1 package white cake mix (regular size)
- 1-1/3 cups water
- 3 large egg whites
- 2 tablespoons canola oil
- 3 strawberry Fruit Roll-Ups, unrolled
- 1 can (16 ounces) vanilla frosting
- 6 pouches strawberry Fruit Snacks

Direction

- Combine the cake mix with the canola oil, water, and egg whites in a large bowl. Whisk the mixture on low speed for 30 seconds. Whisk the mixture on medium speed for 2 minutes.
- Fill the paper-lined muffin cups with the mixture, about half full. Slice each fruit roll into 8 slices. Arrange 1 slice over the batter in each cup. Fill the cups with the remaining batter, about 2/3 full.
- Bake them at 350° for 15 to 20 minutes until the inserted toothpick into the center will come out clean. Let them cool for 10 minutes, and then remove them from the pans. Place them on wire racks and let them cool completely. Use the vanilla frosting to frost the cupcakes. Garnish the cupcakes with Fruit Snacks.

Nutrition Information

- Calories: 207 calories
- Protein: 1g protein.
- Total Fat: 7g fat (2g saturated fat)

- Sodium: 198mg sodium
- Fiber: 0 fiber)
- Total Carbohydrate: 34g carbohydrate (23g sugars
- Cholesterol: 0 cholesterol

248. Bunny Carrot Cakes & Cookies

Serving: 2 dozen cupcakes. | Prep: 45mins | Cook: 35mins | Ready in:

Ingredients

- 1 tube (16-1/2 ounces) refrigerated sugar cookie dough
- 2/3 cup all-purpose flour
- 3-3/4 to 4 cups confectioners' sugar
- 3 tablespoons meringue powder
- 5 to 6 tablespoons warm water
- Red, yellow and green paste food coloring
- Green colored sugar
- 1 package spice cake mix (regular size)
- 1-1/2 cups shredded carrots
- 1 teaspoon ground cinnamon
- 12 ounces white baking chocolate, chopped
- 18 ounces cream cheese, softened
- 3 tablespoons butter, softened
- 4-1/2 teaspoons lemon juice
- Brown and pink candy-coated sunflower kernels
- 1 tablespoon chocolate frosting

Direction

- Start preheating the oven to 375°F. Beat flour and cookie dough together in a big bowl until blended. On a surface lightly scattered with flour, roll the dough out to 1/4-inch thickness. Use floured 3-inch cookie cutters to cut out bunny ears. Roll the leftover dough again, cut out 1 1/2-inch carrots. Put on un-oiled baking sheets, 1-inch apart.
- Bake until firm, 6-8 minutes. Let sit for 2

- minutes, and then transfer onto wire racks to cool.
- Mix warm water, meringue powder, and confectioners' sugar together in a big bowl. Use a portable mixer to whip on high speed for 10-12 minutes, or a stand mixer to whip on low speed for 7-10 minutes until forming peaks. Tint 1/4 cup of icing green, 1/4 cup orange, and 1 cup pink. Put plastic wrap or damp paper towels on the frosting to cover between uses.
- On bunny ears, pipe white outlines, then use water to slightly thin the leftover white icing. Add the thinned icing to fill the ears, let sit for 30 minutes. On the carrots, pipe orange outlines, then fill in the middles. Let sit for 30 minutes.
- Pipe carrot tops with greens, sprinkle colored sugar over. On each carrot, pipe 3 orange lines. Pipe on the inside of the bunny ears with pink icing. Allow to dry at room temperature until firm for a few hours.
- Start preheating the oven to 350°. For the cake batter, prepare following the package instructions. Fold in cinnamon and carrots.
- Fill muffin cups lined with paper until 1/2 full. Bake until a toothpick comes out clean when you insert one into the middle, 18-23 minutes. Transfer from the pans to wire racks to fully cool.
- Melt baking chocolate in a microwave; whisk until smooth. Let cool to room temperature.
- Beat butter and cream cheese together in a big bowl until fluffy and light. Beat in lemon juice and cooled baking chocolate until smooth.
- Generously frost approximately 1/4 cup cream cheese icing onto each cupcake. Right before eating, add candy-coated sunflower kernels for nose and eyes and bunny ears. Pipe the chocolate frosting into a smile.

Nutrition Information

- Calories:
- Protein:
- Total Fat:
- Sodium:
- Fiber:
- Total Carbohydrate:
- Cholesterol:

249.   Bunny Cupcakes

Serving: 2 dozen. | Prep: 30mins | Cook: 0mins | Ready in:

Ingredients

- 1 package yellow cake mix (regular size)
- 1 can (16 ounces) cream cheese frosting, divided
- 8 drops green food coloring
- 12 large marshmallows
- 3/4 cup sweetened shredded coconut, chopped
- 24 miniature pink jelly beans
- 12 miniature red jelly beans
- 24 miniature white jelly beans
- Red shoestring licorice
- 1 to 2 drops red food coloring
- 48 small oval sugar cookies

Direction

- Prepare and bake cupcakes following the directions on the package. Allow to cool on wire racks.
- Mix green food coloring and 1 cup of frosting in a small bowl; frost the cupcake. Put aside remaining frosting. Slice the marshmallows in half; dip the cut ends into coconut immediately. To form rabbits' heads, arrange coconut side up on the cupcakes.
- Chop red and pink jelly beans in half widthwise. Chop white jelly beans in half lengthways. Dab remaining frosting onto cut sides of the pink jelly beans pieces using a toothpick; adhere to the marshmallows to make the eyes. For the nose, attach red jelly beans and for teeth, use white jelly beans.

- To make the whiskers, chop the licorice into 1-inch pieces; stick 4 pieces to each cupcake. Color the frosting pink. Make a small hole in the corner of a resealable plastic bag; put in pink frosting. To make the ears, use frosting to pipe an oval outline toward the center of each cookie; put 2 ears into each cupcake.

Nutrition Information

- Calories:
- Protein:
- Total Fat:
- Sodium:
- Fiber:
- Total Carbohydrate:
- Cholesterol:

250. Buried Surprise Cupcakes

Serving: 2 dozen. | Prep: 40mins | Cook: 20mins | Ready in:

Ingredients

- 1 package red velvet cake mix (regular size)
- 1 package (3.4 ounces) cook-and-serve chocolate pudding mix
- 1-1/4 cups water
- 1/3 cup canola oil
- 3 eggs
- 1/2 cup seedless raspberry spreadable fruit
- 24 Halloween gummy candy body parts or gummy candy finger rings
- 1 can (16 ounces) cream cheese frosting
- 6 to 12 drops purple neon food coloring
- Purple sugar

Direction

- Mix the pudding mixes and cake in a large bowl. Whisk in eggs, oil, and water for half a minute at low speed. Whisk for 2 minutes on medium speed.
- Fill 2/3 full in the paper-lined muffin cups. Bake at 350 degrees until a toothpick comes out clean when inserted into the center, for 18-22 minutes. Let cool for 10 minutes, then transfer from the pans onto wire racks to completely cool.
- Use a sharp knife to slice a 1-inch circle with 1 inch in depth at the top of each cupcake. Remove the tops carefully and put aside. Fill a gummy candy and a teaspoon of spreadable fruit into each; then replace the tops. Tint the frosting; then spread over the cupcakes and dust with purple sugar.

Nutrition Information

- Calories: 269 calories
- Sodium: 219mg sodium
- Fiber: 0 fiber)
- Total Carbohydrate: 43g carbohydrate (32g sugars
- Cholesterol: 26mg cholesterol
- Protein: 2g protein.
- Total Fat: 10g fat (3g saturated fat)

251. Butterfly Cupcakes

Serving: 24 servings | Prep: 25mins | Cook: | Ready in:

Ingredients

- 1 pkg. (3.9 oz.) JELL-O Chocolate Flavor Instant Pudding
- 1 cup cold milk
- 1-1/2 cups thawed COOL WHIP Whipped Topping
- 24 baked cupcakes
- 1/4 cup sprinkles
- decorating gel s or icings (assorted colors)
- 48 pieces black string licorice (2 inch)

Direction

- In a medium bowl, mix the milk and pudding mix using the whisk for 2 minutes. Mix in the COOL WHIP.
- Remove the tops of the cupcakes off. To make the butterfly wings, cut each top in half-crosswise; put aside. Fill the bottom half of each cupcake with a heaping tablespoonful of the pudding mixture. Top the cupcakes with sprinkles.
- Insert in each cupcake with the cut sides of 2 wings, making sure that the outside edges are raised slightly. If desired, style each cupcake with gels. For the antennae, insert the two licorice pieces into each of the cupcakes. Keep them refrigerated.

Nutrition Information

- Calories: 140
- Total Fat: 3.5 g
- Sodium: 230 mg
- Cholesterol: 0 mg
- Protein: 2 g
- Saturated Fat: 1.5 g
- Fiber: 0 g
- Sugar: 17 g
- Total Carbohydrate: 26 g

252. Candy Corn Flower Cupcakes

Serving: 2 dozen. | Prep: 15mins | Cook: 20mins | Ready in:

Ingredients

- 1/2 cup shortening
- 1-1/2 cups sugar
- 1 teaspoon vanilla extract
- 2 cups all-purpose flour
- 3-1/2 teaspoons baking powder
- 1 teaspoon salt
- 1 cup milk
- 4 egg whites
- Frosting of your choice
- Assorted candies

Direction

- Cream the sugar and shortening in a large bowl until fluffy and light. Whisk in vanilla. Combine the baking powder, flour, and salt, and then add the mixture to the creamed mixture, adding it alternately with milk. Make sure to whisk well after every addition. Mix in the egg whites.
- Pour the mixture into the paper-lined muffin cups, filling them half full. Bake them at 350° for 18 to 22 minutes until the inserted toothpick into the center comes out clean. Let them cool for 10 minutes. Remove them from the pans and let them cool on wire racks. Once cool, frost the cupcakes and garnish them as desired.

Nutrition Information

- Calories:
- Protein:
- Total Fat:
- Sodium:
- Fiber:
- Total Carbohydrate:
- Cholesterol:

253. Caramel Apple Cupcakes

Serving: 24 | Prep: 20mins | Cook: 25mins | Ready in:

Ingredients

- 1 (18.25 ounce) package spice cake mix
- 1 1/3 cups water
- 1/3 cup vegetable oil
- 3 eggs
- 1 large Granny Smith apple, cored and chopped
- 35 caramels

- 1/4 cup evaporated milk
- 1/2 cup chopped peanuts
- 24 wooden craft sticks

Direction

- Prepare a 24-cupcake pan with cupcake paper liners and preheat the oven to 175°C or 350°F.
- Add the cake mix in a big bowl, then add in the vegetable oil, eggs and water. Mix with an electric mixer for 30 seconds on low speed, until the mixture is well combined and moistened. Increase the speed to medium, and whisk for 2 more minutes. Add in the chopped apple, stir, and fill cupcake cups. Every cup should be around 2/3 full.
- Bake for around 20 minutes until the cupcakes become lightly brown. An inserted toothpick should come out clean from the middle of a cupcake. Place the cupcakes on a wire rack and let cool.
- When cupcakes have cooled, add evaporated milk and caramels on low heat in a saucepan and cook for 4 minutes. Stir constantly until the mixture is combined and smooth. Pour the caramel topping on the cupcakes. Garnish with chopped peanuts, inserting a wooden stick in every cupcake's center.

Nutrition Information

- Calories: 209 calories;
- Total Carbohydrate: 29.2
- Cholesterol: 25
- Protein: 3.7
- Total Fat: 9.2
- Sodium: 193

254. Chocolate Candy Corn Cupcakes

Serving: 2 dozen. | Prep: 25mins | Cook: 20mins | Ready in:

Ingredients

- 1 package fudge marble cake mix (regular size)
- 1 cup (8 ounces) sour cream
- 2 eggs
- 1/2 cup 2% milk
- 1/3 cup canola oil
- Orange paste food coloring
- 1 carton (8 ounces) frozen whipped topping, thawed
- Chocolate candy corn

Direction

- Use paper liners to line 24 muffin cups.
- Open the cake mix and keep the cocoa packet aside. Whisk the eggs, cake mix, oil, sour cream and milk together in a big bowl for 30 seconds on low speed setting. Adjust the speed setting to medium speed and continue whisking for 2 minutes. In a small bowl, put in 1/2 of the prepared batter mixture and use orange-colored food coloring to color it. Add the contents of the reserved cocoa packet into the remaining 1/2 of the prepared batter mixture.
- Distribute the chocolate batter mixture evenly among each of the prepared cups. Gently put the prepared orange-tinted batter mixture over the chocolate batter without swirling it. Follow the package instructions in baking and cooling down the cupcakes.
- Garnish each of the baked cupcakes with whipped topping and candy corn on top, then serve. Keep any leftovers in the fridge.

Nutrition Information

- Calories:
- Total Carbohydrate:
- Cholesterol:
- Protein:
- Total Fat:
- Sodium:
- Fiber:

255. Chocolate Caramel Cupcakes

Serving: 2 dozen. | Prep: 20mins | Cook: 15mins | Ready in:

Ingredients

- 1 package chocolate cake mix (regular size)
- 24 caramels
- 3/4 cup semisweet chocolate chips
- 1 cup chopped walnuts
- Chocolate frosting and hot caramel ice cream topping
- Additional walnuts, optional

Direction

- Follow package instructions in making the batter for cupcakes. Pour into 24 muffin cups lined with paper up to 1/3 full and put aside the remaining batter. Bake for 7-8 minutes at 350 degrees or until cupcake top is set.
- Push a caramel into each cupcake gently and sprinkle with walnuts and chocolate chips. Pour remaining batter on top. Bake until an inserted toothpick can be removed cleanly without any sticking residue or for 15-20 minutes.
- Leave to cool for 5 minutes before transferring to wire racks from trays to fully cool. Cover with chocolate frosting and top with a drizzle of ice cream. Use additional nuts as a sprinkle if needed.

Nutrition Information

- Calories:
- Protein:
- Total Fat:
- Sodium:
- Fiber:
- Total Carbohydrate:
- Cholesterol:

256. Chocolate Chip Cupcakes

Serving: 2-1/2 dozen. | Prep: 15mins | Cook: 20mins | Ready in:

Ingredients

- 1 package yellow cake mix (regular size)
- 1 package (3.4 ounces) instant vanilla pudding mix
- 1 cup water
- 1/2 cup canola oil
- 4 large eggs
- 1 cup (6 ounces) miniature semisweet chocolate chips
- 1 can (16 ounces) chocolate or vanilla frosting
- Additional miniature semisweet chocolate chips, optional

Direction

- Combine eggs, oil, water, pudding mixes, and cake in a large bowl; beat mixture for half a minute on low speed. Beat for 2 minute on medium speed. Mix in chocolate chips.
- Pour into paper-lined muffin cups to 2/3 full. Bake for 18 to 22 minutes at 375° until a toothpick comes out clean from the center. Allow to cool for 10 minutes before transferring to wire racks to cool entirely. Frost cupcakes. Garnish top with more chips if desired.

Nutrition Information

- Calories: 215 calories
- Cholesterol: 28mg cholesterol
- Protein: 2g protein.
- Total Fat: 10g fat (3g saturated fat)
- Sodium: 199mg sodium
- Fiber: 1g fiber)
- Total Carbohydrate: 30g carbohydrate (21g sugars

257. Chocolate Cookie Cupcakes

Serving: 2 dozen. | Prep: 20mins | Cook: 20mins | Ready in:

Ingredients

- 1 package white cake mix (regular size)
- 1-1/4 cups water
- 1/4 cup canola oil
- 3 large egg whites
- 1 cup Oreo cookie crumbs
- 1 can (16 ounces) vanilla frosting
- Additional Oreo cookie crumbs

Direction

- Mix together egg whites, oil, water and cake mix in a big bowl; beat the mixture for half a minute on low speed. Set the speed on high and beat for 2 minutes. Gently fold cookie crumbs into the mixture. In muffin cups lined with paper, add batter to 2/3 full.
- Bake in 350-degree oven until a toothpick is clean when coming out of the middle, 18 to 22 minutes. Allow to cool for 10 minutes, then transfer from pans to wire racks and finish cooling. Add frosting and sprinkle additional cookie crumbs on top of the cupcakes.

Nutrition Information

- Calories: 227 calories
- Cholesterol: 0 cholesterol
- Protein: 2g protein. Diabetic Exchanges: 2 starch
- Total Fat: 9g fat (2g saturated fat)
- Sodium: 214mg sodium
- Fiber: 1g fiber)
- Total Carbohydrate: 34g carbohydrate (23g sugars

258. Chocolate Cupcakes With Marshmallow Cream Filling

Serving: 1-1/2 dozen. | Prep: 60mins | Cook: 20mins | Ready in:

Ingredients

- 3/4 cup boiling water
- 1/2 cup baking cocoa
- 1/4 cup hot brewed coffee
- 1/2 cup unsalted butter, softened
- 1-1/4 cups sugar
- 2 large eggs
- 2 teaspoons vanilla extract
- 1-1/2 cups cake flour
- 1 teaspoon baking soda
- 1/2 teaspoon salt
- 1/4 teaspoon baking powder
- FILLING:
- 2 teaspoons hot water
- 1/4 teaspoon salt
- 1 jar (7 ounces) marshmallow creme
- 1/2 cup shortening
- 1/2 teaspoon vanilla extract
- 1/3 cup confectioners' sugar
- FROSTING:
- 4 ounces cream cheese, softened
- 3 tablespoons unsalted butter, softened
- 3/4 teaspoon vanilla extract
- 1-1/2 cups confectioners' sugar
- Assorted seasonal sprinkles and candies

Direction

- Mix the coffee, cocoa and boiling water in a small bowl. Mix until cocoa has dissolved; put aside.
- Beat sugar and butter in a big bowl until light and fluffy.
- Put in eggs, one at a time, mixing thoroughly after each addition. Mix in cocoa mixture and vanilla. Mix the baking powder, salt, baking soda and flour; put into whipped mixture just until moistened.
- Put batter in paper-lined muffin tins until 3/4 full. Bake for 18 to 20 mins at 375° or until a

toothpick inserted in the cupcake exits clean. Let cool for 10 minutes before taking out from pans to wire racks to cool entirely.
- Mix salt and hot water; mix until dissolved. Let cool. Whip the vanilla, shortening and marshmallow crème in a big bowl until light and fluffy. Put in the confectioners' sugar and salt mixture gradually. Whip until fluffy.
- Snip a small hole in the corner of a plastic or pastry bag; attach a very small tip. Put marshmallow filling in the bag. Push the tip through the top to fill each cupcake.
- Whip the vanilla, butter and cream cheese in a big bowl until fluffy. Put in confectioners' sugar; whip until smooth. Spread on cupcakes to frost. Top with sprinkles and candies to decorate as desired. Chill the remaining.

Nutrition Information

- Calories: 328 calories
- Total Carbohydrate: 46g carbohydrate (33g sugars
- Cholesterol: 49mg cholesterol
- Protein: 3g protein.
- Total Fat: 15g fat (7g saturated fat)
- Sodium: 211mg sodium
- Fiber: 1g fiber)

259. Chocolate Ganache Peanut Butter Cupcakes

Serving: 2 dozen. | Prep: 55mins | Cook: 20mins | Ready in:

Ingredients

- 2 cups sugar
- 1-3/4 cups all-purpose flour
- 3/4 cup baking cocoa
- 1/2 teaspoon salt
- 1/2 teaspoon baking soda
- 1/2 teaspoon baking powder
- 1 cup buttermilk
- 1 cup strong brewed coffee, room temperature
- 1/2 cup canola oil
- 2 large eggs
- 1 teaspoon vanilla extract
- FILLING:
- 1/2 cup creamy peanut butter
- 3 tablespoons unsalted butter, softened
- 1 cup confectioners' sugar
- 2 to 4 tablespoons 2% milk
- GANACHE:
- 2 cups (12 ounces) semisweet chocolate chips
- 1/2 cup heavy whipping cream
- PEANUT BUTTER FROSTING:
- 1 cup packed brown sugar
- 4 large egg whites
- 1/4 teaspoon salt
- 1/4 teaspoon cream of tartar
- 1 teaspoon vanilla extract
- 2 cups unsalted butter, softened
- 1/3 cup creamy peanut butter

Direction

- Set the oven at 350° and start preheating. Mix together the first 6 ingredients in a large bowl. Whisk together vanilla, eggs, oil, coffee and buttermilk till well-blended; put into the dry ingredients till combined. (The batter should be very thin.) Fill the batter into paper-lined muffin cups, 2/3 full.
- Bake till a toothpick comes out clean when inserted into the center, 18-20 minutes. Allow to cool for 10 minutes; take away from the pans and allow to cool completely on wire racks.
- In a small bowl, cream together confectioners' sugar, butter, peanut butter and enough milk to achieve a piping consistency. In the corner of a plastic bag or a pastry bag, cut a small hole; insert a small round tip. Fill the peanut butter filling into the bag. In the top center of each cupcake, insert a tip; pipe around 1 tablespoon of the filling into each.
- In a small bowl, put chocolate chips. Boil cream in a small saucepan. Spread over the chocolate; whisk till smooth. Dip the top of

each cupcake into the ganache; arrange on wire racks to set.

- In a large heavy saucepan over low heat, mix cream of tartar, salt, egg whites and brown sugar. Beat with a hand mixer on low speed for 1 minute. Keep beating on low over low heat for around 8-10 minutes, till the frosting reaches 160°. Transfer to a large bowl; put in vanilla. Beat on high for around 5 minutes, or till it forms stiff peaks.
- Put in butter, 1 tablespoon per time, beating well after each addition. If the mixture starts to look curdled, put the frosting bowl in another bowl of hot water for a few seconds. Keep putting in butter, beating till smooth. Beat in peanut butter till smooth, 1-2 minutes.
- Put the frosting into a plastic bag or a pastry bag with a large star tip; pipe onto each cupcake. Place in an airtight container in the refrigerator for storage. Before serving, allow to sit at room temperature.

Nutrition Information

- Calories: 498 calories
- Sodium: 196mg sodium
- Fiber: 2g fiber)
- Total Carbohydrate: 50g carbohydrate (39g sugars
- Cholesterol: 69mg cholesterol
- Protein: 6g protein.
- Total Fat: 33g fat (16g saturated fat)

260. Chocolate Dipped Ice Cream Cone Cupcakes

Serving: 2 dozen. | Prep: 40mins | Cook: 15mins | Ready in:

Ingredients

- 1 package French vanilla or yellow cake mix (regular size)
- 24 ice cream cake cones (about 3 inches tall)
- FROSTING:
- 1 cup butter, softened
- 1/2 cup shortening
- 6 cups confectioners' sugar
- 1/4 cup 2% milk
- 2 teaspoons vanilla extract
- GLAZE:
- 4 cups (24 ounces) semisweet chocolate chips
- 1/4 cup shortening
- Colored sprinkles

Direction

- Set the oven at 350° to preheat. Coat 24 mini-muffin cups with cooking spray. In additional mini-muffin cups, stand ice cream cones.
- Prepare cake mix batter following the package directions. Fill 1 tablespoon of the batter into each greased muffin cup. Distribute with scant 2 tablespoons of the leftover batter among each ice cream cones.
- Bake for around 15-20 minutes, until inserting in the center with a knife and it comes out clean. Then let it cool for 5 minutes in pans. Transfer both cone and plain cupcakes to wire racks and let it completely cool.
- To make the frosting: Beat shortening and butter until blended. On medium speed, beat in vanilla, milk, and confectioners' sugar gradually until it forms soft peaks.
- To assemble, on the bottom of each plain cupcake, spread a small amount of frosting, then attach to the top of a cone cupcake. Next, spread on top of the cupcakes with the leftover frosting, rounding the tops to resemble the ice cream scoop. Let it freeze for 5-10 minutes, or until the frosting is firm.
- To make the glaze: Melt shortening and chocolate in a large metal bowl over a simmering water, stir until smooth. Then dip the tops of the cones in the chocolate mixture. Garnish with sprinkles. Then allow to stand until set.

Nutrition Information

- Calories:

- Cholesterol:
- Protein:
- Total Fat:
- Sodium:
- Fiber:
- Total Carbohydrate:

261. Chunky Monkey Cupcakes

Serving: 2 dozen. | Prep: 30mins | Cook: 20mins | Ready in:

Ingredients

- 2 cups mashed ripe bananas (about 5 medium)
- 1-1/2 cups sugar
- 3 large eggs
- 1/2 cup unsweetened applesauce
- 1/4 cup canola oil
- 3 cups all-purpose flour
- 1 teaspoon baking soda
- 1/2 teaspoon baking powder
- 1/2 teaspoon salt
- 1 cup semisweet chocolate chunks
- FROSTING:
- 4 ounces reduced-fat cream cheese
- 1/4 cup creamy peanut butter
- 3 tablespoons butter, softened
- 1 to 1-1/4 cups confectioners' sugar
- Chopped salted peanuts, optional

Direction

- Set the oven to 350 degrees to preheat, and use paper liners to line 24 muffin cups.
- Beat the first 5 ingredients together until combined well. Whisk salt, baking powder, baking soda and flour together in a separate bowl, then beat flour mixture into banana mixture gradually. Fold in chocolate chunks.
- Put into prepped cups until 3/4 full. Bake for 20 to 25 minutes until a toothpick pricked in the center exits clean. Allow to cool in pans for 10 minutes, then transfer to wire racks to let cool through.
- To make frosting, beat together butter, peanut butter and cream cheese until smooth. Beat in enough amount of confectioners' sugar slowly to attain desired consistency. Spread the frosting over cupcakes and sprinkle with peanuts, if you want. Chill the leftovers.

Nutrition Information

- Calories: 250 calories
- Total Fat: 9g fat (4g saturated fat)
- Sodium: 165mg sodium
- Fiber: 2g fiber)
- Total Carbohydrate: 40g carbohydrate (25g sugars
- Cholesterol: 30mg cholesterol
- Protein: 4g protein.

262. Classic Yellow Cupcakes

Serving: 1-1/2 dozen. | Prep: 15mins | Cook: 20mins | Ready in:

Ingredients

- 2/3 cup butter, softened
- 3/4 cup sugar blend
- 3 large eggs
- 1-1/2 teaspoons vanilla extract
- 2-1/4 cups cake flour
- 2 teaspoons baking powder
- 1/4 teaspoon salt
- 3/4 cup fat-free milk
- Fat-free whipped topping, optional
- 1 teaspoon confectioners' sugar

Direction

- Cream the sugar substitute and butter in a large bowl until fluffy and light. Add the eggs, one at a time and whisking after every addition. Mix in the vanilla. Mix the salt, flour,

- and baking powder, and then add the mixture to the creamed mixture alternately with milk, whisking well after every addition.
- Fill the paper-lined muffin cups with the mixture, about 3/4 full. Bake them at 350° for 20 to 25 minutes until browned lightly and the inserted toothpick into the center will come out clean. Let them cool for 5 minutes, and then transfer them onto wire racks. Cool them completely.
- Place a dollop of whipped topping on each top if desired. Sprinkle them with confectioners' sugar.

Nutrition Information

- Calories: 171 calories
- Protein: 3g protein. Diabetic Exchanges: 1-1/2 starch
- Total Fat: 8g fat (4g saturated fat)
- Sodium: 171mg sodium
- Fiber: 0 fiber)
- Total Carbohydrate: 22g carbohydrate (9g sugars
- Cholesterol: 54mg cholesterol

263. Clown Cupcakes

Serving: 2 dozen. | Prep: 02hours00mins | Cook: 20mins | Ready in:

Ingredients

- 1 package yellow cake mix (regular size)
- 3 cans (16 ounces each) vanilla frosting, divided
- Yellow, red and blue paste food coloring
- 24 ice cream sugar cones
- Assorted candies: M&M's miniature baking bits, red shoestring licorice and cherry sour ball candies

Direction

- Follow the package directions to prepare and bake the cake batter for the cupcakes. Let them cool on a wire rack completely. Distribute the 2 cans of frosting among the 3 bowls. Tint the bowls with blue, yellow, and red food coloring.
- To make clown hats, use kitchen scissors or serrated knife to cut 2-inches from the open end of each of the cones. Use the tinted frosting to frost the cones. Style the cones with some baking bits. Arrange them on a waxed paper and allow frosting to set for 30 minutes.
- Use the vanilla frosting to frost the cupcakes. Make sure to leave the cupcake some space for the hat. Use candies to form the clown hair and face. Pipe each cupcake with a matching ruffle. Place the hat carefully onto each cupcake.

Nutrition Information

- Calories:
- Sodium:
- Fiber:
- Total Carbohydrate:
- Cholesterol:
- Protein:
- Total Fat:

264. Cocoa Banana Cupcakes

Serving: 1-1/2 dozen. | Prep: 25mins | Cook: 20mins | Ready in:

Ingredients

- 2 cups all-purpose flour
- 1 cup sugar
- 1/2 cup baking cocoa
- 1 teaspoon baking powder
- 1/2 teaspoon each baking soda and salt
- 2 eggs
- 1-1/4 cups fat-free milk
- 1 cup mashed ripe banana (2 to 3 medium)

- 3 tablespoons canola oil
- 1 teaspoon vanilla extract
- FROSTING:
- 4 ounces reduced-fat cream cheese
- 3 tablespoons fat-free milk
- 2 ounces semisweet chocolate, melted and cooled
- 1 teaspoon vanilla extract
- 2 cups confectioners' sugar
- 1/3 cup baking cocoa

Direction

- Mix all the dry ingredients in a bowl. In a separate bowl, mix the vanilla, eggs, oil, milk, and banana and whisk the mixture into the dry ingredients until just moistened.
- Use the cooking spray to coat the muffin cups or paper liners to line the cups. Fill the cups with the mixture, about 3/4 full. Bake them at 375° for 18 to 20 minutes until the toothpick will come out clean. Let them cool for 5 minutes. Place them on wire racks and let them cool completely.
- Whisk the vanilla, cream cheese, chocolate, and milk until smooth. Mix the cocoa and confectioners' sugar and beat the mixture gradually into the cream cheese mixture. Use this to frost the cupcakes.

Nutrition Information

- Calories: 224 calories
- Total Carbohydrate: 40g carbohydrate (0 sugars
- Cholesterol: 29mg cholesterol
- Protein: 4g protein. Diabetic Exchanges: 2-1/2 starch
- Total Fat: 6g fat (2g saturated fat)
- Sodium: 171mg sodium
- Fiber: 2g fiber)

265. Coconut Orange Cupcakes

Serving: 2 dozen. | Prep: 15mins | Cook: 15mins | Ready in:

Ingredients

- 1 cup sugar
- 2/3 cup vegetable oil
- 2 eggs
- 1 cup orange juice
- 3 cups all-purpose flour
- 1 tablespoon baking powder
- 1 teaspoon baking soda
- 3/4 teaspoon salt
- 1 can (11 ounces) mandarin oranges, drained
- 1 cup vanilla or white chips
- TOPPING:
- 1 cup sweetened shredded coconut
- 1/3 cup sugar
- 2 tablespoons butter, melted

Direction

- Beat the orange juice, sugar, eggs, and oil in a large bowl until well-combined. Combine the salt, baking soda, baking powder, and flour. Whisk the mixture gradually into the orange juice mixture until just moistened. Fold in the chips and oranges.
- Pour the mixture into the paper-lined muffin cups, filling them to 2/3 full. Combine the topping ingredients in a small bowl and sprinkle the mixture all over the cupcakes. Bake them at 375° until golden brown, for about 15 to 20 minutes. Place them on wire racks; cool.

Nutrition Information

- Calories: 238 calories
- Sodium: 209mg sodium
- Fiber: 1g fiber)
- Total Carbohydrate: 32g carbohydrate (15g sugars
- Cholesterol: 22mg cholesterol

- Protein: 3g protein.
- Total Fat: 11g fat (4g saturated fat)

266. Cookie Cupcakes

Serving: 1 dozen. | Prep: 20mins | Cook: 25mins | Ready in:

Ingredients

- 1/2 cup butter, softened
- 6 tablespoons sugar
- 6 tablespoons packed brown sugar
- 1 egg
- 1/2 teaspoon vanilla extract
- 1 cup plus 2 tablespoons all-purpose flour
- 1/2 teaspoon baking soda
- 1/2 teaspoon salt
- FILLING:
- 1/2 cup packed brown sugar
- 1 egg
- 1/8 teaspoon salt
- 1 cup (6 ounces) semisweet chocolate chips
- 1/2 cup chopped walnuts

Direction

- Cream sugars and butter till fluffy and light in a big bowl; beat in vanilla and egg. Mix salt, baking soda and flour; add to creamed mixture slowly. Stir well.
- Into each of the 12 paper-lined muffin cups, put 2 tbsp. dough, filling each halfway. Bake till edges are light brown for 10 minutes at 375°.
- Meanwhile, beat salt, egg and brown sugar till lighter in color for 5 minutes in a small bowl; mix in walnuts and chocolate chips.
- Take partially-baked cupcakes out of oven. In middle of each cupcake, put rounded tbsp. filling. Bake till deep golden brown for 12-14 minutes. Cool for 10 minutes. Transfer from pan onto wire rack; cool.

Nutrition Information

- Calories: 305 calories
- Protein: 4g protein.
- Total Fat: 16g fat (8g saturated fat)
- Sodium: 249mg sodium
- Fiber: 1g fiber)
- Total Carbohydrate: 40g carbohydrate (30g sugars
- Cholesterol: 55mg cholesterol

267. Cream Filled Chocolate Cupcakes

Serving: 3 dozen. | Prep: 20mins | Cook: 15mins | Ready in:

Ingredients

- 2 cups sugar
- 1 cup 2% milk
- 1 cup canola oil
- 1 cup water
- 2 eggs
- 1 teaspoon vanilla extract
- 3 cups all-purpose flour
- 1/3 cup baking cocoa
- 2 teaspoons baking soda
- 1 teaspoon salt
- FILLING:
- 1/4 cup butter, softened
- 1/4 cup shortening
- 2 cups confectioners' sugar
- 3 tablespoons 2% milk
- 1 teaspoon vanilla extract
- Pinch salt
- Chocolate frosting

Direction

- Beat together the sugar, milk, water, oil, vanilla and eggs in a large bowl till well blended. Mix together the salt, cocoa, flour and baking soda; beat into the egg mixture gradually till blended.

- Fill the mixture half full into paper-lined muffin cups. Bake until a toothpick inserted in the middle comes out clean, at 375° for 15-20 minutes. Take out of pans and put onto wire racks to cool thoroughly.
- Beat together the salt, milk, confectioners' sugar, shortening, vanilla and butter in a small bowl for about 5 minutes until fluffy. Put a very small tip into a plastic or pastry bag; pour cream filling in. Thrust the tip through the paper liner's bottom to fill each cupcake. Frost the cupcakes.

Nutrition Information

- Calories: 195 calories
- Sodium: 160mg sodium
- Fiber: 0 fiber)
- Total Carbohydrate: 27g carbohydrate (18g sugars
- Cholesterol: 16mg cholesterol
- Protein: 2g protein.
- Total Fat: 9g fat (2g saturated fat)

268. Cream Filled Cupcakes

Serving: 2 dozen. | Prep: 20mins | Cook: 15mins | Ready in:

Ingredients

- 1 package devil's food cake mix (regular size)
- 2 teaspoons hot water
- 1/4 teaspoon salt
- 1 jar (7 ounces) marshmallow creme
- 1/2 cup shortening
- 1/3 cup confectioners' sugar
- 1/2 teaspoon vanilla extract
- GANACHE FROSTING:
- 1 cup semisweet chocolate chips
- 3/4 cup heavy whipping cream

Direction

- Prepare and bake cake batter using paper-lined muffin cups, as stated by the package directions. Let cool for 5 minutes before transferring from pans to wire racks for totally cooling.
- For filling, in a little bowl, combine salt and water till salt becomes dissolved. Allow to cool. In a small bowl, beat the vanilla, confectioners' sugar, shortening, and marshmallow creme up to fluffy and light; whisk in the salt mixture.
- Cut a tiny hole in the corner of a plastic bag or pastry; put in a round pastry tip. Fill cream filling into the bag. Fill each cupcake by pushing the tip through the bottom of the paper liner.
- In a little bowl, add chocolate chips. In a little saucepan, set cream just to a boil. Spread over chocolate; then whisk until smooth. Allow to cool, while occasionally stirring, to room temperature or till ganache gets a dipping consistency.
- Soak cupcake tops in ganache; let chill for 20 minutes or up till set. Reserve in the refrigerator to store.

Nutrition Information

- Calories: 262 calories
- Protein: 2g protein.
- Total Fat: 15g fat (5g saturated fat)
- Sodium: 223mg sodium
- Fiber: 1g fiber)
- Total Carbohydrate: 29g carbohydrate (20g sugars
- Cholesterol: 32mg cholesterol

269. Creepy Crawly Cupcakes

Serving: 2 dozen. | Prep: 30mins | Cook: 20mins | Ready in:

Ingredients

- 1 package chocolate cake mix (regular size)
- 1 can (16 ounces) chocolate frosting
- 20 Oreo cookies, crushed
- 24 gummy worms, halved

Direction

- Follow the package directions on how to prepare and bake the cake batter for the cupcakes. Let them cool completely.
- Reserve 1 tbsp. of frosting. Use the remaining frosting to frost the cupcakes. Dip each cupcake into the crushed cookies. On the cut end of each of the worm halves, put a dab of the reserved frosting, and then place the two onto each cupcake.

Nutrition Information

- Calories: 282 calories
- Sodium: 266mg sodium
- Fiber: 1g fiber
- Total Carbohydrate: 42g carbohydrate (30g sugars
- Cholesterol: 26mg cholesterol
- Protein: 2g protein.
- Total Fat: 12g fat (3g saturated fat)

270. Cupcake Christmas Tree

Serving: 23 servings. | Prep: 45mins | Cook: 20mins | Ready in:

Ingredients

- 1 package devil's food cake mix (regular size)
- 1-1/2 cups mint chocolate chips
- 6 tablespoons butter, softened
- 2-2/3 cups confectioners' sugar
- 4 to 5 tablespoons milk
- 1/2 teaspoon vanilla extract
- 1/4 teaspoon peppermint extract
- 1 teaspoon baking cocoa
- 1/4 teaspoon green paste food coloring
- Candy-coated milk chocolate miniature kisses
- 2 chocolate stars
- 12 Starburst candies

Direction

- Follow the package instructions on how to prepare the cake batter mix for the cupcakes. Fold the chips into the batter. Pour the batter into the muffin cups lined with foil, filling them up to 2/3 full.
- Let them bake at 350° for 18 to 24 minutes until the inserted toothpick into the center will come out clean. Let them cool for 5 minutes, and then remove them from the pans. Place them on wire racks and let them cool completely.
- Cream the confectioners' sugar and butter in a large bowl for the frosting until fluffy and light. Whisk in the extracts and milk until combined. Pour 2 tbsp. of the mixture into the small bowl and mix in the cocoa. Whisk the green food coloring into the large bowl with the remaining frosting.
- Use the green frosting to frost the 21 cupcakes, styling them like a pyramid to resemble a tree. For the lights, use the miniature kisses to garnish all except the top of the cupcake. Use the chocolate frosting to frost the 2 cupcakes. Arrange the two cupcakes at the base of the tree to make a trunk. Top each cupcake with the chocolate star. You can save the remaining cupcake for future use.
- Roll the 2 yellow Starburst candies using the rolling pin until flat. Use the 2-inch and 1 1/2-inch star-shaped cookie cutters to cut the candies. Arrange the smaller star onto the larger star. Place the star on the cupcake on top of the tree.
- Form the 5 Starburst candies into rectangles with size of 3x3/4-inches for the presents. Slice each rectangle into four 3-inches long strips and arrange two of the strips widthwise onto 1 whole Starburst candy, pressing them at the base until attached.
- Form 2 of the strips into figure eights for the bow. Press the strips in the center and press on

a wrapped candy. Do the same with the remaining 4 whole Starburst candies and strips. Arrange the presents below the cupcake tree.

Nutrition Information

- Calories: 0

271. Cupcake Cones

Serving: about 2 dozen. | Prep: 25mins | Cook: 25mins | Ready in:

Ingredients

- 1/3 cup butter, softened
- 1/2 cup creamy peanut butter
- 1-1/2 cups packed brown sugar
- 2 large eggs
- 1 teaspoon vanilla extract
- 2 cups all-purpose flour
- 2-1/2 teaspoons baking powder
- 1/2 teaspoon salt
- 3/4 cup 2% milk
- 24 ice cream cake cones (about 3 inches tall)
- Frosting of your choice
- Sprinkles or chopped peanuts, optional

Direction

- Cream the brown sugar, butter, and peanut butter in a large bowl until fluffy and light. Whisk in vanilla and eggs. Combine all the dry ingredients and add the mixture to the creamed mixture alternately with milk. Make sure to whisk the mixture well after every addition.
- Set the ice cream cones into the muffin cups. Fill each cone with 3 tbsp. of the batter, filling them to 3/4-inches from the top
- Let them bake at 350° for 25 to 30 minutes until the inserted toothpick into their center will come out clean. Let them cool on wire racks completely. As desired, frost and style the cupcakes.

Nutrition Information

- Calories: 171 calories
- Sodium: 162mg sodium
- Fiber: 1g fiber)
- Total Carbohydrate: 26g carbohydrate (14g sugars
- Cholesterol: 26mg cholesterol
- Protein: 4g protein.
- Total Fat: 6g fat (2g saturated fat)

272. Cupcakes With Peanut Butter Frosting

Serving: 1-1/2 dozen. | Prep: 15mins | Cook: 20mins | Ready in:

Ingredients

- 1 package white cake mix (regular size)
- 18 miniature peanut butter cups
- 1-1/3 cups prepared vanilla frosting
- 2 tablespoons creamy peanut butter

Direction

- For the cake mix, prepare following the package instructions. Spoon into each muffin cup lined with paper with approximately 2 tablespoons of batter. Put 1 peanut butter cup in each; fill with the leftover batter until 2/3 full.
- Bake at 350° until turning light brown and a toothpick will come out clean when you insert it into the cake portion, about 20-25 minutes. Let cool for 10 minutes, and then transfer onto wire racks to fully cool.
- Mix peanut butter and frosting together in a small bowl until smooth. Frost the cupcakes.

Nutrition Information

- Calories: 257 calories
- Sodium: 254mg sodium
- Fiber: 1g fiber)
- Total Carbohydrate: 41g carbohydrate (28g sugars
- Cholesterol: 0 cholesterol
- Protein: 2g protein.
- Total Fat: 9g fat (3g saturated fat)

273. Cupcakes With Whipped Cream Frosting

Serving: 2 dozen. | Prep: 25mins | Cook: 15mins | Ready in:

Ingredients

- 1 package white cake mix (regular size)
- 1-1/4 teaspoons unflavored gelatin
- 5 teaspoons cold water
- 1-1/4 cups heavy whipping cream
- 5 tablespoons confectioners' sugar
- 1/4 teaspoon vanilla extract
- Red and yellow food coloring

Direction

- Follow the package directions to prepare and bake the cake mix for cupcakes. Let the cupcakes cool on the wire racks.
- Sprinkle water with gelatin in a small saucepan. Allow it to stand for a minute until softened. Heat the mixture over low heat while stirring until the gelatin has fully dissolved. Remove it from the heat and let it cool to room temperature.
- Beat the gelatin mixture and cream in a large bowl until it starts to thicken. Add the vanilla and sugar. Beat the mixture until it forms soft peaks. Put 1 cup of the mixture aside for decorating.
- Top the cupcakes with the remaining frostings. Divide the reserved frosting into two equal portions, tinting one portion with yellow and the other with pink.
- Make an outline shape of heart, sunburst or flower on the top of each cupcake using the toothpick. Pipe along the outline using the medium star tip with yellow or pink stars. If desired, fill the shape with the piped stars.

Nutrition Information

- Calories:
- Sodium:
- Fiber:
- Total Carbohydrate:
- Cholesterol:
- Protein:
- Total Fat:

274. Curveball Cupcakes

Serving: 2 dozen. | Prep: 50mins | Cook: 20mins | Ready in:

Ingredients

- 1 package yellow cake mix (regular size)
- 1 can (16 ounces) vanilla frosting
- 1 tube red decorating frosting or gel

Direction

- Follow the package directions to prepare the cake batter for the cupcakes. Pour the batter into the paper-lined muffin cups, filling them to 2/3 full. Bake them at 350° for 20 to 22 minutes until the inserted toothpick will come out clean. Let them cool for 10 minutes. Remove them from the pans and let them cool completely on wire racks.
- Use the vanilla frosting to frost the cupcakes. Use gel or red frosting to decorate some stitch marks onto the cupcakes for it to look like baseballs.

Nutrition Information

- Calories: 220 calories
- Cholesterol: 26mg cholesterol
- Protein: 1g protein.
- Total Fat: 10g fat (3g saturated fat)
- Sodium: 275mg sodium
- Fiber: 0 fiber)
- Total Carbohydrate: 32g carbohydrate (23g sugars

275. Devil's Food Cupcakes With Chocolaty Frosting

Serving: 2 dozen. | Prep: 40mins | Cook: 15mins | Ready in:

Ingredients

- 1 ounce unsweetened chocolate, chopped
- 1 cup hot strong brewed coffee
- 1-3/4 cups sugar
- 2/3 cup canola oil
- 1 large egg
- 2 cups all-purpose flour
- 1/2 cup baking cocoa
- 3 teaspoons baking soda
- 1/2 teaspoon salt
- 1 cup buttermilk
- FROSTING:
- 2 cups (12 ounces) semisweet chocolate chips
- 1-1/2 cups heavy whipping cream
- 1/2 cup light corn syrup
- 1 teaspoon vanilla extract
- Optional decorations: gumdrops, semisweet chocolate chips and regular or Dum Dums lollipops

Direction

- Set oven to 350° to preheat. Line 24 muffin tins with paper liners. Put chocolate in a small bowl. Add hot coffee on top of chocolate; mix until smooth. Let cool to lukewarm.
- Whip coffee mixture, egg, oil and sugar in a big bowl until thoroughly combined. Beat salt, baking soda, cocoa and flour in a separate bowl; put to coffee mixture alternately with buttermilk, mixing well after each addition.
- Put batter in the lined cups, about 2/3 full. Bake for 15-20 minutes or until a toothpick inserted in the middle comes out clean. Let cool in pans for 10 minutes before taking out to wire racks to cool completely.
- To make frosting, put chocolate chips in a big bowl. Heat cream and corn syrup in a small saucepan just to a boil. Add over chocolate; mix using a whisk until smooth. Mix in vanilla. Let cool to room temperature, mixing from time to time. Cover, chill until completely cold.
- Whip chocolate mixture on medium speed until just fluffy (don't overbeat). Spread on top of cupcakes right away. To make the monster eyes, snip both ends of each gumdrop. Stick a chocolate chip to an end; stick gumdrop to lollipop. Attach into cupcakes. Chill cupcakes until ready to serve.

Nutrition Information

- Calories: 308 calories
- Sodium: 233mg sodium
- Fiber: 2g fiber)
- Total Carbohydrate: 40g carbohydrate (29g sugars
- Cholesterol: 29mg cholesterol
- Protein: 3g protein.
- Total Fat: 17g fat (7g saturated fat)

276. Dreamy Orange Cupcakes

Serving: 24 | Prep: 30mins | Cook: 15mins | Ready in:

Ingredients

- 1 (18.25 ounce) package orange cake mix

- 3/4 cup creamy salad dressing (such as Miracle Whip®)
- 1 (1.3 ounce) envelope dry whipped topping mix (such as Dream Whip®)
- 3/4 cup freshly squeezed orange juice
- 3 large eggs
- 2 tablespoons grated orange zest
- 1 (13 ounce) jar marshmallow creme
- 1/2 cup unsalted butter at room temperature
- 1/2 cup vegetable shortening
- 1/2 cup unsalted butter at room temperature
- 1/2 cup vegetable shortening
- 1/4 cup freshly squeezed orange juice
- 1 tablespoon orange zest
- 1/4 teaspoon vanilla extract
- 2 drops orange paste food coloring, or as desired
- 4 cups confectioners' sugar

Direction

- Preheat the oven to 175°C or 350°F. Line paper liners on 2 dozen muffin cups.
- In a big bowl, whip 2 tablespoons of orange zest, 3/4 cup of orange juice, eggs, whipped topping mix, creamy salad dressing and orange cake mix on low speed using electric mixer for a minute, till mixture moisten. Use spatula to scrape down bowl sides, then raise speed to moderate and keep whipping till thoroughly incorporated, for an additional of 2 minutes. Pour batter into prepped cupcake cups, filling it roughly 2/3 full.
- In prepped oven, bake for 15 minutes, till an inserted toothpick into the middle of cupcake gets out clean. Cool for 10 minutes in pans prior to transferring on wire rack to fully cool prior to frosting.
- Prepare cream topping: use an electric mixer to whip half cup of unsalted butter, half cup of shortening and marshmallow crème in bowl till creamy and smooth. Put half-inch thick cream topping layer on top of every cooled cupcake, with knife to smear the topping even. Let roughly half-inch orange cupcake to expose under white layer.
- Prepare orange butter cream: in bowl, whip half cup of shortening and half cup of unsalted butter till fluffy and light. Stir in food coloring, vanilla extract, zest from an orange and quarter cup orange of juice till thoroughly blended. Slowly whip in confectioners' sugar till smooth.
- Turn frosting onto piping bag equipped with one big star tip, and pipe single layer of orange butter cream in a decorative manner, finishing in one peak, on top of cream topping on cupcakes.

Nutrition Information

- Calories: 411 calories;
- Total Carbohydrate: 53.5
- Cholesterol: 47
- Protein: 2
- Total Fat: 21.4
- Sodium: 278

277. Easter Basket Cupcakes

Serving: 2-1/2 dozen. | Prep: 35mins | Cook: 20mins | Ready in:

Ingredients

- 4 large eggs
- 1 cup sugar
- 1 cup packed brown sugar
- 1 cup canola oil
- 3 teaspoons vanilla extract
- 3 cups all-purpose flour
- 2 teaspoons baking powder
- 2 teaspoons ground cinnamon
- 1 teaspoon salt
- 1 teaspoon baking soda
- 1/2 teaspoon ground ginger
- 1/4 teaspoon ground nutmeg
- 3/4 cup buttermilk
- 1 pound carrots, grated
- 2 cups chopped walnuts, toasted

- 1 can (8 ounces) crushed pineapple, drained
- 1 cup sweetened shredded coconut
- FROSTING/DECORATIONS:
- 1 package (8 ounces) cream cheese, softened
- 1/2 cup butter, softened
- 1 teaspoon grated orange zest
- 1 teaspoon vanilla extract
- 4 cups confectioners' sugar
- 1 teaspoon water
- 2 to 4 drops food coloring
- 3 cups sweetened shredded coconut
- Optional candies: jelly beans, bunny Peeps candy and Sour Punch straws

Direction

- Set the oven to 350° and start preheating. Use paper lines to line 30 muffin cups. Beat vanilla, oil, sugars and eggs until well blended in a large bowl. Whisk nutmeg, ginger, baking soda, salt, cinnamon, baking powder and flour in another bowl; add to egg mixture alternately with buttermilk; after each addition, beat well. Stir in coconut, pineapple, walnuts and carrots.
- Fill prepared cups 3/4 full. Bake 20-25 minutes or until the inserted toothpick in the center comes out clean. Allow to cool in pan for 10 minutes before transferring to wire racks to completely cool.
- Beat butter and cream cheese until blended in a large bowl. Beat in vanilla and orange zest. Beat in confectioners' sugar gradually until smooth. Frost cupcakes.
- Mix food coloring and water in a large resealable plastic bag; add coconut. Seal bag, shake until coconut is tinted evenly. Top over cupcakes. Garnish with candies as preferred. Chill in the fridge until serving.

Nutrition Information

- Calories: 420 calories
- Total Fat: 24g fat (9g saturated fat)
- Sodium: 253mg sodium
- Fiber: 2g fiber)
- Total Carbohydrate: 50g carbohydrate (36g sugars
- Cholesterol: 45mg cholesterol
- Protein: 5g protein.

278. Elf Cupcakes

Serving: 22 cupcakes. | Prep: 45mins | Cook: 15mins | Ready in:

Ingredients

- 2/3 cup butter, softened
- 1-3/4 cups sugar
- 1-1/2 teaspoons vanilla extract
- 2 large eggs
- 2-1/2 cups all-purpose flour
- 2-1/2 teaspoons baking powder
- 1/2 teaspoon salt
- 1-1/4 cups 2% milk
- FROSTING:
- 3/4 cup butter, softened
- 3/4 cup shortening
- 1-1/2 teaspoons clear vanilla extract
- 6 cups confectioners' sugar
- 4 to 6 tablespoons 2% milk
- DECORATIONS:
- 44 miniature candy canes
- Pastel miniature marshmallows
- Candy cane kisses

Direction

- Set the oven to 350° for preheating. Use paper liners to line the 22 muffin cups.
- Cream the sugar and butter until fluffy and light. Whisk in vanilla and eggs, adding them one at a time. In a separate bowl, whisk the salt, flour, and baking powder. Add the mixture to the creamed mixture alternately with the milk while whisking well.
- Pour the mixture into the prepared cups, filling them 2/3 full. Bake them for 15 to 20 minutes until the inserted toothpick into the center comes out clean. Let them cool in pans

for 10 minutes, and then remove them to wire racks. Let them cool completely.
- Whisk the vanilla, butter, and shortening for the frosting until blended. Beat in enough amount of milk and confectioners' sugar until the desired spreading consistency was reached. Drizzle mixture over the cupcakes.
- To style the cupcakes, break the curved ends of the candy canes, reserving the straight portions for the elf legs. Slice the lime or strawberry marshmallows in half diagonally and attach them to the legs for the shoes. Insert the legs to the frosting. For the ears, slice the orange marshmallows in half diagonally. For the elf heads, insert the orange marshmallows and kisses.

Nutrition Information

- Calories: 422 calories
- Sodium: 218mg sodium
- Fiber: 0 fiber)
- Total Carbohydrate: 60g carbohydrate (49g sugars
- Cholesterol: 50mg cholesterol
- Protein: 3g protein.
- Total Fat: 19g fat (10g saturated fat)

279. Fancy Cream Cupcakes

Serving: 22 cupcakes. | Prep: 25mins | Cook: 15mins | Ready in:

Ingredients

- 1/2 cup shortening
- 1-1/2 cups sugar
- 4 egg whites
- 1 teaspoon vanilla extract
- 2 cups all-purpose flour
- 3-1/2 teaspoons baking powder
- 1 teaspoon salt
- 1 cup 2% milk
- 1 cup heavy whipping cream
- 2 tablespoons confectioners' sugar
- 4 to 5 drops red food coloring, optional
- 1/4 teaspoon almond extract

Direction

- Cream the sugar and shortening in a large bowl until fluffy and light. Add the egg whites, one at a time and whisking well after every addition. Mix in vanilla. Mix the salt, flour, and baking powder, and then add the mixture to the creamed mixture alternately with milk, making sure to beat well after every addition.
- Fill the foil or paper-lined muffin cups with the batter, about 2/3 full. Bake them at 350° for 15 to 20 minutes until the inserted toothpick into the center will come out clean. Let them cool for 10 minutes, and then transfer them to wire racks. Let them cool completely.
- For the filling, whisk the cream in a chilled small bowl until it starts to thicken. Whisk in confectioners' sugar gradually and if desired, food coloring until it forms stiff peaks. Mix in almond extract.
- Make a 1-inch cone shape from the center of each cupcake, and then put the cone aside. Pour the filling into the indentation. Cut each of the cones in half, starting from the top to bottom. For the butterfly wings, arrange the two halves onto the filling. Pipe a thin strip of the filling between the wings for the butterfly's body if desired.

Nutrition Information

- Calories: 185 calories
- Fiber: 0 fiber)
- Total Carbohydrate: 24g carbohydrate (15g sugars
- Cholesterol: 16mg cholesterol
- Protein: 2g protein.
- Total Fat: 9g fat (4g saturated fat)
- Sodium: 191mg sodium

280. Frosted Banana Cupcakes

Serving: 1-1/2 dozen. | Prep: 25mins | Cook: 20mins | Ready in:

Ingredients

- 1/2 cup shortening
- 1-1/2 cups sugar
- 2 eggs
- 1 cup mashed ripe bananas (about 2 medium)
- 1 teaspoon vanilla extract
- 2 cups all-purpose flour
- 3/4 teaspoon baking soda
- 1/2 teaspoon baking powder
- 1/2 teaspoon salt
- 1/2 cup buttermilk
- LEMON BUTTER FROSTING:
- 2 cups confectioners' sugar
- 1/3 cup butter, softened
- 3 tablespoons mashed ripe banana
- 1 tablespoon lemon juice

Direction

- Cream sugar and shortening in a large bowl until fluffy and light. Put in the eggs, 1 at a time; after each addition, beat well. Next, beat in vanilla and bananas. Mix salt, baking powder, baking soda, and flour; add alternately with buttermilk into the creamed mixture, after each addition, beat well.
- Fill 2/3 full into the paper-lined muffin cups. Then bake for 18-22 minutes at 375°, or until inserting in the center with a toothpick and it comes out clean. Then let it cool for around 10 minutes before transferring from the pan to a wire rack to completely cool.
- Combine the frosting ingredients in a small bowl; beat until fluffy and light. Frost the cupcakes.

Nutrition Information

- Calories: 270 calories
- Sodium: 168mg sodium
- Fiber: 1g fiber)
- Total Carbohydrate: 44g carbohydrate (32g sugars
- Cholesterol: 33mg cholesterol
- Protein: 3g protein.
- Total Fat: 10g fat (4g saturated fat)

281. Fruit Filled Cupcakes

Serving: about 2 dozen. | Prep: 30mins | Cook: 25mins | Ready in:

Ingredients

- 1 package strawberry cake mix (regular size)
- 2 cups (16 ounces) sour cream
- 2 large eggs
- 1/3 cup strawberry preserves
- 1 can (16 ounces) vanilla frosting, divided
- Red food coloring, optional
- Red nonpareils and pink jimmies, optional

Direction

- Combine eggs, sour cream and cake mix in a large bowl. Beat for half a minute on low speed; beat for 2 mins on medium.
- Place 27 foil or paper liners in standard muffin or heart-shaped tins. (If you use the standard tins, tuck a 1/2-inch foil marble or ball between liner and cup to shape the heart form.) Fill batter into cups by half full. Create an indentation in middle of each with the end of wooden spoon handle and fill it with half a teaspoon of the preserves. Add the remaining batter on top.
- Bake for 22 to 27 mins at 350, or until a toothpick comes out clean when inserted in cake portion. Let it cool 10 mins then remove from the pan to cool completely on a wire rack.
- Put a third of frosting in small bowl, if desired. Add red food coloring to tint pink. Frost the cupcakes with the white frosting. Pipe the edges with the pink frosting, if desired.

Garnish with jimmies and nonpareils if desired.

Nutrition Information

- Calories: 205 calories
- Total Fat: 8g fat (4g saturated fat)
- Sodium: 173mg sodium
- Fiber: 0 fiber
- Total Carbohydrate: 30g carbohydrate (23g sugars
- Cholesterol: 28mg cholesterol
- Protein: 2g protein.

282. Fun Party Cupcakes

Serving: 2 dozen. | Prep: 60mins | Cook: 20mins | Ready in:

Ingredients

- 1 package cake mix of your choice (regular size)
- 1 can (16 ounces) vanilla frosting
- Green gel food coloring or color of your choice, optional
- Assorted candies of your choice: Pretzel sticks, Tic Tacs, Life Savers, red string licorice, Tart'n'Tinys, Chuckles, and Peanut M&M's

Direction

- Prepare cake batter following the package directions. Fill 2/3 full into the paper-lined or greased muffin cups.
- Bake for 18-24 minutes at 350°, or until inserting in the center with a toothpick and it comes out clean. Before transferring from pans to wire racks, let it cool for around 5 minutes; then allow it to completely cool.
- If desired, use food coloring to tint the frosting. Frost the cupcakes and garnish as desired.

Nutrition Information

- Calories: 202 calories
- Protein: 2g protein.
- Total Fat: 8g fat (2g saturated fat)
- Sodium: 189mg sodium
- Fiber: 0 fiber
- Total Carbohydrate: 30g carbohydrate (21g sugars
- Cholesterol: 23mg cholesterol

283. Gluten Free Chocolate Cupcakes

Serving: 1 dozen. | Prep: 15mins | Cook: 20mins | Ready in:

Ingredients

- 2 cups gluten-free oat flour
- 1 cup sugar
- 1/4 cup baking cocoa
- 1 teaspoon baking soda
- 1/2 teaspoon salt
- 1 cup water
- 1/3 cup canola oil
- 1 teaspoon cider vinegar
- 1/2 teaspoon vanilla extract
- 2 teaspoons confectioners' sugar

Direction

- Mix salt, baking soda, cocoa, sugar, and flour together in a big bowl. Mix vanilla, vinegar, oil, and water together in a separate bowl. Mix into the dry ingredients until barely moist.
- Fill muffin cups lined with papers until 3/4 full. Bake at 350° until a toothpick will come out clean when you insert it into the middle, about 20-25 minutes. Leave in the pans to cool for 10 minutes, and then transfer from the pan to a wire rack to fully cool. Dust confectioners' sugar over.

Nutrition Information

- Calories: 187 calories
- Protein: 2g protein. Diabetic Exchanges: 2 starch
- Total Fat: 8g fat (1g saturated fat)
- Sodium: 203mg sodium
- Fiber: 2g fiber)
- Total Carbohydrate: 29g carbohydrate (17g sugars
- Cholesterol: 0 cholesterol

284. Golden Orange Cupcakes

Serving: 15 cupcakes. | Prep: 20mins | Cook: 20mins | Ready in:

Ingredients

- 1/2 cup shortening
- 1 cup sugar
- 4 egg yolks
- 1 teaspoon vanilla extract
- 1 teaspoon orange extract
- 2 cups cake flour
- 1-1/2 teaspoons baking powder
- 1/2 teaspoon salt
- 1/8 teaspoon baking soda
- 1/3 cup water
- 1/3 cup orange juice
- Orange Buttercream Frosting or frosting of your choice

Direction

- Cream the sugar and shortening in a large bowl until light and fluffy. Add the egg yolks, one at a time and whisking well after every addition. Mix in the extracts.
- Combine the baking soda with salt, flour, and baking powder. Add the mixture to the creamed mixture alternately with orange juice and water, whisking the mixture well after every addition.
- Pour the mixture into the paper-lined muffin cups, filling them 2/3 full. Bake them at 350° for 20 to 25 minutes until the inserted toothpick into the center will come out clean. Let them cool for 10 minutes. Transfer them onto wire racks and let them cool completely, then frost the cupcakes.

Nutrition Information

- Calories: 197 calories
- Cholesterol: 57mg cholesterol
- Protein: 2g protein.
- Total Fat: 8g fat (2g saturated fat)
- Sodium: 108mg sodium
- Fiber: 0 fiber)
- Total Carbohydrate: 28g carbohydrate (14g sugars

285. Hidden Treasure Cupcakes

Serving: 24 servings. | Prep: 60mins | Cook: 20mins | Ready in:

Ingredients

- 1 package chocolate cake mix (regular size)
- 1/4 cup strawberry pie filling
- 24 Swiss cake rolls
- 1 can (16 ounces) vanilla frosting
- Blue food coloring, optional
- Assorted candies: Jolly Ranchers, Nerds, skull and fish hard candies
- Yellow food coloring, optional

Direction

- Prepare the cake mix following the package instructions. Fill half full into the paper-lined muffin cups. Drop half a teaspoon of pie filling in middle of each. Add the remaining batter on top.

- Bake for 18 to 22 mins at 350°, or until a toothpick comes out clean when inserted into the cake portion. Let it cool 10 then remove from the pan to cool completely on wire racks.
- In the meantime, slice the cake rolls lengthwise (but do not cut through). Put aside. In a small bowl, add 2 tablespoons of the frosting. Put aside. If desired, tint blue food coloring into the remaining frosting; then frost the cupcakes.
- Arrange a cake roll on each cupcake. Garnish with the assorted candies. If desired, tint yellow food coloring into the reserved frosting; put into resealable plastic bag. Slice a small hole in a corner of the bag; then pipe latches onto the chests.

Nutrition Information

- Calories:
- Sodium:
- Fiber:
- Total Carbohydrate:
- Cholesterol:
- Protein:
- Total Fat:

286. Holiday Gingerbread Cupcakes

Serving: 21 cupcakes. | Prep: 25mins | Cook: 20mins | Ready in:

Ingredients

- 2/3 cup sugar
- 1/2 cup canola oil
- 2 egg whites
- 1 egg
- 1 cup unsweetened applesauce
- 1 cup molasses
- 1-1/2 cups all-purpose flour
- 1 cup whole wheat flour
- 2-1/2 teaspoons baking soda
- 1 teaspoon ground ginger
- 1 teaspoon ground cinnamon
- 1 teaspoon ground allspice
- 1/2 teaspoon salt
- 1-1/3 cups reduced-fat whipped topping

Direction

- Beat egg whites, sugar, egg and oil until blended well in a big bowl. Mix in molasses and applesauce; mix well. In a small bowl, combine the baking soda, flours, cinnamon, ginger, salt and allspice; beat into applesauce mixture gradually until blended.
- Fill about two-thirds full of the paper-lined muffin cups. Bake at 350° for around 18 for 22 minutes or until a toothpick inserted in the center comes out clean. Allow 10 minutes for cooling before taking away from pans to wire racks to completely cool.
- Use 1 tablespoon whipped topping to top each cupcake just before serving.

Nutrition Information

- Calories: 189 calories
- Cholesterol: 10mg cholesterol
- Protein: 2g protein. Diabetic Exchanges: 2 starch
- Total Fat: 6g fat (1g saturated fat)
- Sodium: 221mg sodium
- Fiber: 1g fiber)
- Total Carbohydrate: 32g carbohydrate (17g sugars

287. Lady Bug Chocolate Cupcakes

Serving: 14 cupcakes. | Prep: 30mins | Cook: 25mins | Ready in:

Ingredients

- 1/2 cup butter, softened

- 1 cup sugar
- 1 large egg
- 1 teaspoon vanilla extract
- 1-1/2 cups all-purpose flour
- 1/2 cup baking cocoa
- 1 teaspoon baking soda
- 1/4 teaspoon salt
- 1/2 cup buttermilk
- 1/2 cup strong brewed coffee
- Chocolate wafer cookies
- 1 can (16 ounces) dark chocolate fudge frosting
- Red jimmies
- Black jelly beans, shoestring licorice and nonpareils; white hard candies

Direction

- Cream sugar and butter in a small bowl until the mixture is fluffy and light. Beat in vanilla and egg. Mix salt, baking soda, cocoa and flour; put into creamed mixture gradually and alternately with coffee and buttermilk, beat well after every addition.
- Pour into muffin cups lined with papers, filling two-thirds. Bake for 25-30 minutes at 350 o or until a toothpick comes out clean when inserted in the center. Let it cool for 10 minutes before transferring from pans to wire racks to cool completely.
- To make the wings of the lady bug, put chocolate wafers in the microwave and process for a few seconds so that they are slightly softened. Chop each chocolate wafer in half using a serrated knife. Remove the tips to make room for the lady bug's face; keep remaining wafer pieces to shore up wings. Frost both of the wings, dunk in red jimmies. Chop black jelly beans in half; stick as spots on the wings. Put aside.
- To make the antennae, chop licorice into 1-inch pieces. Dunk 1 end into the frosting, roll over black nonpareils; put aside to dry.
- For assembling, frost the cupcake with chocolate icing. Put decorated wings onto the cupcakes; to prop up the wings, place reserved wafer piece under wing tip if you like. Attach the antennae and use white hard candy for eyes. For eyeballs, pipe a little frosting dot. For the mouth, use a big curved red Jimmie and 2 small ones.

Nutrition Information

- Calories:
- Fiber:
- Total Carbohydrate:
- Cholesterol:
- Protein:
- Total Fat:
- Sodium:

288. Lemon Butterfly Cupcakes

Serving: 14 cupcakes. | Prep: 35mins | Cook: 20mins | Ready in:

Ingredients

- 1/2 cup butter, softened
- 1 cup sugar
- 2 eggs
- 1 teaspoon vanilla extract
- 1-3/4 cups cake flour
- 1-3/4 teaspoons baking powder
- 1/2 teaspoon salt
- 1/2 cup milk
- FILLING:
- 1-3/4 cups cold milk
- 1 package (3.4 ounces) instant lemon pudding mix
- 28 pieces shoestring licorice (2 inches), optional
- 1 teaspoon confectioners' sugar

Direction

- Beat butter with sugar in a large mixing bowl until fluffy and light. Put in eggs, one by one, beating well between additions. Whisk in vanilla. Mix salt, baking powder, and flour

together; pour alternately with milk into creamed mixture, beating well between additions.
- Pour batter into paper-lined muffin cups to 2/3 full. Bake for 18 to 22 minutes at 350° until a toothpick comes out clean from the center. Allow to cool in pans for 10 minutes before transferring to wire racks to cool entirely.
- In the meantime, prepare filling. Beat pudding mix and milk in a small mixing bowl for 2 minutes. Allow to sit until soft-set, about 2 minutes.
- Cut a 1-inch cone-shaped piece with 1 inch deep from the middle of each cupcake using a sharp knife. Remove carefully and put to one side. Fill pudding mixture into cavity.
- To make wings, cut the reserved cone pieces in half vertically; place over the filling with points touching. Insert licorice for antennae, if desired. Sprinkle with confectioners' sugar. Chill leftovers.

Nutrition Information

- Calories: 235 calories
- Sodium: 292mg sodium
- Fiber: 0 fiber)
- Total Carbohydrate: 36g carbohydrate (22g sugars
- Cholesterol: 51mg cholesterol
- Protein: 4g protein.
- Total Fat: 9g fat (5g saturated fat)

289. Lemon Cupcakes With Strawberry Frosting

Serving: 2 dozen. | Prep: 20mins | Cook: 25mins | Ready in:

Ingredients

- 1 package white cake mix (regular size)
- 1/4 cup lemon curd
- 3 tablespoons lemon juice
- 3 teaspoons grated lemon peel
- 1/2 cup butter, softened
- 3-1/2 cups confectioners' sugar
- 1/4 cup seedless strawberry jam
- 2 tablespoons 2% milk
- 1 cup sliced fresh strawberries

Direction

- Use paper liners to line 24 muffin cups. Following the package instructions, prepare cake mix batter properly, reducing water by 1 tablespoon; include lemon peel, lemon juice and lemon curd before combining the batter. Fill around 2/3 full into the prepared cups. Following the package directions, bake and cool the cupcakes properly.
- Beat milk, jam, confectioners' sugar and butter in a large bowl till smooth. Frost the cooled cupcakes; arrange strawberries on top. Place any leftovers in the refrigerator.

Nutrition Information

- Calories: 219 calories
- Protein: 1g protein. Diabetic Exchanges: 1-1/2 starch
- Total Fat: 7g fat (3g saturated fat)
- Sodium: 171mg sodium
- Fiber: 0 fiber)
- Total Carbohydrate: 23g carbohydrate (29g sugars
- Cholesterol: 13mg cholesterol

290. Lemon Tea Cakes

Serving: Makes 36 3-inch (8-cm) madeleines | Prep: | Cook: | Ready in:

Ingredients

- 4 eggs
- 1 cup (200 g) sugar
- Grated zest of 2 lemons

- 1 3/4 cups (225 g) all-purpose flour (do not use unbleached flour)
- 3/4 cup (6 ounces; 185 g) unsalted butter, melted and cooled
- 1 tablespoon (1/2 ounce; 15 g) unsalted butter, for buttering madeleine tins (see above)

Direction

- Use an electric mixer/whisk to beat sugar and eggs till lemon colored in a big bowl. Add zest. Fold in flour and then 3/4 cup of melted butter.
- Refrigerate batter for 1 hour, covered.
- Preheat an oven to 190°C/375°F.
- Butter madeleine tins. Add batter; fill each well to 3/4 full. Bake till madeleines are golden brown for 10-12 minutes.
- As soon as it's baked, remove madeleines from tins; cool on wire rack. Immediately wash tins with hot water and stiff brush without detergent to retain the seasoning. Best eaten immediately after cooling; you may store in airtight container in an airtight container for a few days.

Nutrition Information

- Calories: 56
- Total Fat: 1 g(2%)
- Saturated Fat: 0 g(2%)
- Sodium: 7 mg(0%)
- Fiber: 0 g(1%)
- Total Carbohydrate: 11 g(4%)
- Cholesterol: 19 mg(6%)
- Protein: 1 g(3%)

291. Little Holiday Cakes

Serving: 2 dozen. | Prep: 20mins | Cook: 15mins | Ready in:

Ingredients

- Pastry for double-crust pie (9 inches)
- 1/2 cup seedless raspberry jam
- 1 package red velvet cake mix (regular size)
- 1 can (16 ounces) vanilla frosting
- Red and green sprinkles

Direction

- Roll pastry until having 1/8-inch thickness. Slice 24 circles, about 2 1/2-inch each. Press 1/2-inch up the sides and onto the bottom of oil-coated muffin cups. Put 1 teaspoon jam on top of each and put aside.
- Make cake mix batter for cupcakes following the package instructions. Fill the prepared muffin cups until 3/4 full.
- Bake at 350° until a toothpick will come out clean when you insert it into the middle, 14 to 16 mins. Let cool for 10 minutes, and then transfer from the pans to wire racks to fully cool. Use vanilla frosting to frost and sprinkles to garnish.

Nutrition Information

- Calories:
- Fiber:
- Total Carbohydrate:
- Cholesterol:
- Protein:
- Total Fat:
- Sodium:

292. Marshmallow Filled Banana Cupcakes

Serving: 1-1/2 dozen. | Prep: 40mins | Cook: 20mins | Ready in:

Ingredients

- 3/4 cup shortening
- 1-1/2 cups sugar
- 2 large eggs
- 1 cup mashed ripe bananas (about 2 medium)

- 1 teaspoon vanilla extract
- 2 cups all-purpose flour
- 1 teaspoon baking soda
- 1/4 teaspoon salt
- 1/4 cup buttermilk
- FILLING:
- 1 cup butter, softened
- 2 cups marshmallow creme
- 1-1/2 cups confectioners' sugar
- Additional confectioners' sugar

Direction

- Set the oven to 375° for preheating. Use paper or foil liners to line the 18 muffin cups.
- Cream the sugar and shortening in a large bowl until fluffy and light. Add the eggs, one at a time and whisk the mixture well every after addition. Whisk in vanilla and bananas. In a separate bowl, beat the salt, flour, and baking soda, and then add the mixture into the creamed mixture, adding it alternately with the buttermilk. Make sure to whisk the mixture every after addition.
- Distribute the mixture among the prepared cups, filling them 2/3 full. Bake them for 18 to 22 minutes or until the inserted toothpick into the center comes out clean. Let them cool in pans for 10 minutes, and then transfer them onto wire racks. Let them cool completely.
- For the filling, whisk the butter, confectioners' sugar, and marshmallow crème in a large bowl until smooth. Slice a 1-inch circle with 1-inch deep on top of each cupcake using the sharp knife. Remove the cut portions carefully, and then put them aside. Pour 1 tsp. of filling into each cavity. Replace the tops and press them down lightly. Pipe or dollop the remaining filling over the tops and dust them with more confectioners' sugar.

Nutrition Information

- Calories: 373 calories
- Sodium: 195mg sodium
- Fiber: 1g fiber)
- Total Carbohydrate: 49g carbohydrate (35g sugars
- Cholesterol: 50mg cholesterol
- Protein: 2g protein.
- Total Fat: 19g fat (9g saturated fat)

293. Mice Cupcakes

Serving: 2 dozen. | Prep: 45mins | Cook: 20mins | Ready in:

Ingredients

- 1 package chocolate cake mix (regular size)
- 2 cans (16 ounces each) vanilla frosting
- 48 vanilla wafers
- Red Hots, red gumdrops and red shoestring licorice

Direction

- Prepare cake batter and bake following the instruction of the package for cupcakes, using paper- or foil- lined muffin tins. To cool completely, take away from pans to wire racks.
- Frost vanilla frosting over cupcakes generously. For ears, on each cupcake, position two vanilla wafers. For eyes, add Red Hots and use gumdrops for noses. For whiskers, insert short pieces of licorice and use longer pieces for tails.

Nutrition Information

- Calories:
- Total Carbohydrate:
- Cholesterol:
- Protein:
- Total Fat:
- Sodium:
- Fiber:

294. Mini Choco Cupcakes

Serving: 24 regular or 48 mini cupcakes. | Prep: 20mins | Cook: 15mins | Ready in:

Ingredients

- 2-1/2 cups all-purpose flour
- 2-1/2 teaspoons baking powder
- 1/2 teaspoon salt
- 1 cup butter, softened
- 1-1/2 cups sugar
- 1-1/2 teaspoons vanilla extract
- 4 large eggs
- 1 cup whole milk
- 1 cup semisweet mini chocolate chips
- Confectioners' sugar

Direction

- Sift salt, baking powder, and flour in a medium bowl; put aside. In a large bowl, beat sugar and butter. Add vanilla. Put in eggs, 1 at a time; after each addition, beat well. Pour milk and add dry ingredients alternately, starting and finishing with the dry ingredients; keep beating well after each addition. Next, stir in chocolate chips. Use baking papers to line mini or regular muffin cups. Fill each 2/3 full. Then bake for 14-16 minutes at 400°, or until the muffins tests are done. Allow to cool down. Dust with confectioners' sugar.

Nutrition Information

- Calories: 217 calories
- Total Fat: 11g fat (6g saturated fat)
- Sodium: 185mg sodium
- Fiber: 1g fiber)
- Total Carbohydrate: 28g carbohydrate (17g sugars
- Cholesterol: 57mg cholesterol
- Protein: 3g protein.

295. Mint Brownie Cupcakes

Serving: 10 cupcakes. | Prep: 25mins | Cook: 15mins | Ready in:

Ingredients

- 1/2 cup mint chocolate chips
- 1/2 cup butter, cubed
- 1/2 cup sugar
- 2 eggs
- 1/2 cup all-purpose flour
- TOPPING:
- 2 cups miniature marshmallows
- 1/3 cup 2% milk
- 1/2 teaspoon peppermint extract
- Green or red food coloring, optional
- 3/4 cup heavy whipping cream, whipped
- Additional chocolate chips, optional

Direction

- Melt and stir butter and chips until smooth in a big microwave-safe bowl. Let sit until cool, then stir in eggs and sugar. Whisk flour slowly into chocolate mixture until smooth.
- Pour the mixture into muffin cups lined with paper, 2/3 full. Bake for 15-20 minutes at 350 degrees until a toothpick poked in the middle comes out with no crumbs attached. Take out of the pan and transfer to a wire rack to cool.
- Stir to melt milk and marshmallows over low heat until smooth in a large saucepan. Turn off the heat and whisk in food coloring and extract if preferred.
- Pour into a bowl and leave in the fridge to cool for 15 minutes. Fold whipped cream into the mixture. Spread on the top of cupcakes. Let chill in the fridge for at least 60 minutes. Scatter with chocolate chips as desired. Preserve in the fridge.

Nutrition Information

- Calories: 311 calories
- Protein: 4g protein.
- Total Fat: 20g fat (12g saturated fat)

- Sodium: 94mg sodium
- Fiber: 1g fiber)
- Total Carbohydrate: 31g carbohydrate (23g sugars
- Cholesterol: 91mg cholesterol

296. Monkey Cupcakes

Serving: 2 dozen. | Prep: 30mins | Cook: 20mins | Ready in:

Ingredients

- 1 package chocolate cake mix (regular size)
- 1 can (16 ounces) chocolate frosting
- 24 vanilla wafers
- Black and red decorating gel
- 48 pastel blue and/or green milk chocolate M&M's
- 12 Nutter Butter cookies

Direction

- Follow the package directions on how to prepare and bake the batter for the cupcakes. Allow the cupcakes to cool completely.
- Reserve 1/4 cup of the frosting. Use the remaining frosting to frost the cupcakes. Remove and discard a fourth of each of the vanilla wafers using the serrated knife. Arrange the wafer onto each cupcake for the face. The rounded edge of the wafer must be positioned near the edge of the cupcake. For the nostrils, create some dots using the black gel. Use the red gel to create the mouths.
- For the eyes, arrange M&M's on top of the wafers. For the pupils, add some dots of black gel. For the hair, pipe the reserved frosting using a #16-star tip. Separate the cookies carefully, and then cut each cookie into half. Form its ears by arranging one cookie onto each cupcake's side.

Nutrition Information

- Calories: 265 calories
- Sodium: 247mg sodium
- Fiber: 1g fiber)
- Total Carbohydrate: 36g carbohydrate (24g sugars
- Cholesterol: 27mg cholesterol
- Protein: 3g protein.
- Total Fat: 12g fat (4g saturated fat)

297. Mortarboard Cupcakes

Serving: 1-1/2 dozen. | Prep: 20mins | Cook: 20mins | Ready in:

Ingredients

- 3 cups all-purpose flour
- 2 cups sugar
- 3/4 cup baking cocoa
- 2 teaspoons baking soda
- 1 teaspoon salt
- 2 cups water
- 2/3 cup canola oil
- 2 tablespoons white vinegar
- 2 teaspoons vanilla extract
- FROSTING:
- 1/2 cup butter, softened
- 1/2 cup shortening
- 1 teaspoon vanilla extract
- 4 cups confectioners' sugar
- 3 tablespoons milk
- Food coloring
- 9 whole graham crackers, halved
- 18 milk chocolate M&M's
- Black shoestring licorice, cut into 36 pieces (3 inches each)

Direction

- Mix the first 5 ingredients in a large bowl. Combine the oil, water, vanilla, and vinegar in a separate bowl and whisk the mixture into the dry ingredients until just blended.
- Pour the mixture into the greased muffin cups, filling them up to 2/3 full. Bake them at 350°

for 20-25 minutes until the inserted toothpick into the center will come out clean. Let them cool for 10 minutes before transferring to wire racks.
- Cream the vanilla, butter, and shortening in a large bowl until fluffy and light. Pour in confectioners' sugar alternately with milk. Make sure to whisk the mixture well after every addition. If desired, add some food coloring.
- Level the cupcakes' tops off first before frosting their bottoms and sides. Arrange them onto the serving platter or covered board, upside down. Place 1 frosted graham crackers onto each of the cupcakes. Decorate the centers of each of the crackers that have two pieces of licorice with an M&M's candy for the tassel.

Nutrition Information

- Calories:
- Protein:
- Total Fat:
- Sodium:
- Fiber:
- Total Carbohydrate:
- Cholesterol:

298. Out Of This World Cupcakes

Serving: 2 dozen. | Prep: 15mins | Cook: 20mins | Ready in:

Ingredients

- 1 package yellow cake mix (regular size)
- 1 can (16 ounces) vanilla frosting
- Paste food coloring of your choice, optional
- Decorating gel
- Assorted toppings: sprinkles, sour straws and licorice

Direction

- Follow the package directions on how to prepare the cake batter for the cupcakes.
- Pour the batter into the greased or paper-lined muffin cups, filling them 2/3 full. Bake them at 350° for 18 to 24 minutes or until the inserted toothpick into the center comes out clean. Let them cool for 5 minutes. Remove them from the pans and place them onto a wire rack to cool completely.
- Use the food coloring of your choice to tint the frosting. Use it to frost the cupcakes. If desired, decorate each with assorted toppings and decorating gel.

Nutrition Information

- Calories: 174 calories
- Total Carbohydrate: 30g carbohydrate (21g sugars
- Cholesterol: 0 cholesterol
- Protein: 1g protein.
- Total Fat: 5g fat (2g saturated fat)
- Sodium: 174mg sodium
- Fiber: 1g fiber)

299. Owl Tree

Serving: 21 cupcakes and 6 mini cupcakes. | Prep: 60mins | Cook: 20mins | Ready in:

Ingredients

- 1 package chocolate fudge cake mix (regular size)
- 1 cup water
- 1/2 cup canola oil
- 1/4 cup brewed coffee, room temperature
- 3 large eggs
- 1 cup (6 ounces) miniature semisweet chocolate chips
- FROSTING AND DECORATIONS:
- 1 can (16 ounces) chocolate frosting, divided
- 1 teaspoon black paste food coloring
- 12 mini Oreo cookies

- Brown and yellow milk chocolate M&M's
- 3-3/4 cups confectioners' sugar
- 1/2 cup butter, softened
- 1/2 cup shortening
- 1/4 to 1/3 cup water

Direction

- Preheat the oven to 350 degrees. Put paper liners on 6 mini-muffin cups and 21 muffin cups.
- On low speed, beat eggs, cake mix, coffee, oil, and water for half a minute in a big bow. Turn to medium speed then beat for 2mins. Fold in chocolate chips. Transfer the batter on prepared cups until 2/3 full. Bake the regular-sized cupcakes for 18-22mins and the mini cupcakes for 10-12mins until an inserted toothpick in the middle comes out without residue. Cool cupcakes for 10mins in the pans then move to wire racks to completely cool.
- In a small bowl, put 1 1/3 cups chocolate frosting; use food coloring to tint black. Make a small hole at the corner of a food-safe plastic bag or in the tip of a pastry bag; attach #125 or any big petal or even pastry tip. Put the black frosting into the bag; set aside.
- Use some of remaining chocolate frosting to frost the mini cupcakes. Separate the Oreo cookies, leaving the cream filling on one cookies' side. To make eyes, put the filling sides of the Oreos with the cream-side up on the frosted cupcakes. Attach the brown M&M's with chocolate frosting.
- For ears, cut the plain sides of the Oreos into triangles; attach above the eyes. In another pastry bag, put #16 or any star pastry tip. Put the rest of the chocolate frosting into the bag. Pipe feathers around the eyes and on the ears. For the beaks, put yellow M&M's between eyes.
- Whisk shortening, butter, confectioners' sugar, and just enough water to achieve spreading consistency in a big bowl; frost the big cupcakes. On a covered cake board, put the cupcakes side by side.
- Make branches and tree trunk by piping black frosting across tops of the cupcakes. Arrange the owl cupcakes on the branches.

Nutrition Information

- Calories: 389 calories
- Sodium: 261mg sodium
- Fiber: 1g fiber)
- Total Carbohydrate: 49g carbohydrate (38g sugars
- Cholesterol: 36mg cholesterol
- Protein: 2g protein.
- Total Fat: 21g fat (7g saturated fat)

300.   Patriotic Cupcake Cones

Serving: 2 dozen. | Prep: 40mins | Cook: 20mins | Ready in:

Ingredients

- 1/2 cup shortening
- 1-1/2 cups sugar
- 2 eggs
- 1 bottle (1 ounce) red food coloring
- 3 teaspoons white vinegar
- 1 teaspoon butter flavoring
- 1 teaspoon vanilla extract
- 2-1/2 cups cake flour
- 1/4 cup baking cocoa
- 1 teaspoon baking soda
- 1 teaspoon salt
- 1 cup buttermilk
- 24 ice cream cake cones (about 3 inches tall)
- FROSTING:
- 1-1/2 cups shortening
- 1-1/2 teaspoons vanilla extract
- 6 cups confectioners' sugar
- 4 to 5 tablespoons milk
- Blue jimmies

Direction

- Cream the sugar and shortening in a large bowl until fluffy and light. Add the eggs, one at a time and whisking well every after addition. Whisk in the vanilla, vinegar, food coloring, and butter flavoring. Combine the baking soda, flour, salt, and cocoa, and then add this mixture to the creamed mixture alternately with the buttermilk, whisking the mixture well every after addition. Spread the batter into each of the cake cones, filling them up to within 3/4-inches of the top. Set them in ungreased muffin cups.
- Bake them at 350° for 20 to 25 minutes or until the inserted toothpick into the center will come out clean. Let them cool completely.
- Beat the vanilla and shortening in a large bowl until fluffy. Add the confectioners' sugar gradually. Beat the mixture until smooth. Pour in milk, enough to achieve the desired spreading consistency.
- Slice a small hole into the corner of a plastic bag. Insert the large star tip into the hole and fill the bag with the frosting. Pipe the frosting onto the cupcakes and sprinkle them with the jimmies.

Nutrition Information

- Calories: 396 calories
- Protein: 3g protein.
- Total Fat: 17g fat (4g saturated fat)
- Sodium: 175mg sodium
- Fiber: 1g fiber)
- Total Carbohydrate: 58g carbohydrate (42g sugars
- Cholesterol: 18mg cholesterol

301. Patriotic Cupcakes

Serving: 24 servings | Prep: 20mins | Cook: |Ready in:

Ingredients

- 1 pkg. (2-layer size) white cake mix
- 1/4 cup dry JELL-O Berry Blue Flavor Gelatin (from 3-oz. pkg.)
- 1/4 cup dry JELL-O Strawberry Flavor Gelatin (from 3-oz. pkg.)
- 1 container (16 oz.) ready-to-spread vanilla frosting
- 1 cup thawed COOL WHIP Whipped Topping
- 2 pkg. (0.33 oz. each) strawberry popping candy
- 24 pieces string licorice (2 inch each)

Direction

- Follow the package directions on how to prepare the cake batter. Pour half of it into the separate bowl.
- Mix the different flavors of dry gelatin mix into each bowl with the batter. Scoop on the 24 paper-lined muffin cups with the berry blue batter evenly. Top each with the strawberry batter. Follow the package directions on how to bake these for cupcakes. Let them cool completely.
- Scoop the frosting into a medium bowl, and then add the cool whip. Whisk the mixture until blended. Pipe the mixture onto the cupcakes. Sprinkle each with popping candy, and then insert the licorice 'wicks'.

Nutrition Information

- Calories: 210
- Fiber: 0 g
- Total Carbohydrate: 34 g
- Cholesterol: 0 mg
- Protein: 2 g
- Total Fat: 7 g
- Saturated Fat: 2 g
- Sodium: 190 mg
- Sugar: 25 g

302. Patriotic Ice Cream Cupcakes

Serving: 3 dozen. | Prep: 30mins | Cook: 15mins |Ready in:

Ingredients

- 1 package red velvet cake mix (regular size)
- 1-1/2 quarts blue moon ice cream, softened if necessary
- 1 jar (7 ounces) marshmallow creme
- 3 cups heavy whipping cream
- Red, white and blue sprinkles

Direction

- Set the oven to 350° for preheating. Use the paper liners to line 36 of the muffin cups.
- Follow the package guide to prepare the cake batter. Pour the batter into the prepared cups, filling them 1/3 full. Bake them for 11 to 14 minutes until the inserted toothpick into the center will come out clean. Allow them to cool for 10 minutes. Remove them from the pans and place them on wire racks. Let them cool completely.
- Spread the cupcakes with ice cream quickly. Freeze the cupcakes for at least 1 hour until firm.
- Add the whipping cream to the large bowl filled with marshmallow crème. Whisk the mixture until well-blended and it forms stiff peaks. Pipe or spread the mixture all over the cupcakes. Garnish the cupcakes with the sprinkles. You can freeze them until firm or serve them right away.

Nutrition Information

- Calories: 220 calories
- Sodium: 139mg sodium
- Fiber: 0 fiber
- Total Carbohydrate: 21g carbohydrate (16g sugars
- Cholesterol: 46mg cholesterol
- Protein: 4g protein.
- Total Fat: 13g fat (6g saturated fat)

303. Peanut & Banana Cupcakes

Serving: 1-1/2 dozen. | Prep: 25mins | Cook: 20mins | Ready in:

Ingredients

- 1/2 cup butter, softened
- 1 cup sugar
- 2 eggs
- 1-1/4 cups mashed ripe bananas (2-3 medium)
- 1/4 cup buttermilk
- 2 teaspoons vanilla extract
- 2 cups cake flour
- 1-1/2 teaspoons baking powder
- 1/4 teaspoon baking soda
- 1/8 teaspoon salt
- 1 cup chopped lightly salted dry roasted peanuts
- FROSTING:
- 2 cups confectioners' sugar
- 1 cup creamy peanut butter
- 1/2 cup butter, softened
- 2 teaspoons vanilla extract
- 3 to 4 tablespoons 2% milk
- 1 cup chopped lightly salted dry roasted peanuts

Direction

- Cream the sugar and butter in a large bowl until fluffy and light. Add the eggs, one at a time and whisking well after every addition. Combine the vanilla, bananas, and buttermilk. Mix the baking soda, salt, flour, and baking powder and pour the mixture alternately with the banana mixture into the creamed mixture, stirring well after every addition. Mix in the peanuts.
- Fill the paper-lined muffin cups with the batter, about 2/3 full. Bake them at 350° for 18 to 22 minutes until the inserted toothpick into

the center will come out clean. Let them cool for 10 minutes. Remove them from the pans and place them on wire racks. Let them cool completely.
- Beat the butter, confectioners' sugar, and peanut butter in a big bowl until fluffy. Mix in the vanilla and enough amount of milk until the desired consistency is reached. Use this to frost the cupcakes. Sprinkle the cupcakes with the peanuts. Refrigerate the cupcakes.

Nutrition Information

- Calories: 439 calories
- Total Fat: 26g fat (9g saturated fat)
- Sodium: 271mg sodium
- Fiber: 3g fiber)
- Total Carbohydrate: 46g carbohydrate (28g sugars
- Cholesterol: 51mg cholesterol
- Protein: 10g protein.

304. Peanut Butter & Jelly Cupcakes

Serving: 2 dozen. | Prep: 45mins | Cook: 15mins | Ready in:

Ingredients

- 1 package yellow cake mix (regular size)
- 3 large eggs
- 1 cup 2% milk
- 1/2 cup butter, melted
- 1-1/2 teaspoons vanilla extract
- 1 cup peanut butter chips
- FROSTING:
- 1-1/2 cups butter, softened
- 1-1/2 teaspoons vanilla extract
- 6 cups confectioners' sugar
- 2 to 3 tablespoons heavy whipping cream
- 1/3 cup strawberry spreadable fruit
- 1/2 cup peanut butter
- Additional peanut butter chips

Direction

- Start preheating the oven to 350°. Line paper liners on the 24 muffin cups. Combine vanilla, butter, milk, eggs and cake mix in a large bowl; beat for half a minute on low speed. Beat for 2 mins on medium. Stir in the peanut butter chips. Fill 3/4 full into the prepared cups. Bake until a toothpick comes out clean when inserted in the middle, or about 15 to 18 mins. Cool 10 mins in pans then transfer to cool completely on wire racks.
- Beat vanilla and butter in a large bowl until blended. Beat in confectioners' sugar with enough cream, alternately to reach the spreading consistency. Beat for 5 mins on medium-high until fluffy. Put 1-1/2 cups frosting in a small bowl; mix in the spreadable fruit. Put the peanut butter to the remaining frosting then beat until blended.
- Slice a small hole in a corner of a food-safe plastic bag or in a tip of a pastry bag; insert #5 round pastry tip. Place the strawberry frosting into bag. Poke a hole through the bottom of paper liner with the wooden or metal skewer. Insert tip through hole. Then pipe some strawberry filling into the cupcakes. Pipe the peanut butter frosting over the cupcakes, using another pastry bag and #12 round pastry tip. Pipe the remaining strawberry frosting over tops, if desired; scatter with more chips.

Nutrition Information

- Calories:
- Sodium:
- Fiber:
- Total Carbohydrate:
- Cholesterol:
- Protein:
- Total Fat:

305. Peanut Butter Cup Cupcakes

Serving: 18 servings | Prep: 15mins | Cook: |Ready in:

Ingredients

- 18   peanut butter cup miniature s
- 1 pkg. (2-layer size) yellow cake mix
- 1 pkg. (3.4 oz.) JELL-O Vanilla Flavor Instant Pudding
- 1 tub (8 oz.) COOL WHIP Whipped Topping , thawed
- 2 Tbsp. multi-colored sprinkles

Direction

- Fill each of the 18 paper-lined muffin cups with one peanut butter cup.
- Follow the package directions to prepare the cake batter. Add the dry pudding mix and whisk the mixture thoroughly. Pour the mixture into the muffin cups.
- Follow the package directions to bake the cupcakes. Let the cupcakes cool completely.
- Use the COOL WHIP to frost the cupcakes. Place the sprinkles on top of the cupcakes.

Nutrition Information

- Calories: 160
- Fiber: 0 g
- Saturated Fat: 4 g
- Sodium: 125 mg
- Sugar: 13 g
- Total Carbohydrate: 16 g
- Cholesterol: 30 mg
- Total Fat: 10 g
- Protein: 2 g

306. Peanut Butter Filled Brownie Cupcakes

Serving: 1 dozen. | Prep: 15mins | Cook: 15mins |Ready in:

Ingredients

- 1 package fudge brownie mix (8-inch square pan size)
- 1/2 cup miniature semisweet chocolate chips
- 1/3 cup creamy peanut butter
- 3 tablespoons cream cheese, softened
- 1 large egg
- 1/4 cup sugar
- Confectioners' sugar

Direction

- Start preheating the oven to 350°. For the brownie batter, prepare it by following the package instructions; mix in chocolate chips. To prepare the filling, whisk sugar, egg, cream cheese, and peanut butter in a small bowl until smooth.
- Pour the batter into the muffin cups lined with paper until 1/3 full. Drop the middle of each cupcake with teaspoonfuls of the filling. Use the remaining batter to cover the filling.
- Bake until a toothpick will come out clean once you insert it into the brownie portion, about 15-20 minutes. Let it cool for 10 minutes, and then transfer from the pan onto a wire rack to fully cool. Dust confectioners' sugar over the top. Put in the fridge to store.

Nutrition Information

- Calories: 328 calories
- Protein: 5g protein.
- Total Fat: 18g fat (5g saturated fat)
- Sodium: 201mg sodium
- Fiber: 2g fiber)
- Total Carbohydrate: 39g carbohydrate (27g sugars
- Cholesterol: 40mg cholesterol

307. Picnic Cupcakes

Serving: 24 servings. | Prep: 20mins | Cook: 20mins | Ready in:

Ingredients

- 1 package chocolate or yellow cake mix (regular size)
- FILLING:
- 1 package (8 ounces) cream cheese, softened
- 1 large egg, lightly beaten
- 1/3 cup sugar
- 1 cup (6 ounces) semisweet chocolate chips

Direction

- Follow the package directions to prepare the cake mix batter for the cupcakes. Pour the batter into the 24 paper-lined muffin cups, filling them 2/3 full.
- Whisk the sugar, cream cheese, and egg in a small bowl until smooth. Fold the chips into the mixture.
- Drop the mixture by tablespoonfuls into the batter. Bake them at 350° for 20 minutes until the inserted toothpick into the cupcake comes out clean.

Nutrition Information

- Calories: 197 calories
- Fiber: 1g fiber)
- Total Carbohydrate: 25g carbohydrate (17g sugars
- Cholesterol: 41mg cholesterol
- Protein: 3g protein.
- Total Fat: 10g fat (4g saturated fat)
- Sodium: 203mg sodium

308. Pumpkin Caramel Cupcakes

Serving: 2 dozen. | Prep: 25mins | Cook: 20mins | Ready in:

Ingredients

- 1 package yellow cake mix (regular size)
- 1 can (15 ounces) solid-pack pumpkin
- 2/3 cup water
- 1/4 cup maple syrup
- 3 large eggs
- 4 teaspoons sugar
- 4 teaspoons ground cinnamon
- Dash salt
- 1 carton (16 ounces) caramel apple dip
- Chocolate frosting and decorating icing, optional

Direction

- Preheat the oven to 350°F. Prepare 24 muffin cups lined with paper liners. Mix well the first 8 ingredients. Beat the mixture for 30 seconds on low speed first, then beat on medium speed for 2 minutes.
- Fill the muffin cups up to about three-fourths full. Bake for 18 to 22 minutes then insert a toothpick in the middle of the cupcake to check doneness, the toothpick should come out clean. Cool the cupcakes in the muffin pans for ten minutes then remove to cool completely on wire racks.
- Coat the cupcakes with the caramel apple dip. Put decorating icing and frosting if preferred. Keep the leftovers in the fridge.

Nutrition Information

- Calories: 178 calories
- Protein: 2g protein.
- Total Fat: 5g fat (2g saturated fat)
- Sodium: 242mg sodium
- Fiber: 1g fiber)
- Total Carbohydrate: 31g carbohydrate (22g sugars

- Cholesterol: 26mg cholesterol

309. Pumpkin Cupcakes

Serving: Makes 24 servings, 1 cupcake each. | Prep: 15mins | Cook: | Ready in:

Ingredients

- 1 pkg. (2-layer size) white cake mix
- 1/4 cup plus 2 Tbsp. KOOL-AID Orange Flavor Sugar-Sweetened Drink Mix, divided
- 1 container (16 oz.) ready-to-spread vanilla frosting
- 1 Tbsp. decorating icing
- assorted Halloween candies

Direction

- Follow the package instructions in preparing the cake batter then add in 1/4 cup of the dry drink mix and mix everything together until blended. Line 24 pieces of medium-sized muffin cups with paper, then pour the prepared cake batter mixture evenly among the 24 prepared muffin cups.
- Follow the package instructions in baking the cupcakes and let the baked cupcakes fully cool down.
- Combine 1 tablespoon of the remaining dry drink mix and the frosting together and spread it evenly over each of the cupcakes. Use the decorating icing, candies and the remaining 1 tablespoon of dry drink mix to decorate the cupcakes however you like to make them look like jack-o'-lanterns or pumpkins.

Nutrition Information

- Calories: 220
- Protein: 1 g
- Sodium: 220 mg
- Fiber: 0 g
- Total Carbohydrate: 42 g

- Cholesterol: 0 mg
- Total Fat: 6 g
- Saturated Fat: 1 g
- Sugar: 33 g

310. Rainbow Cupcakes

Serving: 24 | Prep: 20mins | Cook: 15mins | Ready in:

Ingredients

- 2 1/2 cups all-purpose flour
- 2 teaspoons baking powder
- 1/2 teaspoon baking soda
- 1/2 teaspoon salt
- 1/2 cup milk
- 1/2 cup vegetable oil
- 1 teaspoon vanilla extract
- 1/2 cup butter
- 1 cup white sugar
- 3 eggs, room temperature
- red food coloring
- blue food coloring
- green food coloring
- yellow food coloring

Direction

- Set oven temperature to 350 degrees F (175 degrees C) and leave aside to preheat. Use paper baking cups as lining for two 12-cup muffin trays. Mix baking powder, flour, salt, and baking soda in a big bowl and stir together. Add vegetable oil, vanilla extract, and milk into a separate bowl and whisk together until even. Leave aside for later.
- Mix sugar and butter in a big bowl and beat using an electric mixer until fluffy and light. The mixture should have an obvious lighter color in appearance. Break the eggs, which are at room temperature, into the butter mix, one at a time, complete blending each egg before adding the next one. Alternate the mixing process of the flour mixture with milk mixture and continue until combined evenly.

- Separate the cake batter into four different bowls. Drip food coloring into one bowl of batter and stir, adding more to obtain the desired color. Repeat the process with the remaining bowls of batter.
- Scoop a small amount of batter from each bowl using a different spoon for each variant of batter, and press into the cupcake liners up to 1/2 or 3/4 full. Avoid mixing the batter once placed inside the cupcake liner. Bake for around 15-20 minutes in the preheated oven until an inserted toothpick can be removed from the cake without any residue on it.

Nutrition Information

- Calories: 166 calories;
- Total Fat: 9.3
- Sodium: 154
- Total Carbohydrate: 18.7
- Cholesterol: 34
- Protein: 2.3

311. Root Beer Cupcakes

Serving: 1 dozen. | Prep: 15mins | Cook: 20mins | Ready in:

Ingredients

- 1/2 cup butter, softened
- 1 cup packed brown sugar
- 2 large eggs
- 2 cups all-purpose flour
- 1 teaspoon baking powder
- 1/8 teaspoon baking soda
- 1/8 teaspoon ground cinnamon
- 1/8 teaspoon ground allspice
- 1 cup root beer
- 1-1/2 cups whipped topping
- 12 root beer barrel candies, crushed

Direction

- Cream the brown sugar and butter in a large bowl until fluffy and light. Add the eggs, one at a time. Make sure to whisk the mixture after every addition. Combine the allspice, baking powder, flour, cinnamon, and baking soda, and then gradually add this mixture to the creamed mixture, adding it alternately with the root beer. Make sure to whisk the mixture after every addition.
- Pour the mixture into the paper-lined muffin cups, filling them 2/3 full. Bake them at 350° for 18 to 22 minutes. The inserted toothpick into the cupcakes must come out clean. Let them cool for 10 minutes. Remove them from the pan and let them cool on a wire rack completely.
- Combine the crushed candies and whipped topping and use this mixture to frost the cupcakes right before serving. Refrigerate any leftovers.

Nutrition Information

- Calories: 279 calories
- Cholesterol: 56mg cholesterol
- Protein: 3g protein.
- Total Fat: 10g fat (7g saturated fat)
- Sodium: 144mg sodium
- Fiber: 1g fiber)
- Total Carbohydrate: 44g carbohydrate (26g sugars

312. Rudolph Cupcakes

Serving: 2 dozen. | Prep: 20mins | Cook: 25mins | Ready in:

Ingredients

- 1 package white cake mix (regular size
- 1 can (16 ounces) chocolate frosting
- 24 each brown and blue M&M's minis
- 24 miniature marshmallows, halved
- 24 red jelly beans

- 24 miniature vanilla wafers
- 48 miniature pretzels

Direction

- Follow instructions on cupcake package to prepare and bake cake mix.
- Put aside 2 to 3 teaspoons of frosting; spread the rest of the frosting onto cooled cupcakes. Press a mini M&M's into each half of the marshmallow with the rest of the frosting to make eyes. Set 2 eyes on each cupcake. On cupcake, attach a jelly bean over each vanilla wafer to make nose. Insert pretzels into cupcakes to make antlers.

Nutrition Information

- Calories:
- Protein:
- Total Fat:
- Sodium:
- Fiber:
- Total Carbohydrate:
- Cholesterol:

313. Santa Cupcakes

Serving: about 1-1/2 dozen. | Prep: 30mins | Cook: 20mins | Ready in:

Ingredients

- 1 package white cake mix (regular size)
- 1 can (16 ounces) vanilla frosting (about 1-2/3 cups)
- Red gel or paste food coloring
- Miniature marshmallows
- Brown M&M's minis
- Red Hots
- Red jimmies
- Sweetened shredded coconut

Direction

- Follow the package directions to prepare and bake the cake mix for the cupcakes, filling muffin cups lined with paper until 2/3 full. Let them cool in pans for 10 minutes, and then transfer them onto wire racks to cool completely.
- Use food coloring to tint two-thirds cup of frosting. Fill the food-safe plastic bag with 3 tbsp. of the white frosting. Make a 1/4-inch hole in one corner of the bag and reserve it for piping.
- Cover 2/3 of each cupcake with the remaining white frosting. For the hats, cover the remaining 1/3 of the cupcake with the red frosting. Using white frosting, pipe fur trim, and then add the marshmallows for their pom-poms. Garnish them with Red Hots, jimmies, and M&M's for their faces. For the beards, add the coconut.

Nutrition Information

- Calories: 276 calories
- Protein: 2g protein.
- Total Fat: 12g fat (2g saturated fat)
- Sodium: 249mg sodium
- Fiber: 0 fiber)
- Total Carbohydrate: 40g carbohydrate (28g sugars
- Cholesterol: 31mg cholesterol

314. Slime Filled Cupcakes

Serving: 2 dozen. | Prep: 30mins | Cook: 20mins | Ready in:

Ingredients

- 1 package chocolate cake mix (regular size)
- FILLING:
- 1/4 cup shortening
- 3 tablespoons butter, softened
- 2 cups confectioners' sugar
- 2 tablespoons milk

- 8 drops green food coloring, optional
- FROSTING:
- 1/2 cup butter, softened
- 4 ounces cream cheese, softened
- 2 cups confectioners' sugar
- 1/4 cup baking cocoa
- 2 tablespoons milk
- GLAZE:
- 1/2 cup confectioners' sugar
- 1 tablespoon milk
- 6 drops green food coloring

Direction

- Follow the package instructions to prepare the cake mix batter. Pour the batter into 24 paper-lined muffin cups. Let them bake at 375° oven for 20 to 22 minutes until the toothpick comes out very clean. Let them cool for 5 minutes. Remove them from the pans and place them on wire racks. Let them cool completely.
- Cream the milk, food coloring, shortening, confectioners' sugar, and butter for the filling until fluffy and light. Make a tiny hole into the plastic or pastry bag's corner. Insert the #7-round tip into the hole. Fill the bag with the filling. Fill the cupcakes with the filling by pushing the tip through the bottoms of the paper liners. Once the cupcakes are full, their tops will start to expand.
- Mix the frosting ingredients in a small bowl. Use the frosting to frost the cupcakes. Mix all the glaze ingredients and drizzle mixture all over the frosting.

Nutrition Information

- Calories:
- Sodium:
- Fiber:
- Total Carbohydrate:
- Cholesterol:
- Protein:
- Total Fat:

315. St. Patrick's Day Cupcakes

Serving: 1 dozen. | Prep: 15mins | Cook: 20mins | Ready in:

Ingredients

- 1-3/4 cups all-purpose flour
- 2/3 cup sugar
- 1 package (3.4 ounces) instant pistachio pudding mix
- 2 teaspoons baking powder
- 1/2 teaspoon salt
- 2 eggs
- 1-1/4 cups 2% milk
- 1/2 cup canola oil
- 1 teaspoon vanilla extract
- Green food coloring, optional
- Cream cheese frosting

Direction

- Mix together salt, baking powder, pudding mix, sugar and flour in a big bowl. Beat together vanilla, oil, milk and eggs in a small bowl, then put into dry mixture and mix until combined.
- Fill batter into muffin cups lined with paper until 3/4 full, then bake at 375 degrees until a toothpick exits clean after being inserted into the center, about 18 to 22 minutes. Allow to cool about 10 minutes prior to transferring from pan to a wire rack to cool thoroughly. Put into frosting with food coloring if wanted, then frost cupcakes.

Nutrition Information

- Calories: 250 calories
- Total Fat: 11g fat (2g saturated fat)
- Sodium: 301mg sodium
- Fiber: 0 fiber)
- Total Carbohydrate: 34g carbohydrate (18g sugars
- Cholesterol: 39mg cholesterol
- Protein: 4g protein.

316. St. Patrick's Day Pistachio Cupcakes

Serving: about 1-1/2 dozen. | Prep: 15mins | Cook: 20mins | Ready in:

Ingredients

- 1-3/4 cups all-purpose flour
- 2/3 cup sugar
- 1 package (3.4 ounces) instant pistachio pudding mix
- 2-1/2 teaspoons baking powder
- 1/2 teaspoon salt
- 2 eggs
- 1-1/2 cups milk
- 1/2 cup vegetable oil
- 1 teaspoon vanilla extract
- 3/4 cup miniature semisweet chocolate chips
- 1 cup cream cheese frosting
- Green sprinkles and/or chocolate jimmies

Direction

- Mix together salt, baking powder, pudding mix, sugar and flour in a big bowl. Mix together vanilla, oil, milk and eggs in a separate bowl, then stir into dry mixture until blended. Fold in chocolate chips.
- Fill the mixture into muffin cups lined with paper or foil until 2/3 full. Bake at 375 degrees until a toothpick exits clean, about 18 to 20 minutes. Allow to cool about 5 minutes prior to transferring from pans to wire racks to cool thoroughly. Frost cake and garnish as preferred.

Nutrition Information

- Calories: 270 calories
- Fiber: 1g fiber)
- Total Carbohydrate: 38g carbohydrate (26g sugars
- Cholesterol: 26mg cholesterol
- Protein: 3g protein.
- Total Fat: 12g fat (3g saturated fat)
- Sodium: 245mg sodium

317. Strawberry Muffin Cones

Serving: 20 servings. | Prep: 20mins | Cook: 20mins | Ready in:

Ingredients

- 2 cups all-purpose flour
- 1/2 cup sugar
- 2 teaspoons baking powder
- 1/2 teaspoon baking soda
- 1/2 teaspoon salt
- 2 large eggs
- 3/4 cup (6 ounces) strawberry yogurt
- 1/2 cup canola oil
- 1 cup chopped fresh strawberries
- 20 cake ice cream cones (about 3 inches tall)
- 1 cup (6 ounces) semisweet chocolate chips
- 1 tablespoon shortening
- Colored sprinkles

Direction

- Mix together the first 5 ingredients in a large bowl. Beat strawberries, oil, yogurt and eggs in another bowl; mix into the dry ingredients just till moistened.
- In muffin cups, place ice cream cones; using a spoon, transfer into each cone with 2 heaping tablespoons of the batter. Bake at 375° till a toothpick comes out clean when inserted into the center, or for 19-21 minutes. Allow to cool completely.
- Melt shortening and chocolate chips in a microwave; mix till smooth. Dip the muffin tops into the chocolate; drip off excess. Decorate with sprinkles.

Nutrition Information

- Calories: 253 calories
- Fiber: 1g fiber
- Total Carbohydrate: 33g carbohydrate (16g sugars
- Cholesterol: 29mg cholesterol
- Protein: 4g protein.
- Total Fat: 13g fat (3g saturated fat)
- Sodium: 196mg sodium

318. Strawberry Surprise Cupcakes

Serving: 2 dozen. | Prep: 25mins | Cook: 25mins | Ready in:

Ingredients

- 1 package strawberry cake mix (regular size)
- 2 cups (16 ounces) sour cream
- 2 large eggs
- 1/4 cup strawberry preserves
- 1 can (16 ounces) vanilla frosting
- Halved fresh strawberries

Direction

- Start preheating the oven to 350°. Line paper liners on 24 muffin cups. Combine eggs, sour cream and cake mix in a large bowl. Beat for half a minute on low speed. Beat for 2 mins on medium.
- Fill 1/2 full the prepared cups. Drop half a teaspoon of the preserves into middle of each cupcake; add the remaining batter to cover.
- Bake until a toothpick comes out clean when inserted in cake portion, about 22 to 27 mins. Let cool in pans for 10 mins. Then discard and cool completely on wire racks.
- Pipe the frosting over the cupcakes. Add on top of each with a strawberry half.

Nutrition Information

- Calories: 228 calories

- Protein: 2g protein.
- Total Fat: 10g fat (5g saturated fat)
- Sodium: 194mg sodium
- Fiber: 0 fiber)
- Total Carbohydrate: 33g carbohydrate (24g sugars
- Cholesterol: 31mg cholesterol

319. Sunshine Cupcakes

Serving: 24 | Prep: 30mins | Cook: | Ready in:

Ingredients

- Cupcakes
- 1 cup egg whites (7 to 9 large)
- ¾ cup sifted cake flour
- 1 cup sugar (see Tip)
- 2 teaspoons vanilla
- 1 teaspoon cream of tartar
- 3 egg yolks
- Halved or quartered fresh strawberries (optional)
- Orange and/or lemon peel strips (optional)
- Lemon Fluff
- ½ 8-ounce container frozen light-whipped dessert topping, thawed
- ½ teaspoon finely shredded lemon peel
- 1 tablespoon lemon juice

Direction

- Let the egg whites stand in a huge bowl at room temperature for half an hour. In the meantime, sift 1/2 cup of sugar and cake flour 3 times. Use the paper bake cups to line 24 2 1/2-inches muffin cups; put aside.
- Set the oven to 375°F for preheating. Add the cream of tartar and vanilla to the egg whites. Use an electric mixer to beat the mixture at high speed until it forms soft peaks that can curl the tips. Add the remaining 1/2 cup of sugar gradually, whisking well until it forms stiff peaks, also, tips will stand straight. Sift 1/4 of the flour mixture over the egg white

mixture, folding the mixture carefully. Do the same procedure of sifting and folding using the remaining flour mixture, adding 1/4 of the flour mixture at a time. Pour half of the egg white mixture into separate bowl; put them aside.

- Beat the egg yolks in a medium bowl using the electric mixer with a speed of high for 5 minutes until lemon-colored and thick. Fold the egg yolk mixture into one portion of the egg white mixture. Pour dollops of white and yellow batters into the paper bake cups alternately. Make sure that the cups are filled 2/3 full. Use a narrow metal spatula or knife to cut through the batter.
- Bake them for 10-12 minutes until the cupcakes will spring back when touched lightly near the middle. Remove them from the cups and let them cool completely on a wire rack.
- Fold 1/2 of the 8-oz container frozen light whipped dessert topping (thawed) in a medium bowl together with 1 tbsp. of lemon juice and 1/2 tsp. of the finely shredded lemon peel until just blended.
- Frost cupcakes with Lemon Fluff. Garnish them with orange and/or lemon peel strips and raspberries if desired. Place the cupcakes inside the fridge.

Nutrition Information

- Calories: 72 calories;
- Total Carbohydrate: 14
- Sugar: 9
- Protein: 2
- Sodium: 18
- Fiber: 0
- Cholesterol: 23
- Total Fat: 1
- Saturated Fat: 1

320. Surprise Cupcakes

Serving: 3 dozen. | Prep: 20mins | Cook: 15mins | Ready in:

Ingredients

- 1 cup shortening
- 2 cups sugar
- 2 eggs
- 2 teaspoons vanilla extract
- 3-1/2 cups all-purpose flour
- 5 teaspoons baking powder
- 1 teaspoon salt
- 1-1/2 cups 2% milk
- 3/4 cup strawberry or grape jelly
- Frosting of your choice
- Colored sprinkles, optional

Direction

- Cream sugar and shortening in a large bowl until fluffy and light. Put in the eggs, 1 at a time; beat well after each addition. Beat in the vanilla. Mix salt, baking powder and flour. Put into creamed mixture alternately with the milk and beat well after each addition.
- Fill 1/2 full 36 paper-lined muffin cups. Drop teaspoonfuls of jelly into middle of each.
- Bake for 15 to 20 mins at 375°, until a toothpick comes out clean when inserted in the cupcake. Let cool for 10 mins. Discard from the pans to cool completely on wire racks. Frost the cupcakes. If desired, garnish with sprinkles.

Nutrition Information

- Calories: 164 calories
- Protein: 2g protein.
- Total Fat: 6g fat (2g saturated fat)
- Sodium: 130mg sodium
- Fiber: 0 fiber)
- Total Carbohydrate: 25g carbohydrate (15g sugars
- Cholesterol: 13mg cholesterol

321. Truffle Filled Cupcakes

Serving: 1-1/2 dozen. | Prep: 60mins | Cook: 20mins | Ready in:

Ingredients

- 3/4 cup dark chocolate chips
- 1/3 cup heavy whipping cream
- 1 package white cake mix (regular size)
- 1-1/4 cups water
- 3 large egg whites
- 1/3 cup canola oil
- 1/2 teaspoon orange paste food coloring
- FROSTING:
- 1/2 cup butter, softened
- 3-3/4 cups confectioners' sugar
- 1 teaspoon vanilla extract
- 1/4 teaspoon salt
- 2 ounces unsweetened chocolate, melted
- 4 to 5 tablespoons evaporated milk
- Assorted decorations: regular and Mega M&M's, Laffy Taffy, Candy Corn, Mega Buttons, Oreo Cookies, sprinkles, pretzels, marshmallows and edible pens

Direction

- Pour all the chocolate chips in a small bowl. Boil the cream in a small saucepan. Pour the cream into the chocolate and let it stand for 5 minutes. Let it cool to room temperature while occasionally stirring it. Cover and refrigerate the mixture until firm.
- Set the oven to 350° for preheating. Use paper liners to line 18 muffin cups. Combine the water, oil, food coloring, cake mix, and egg whites in a large bowl. Beat the mixture on low speed for 30 seconds. Whisk the mixture on medium speed for 2 minutes.
- Pour the mixture into the prepared cups, filling them up to 3/4 full. Top the mixture with 2 tsp. of the chocolate mixture. Bake them until their tops spring back when touched lightly, about 18 to 22 minutes. Let them cool in pans for 10 minutes. Transfer them to wire racks and let them cool completely.
- Whisk the salt, vanilla, butter, and confectioners' sugar in a small bowl for the frosting until smooth. Whisk in the melted butter and add enough milk until the desired consistency was reached. Use it to frost the cupcakes and decorate them as desired.

Nutrition Information

- Calories:
- Sodium:
- Fiber:
- Total Carbohydrate:
- Cholesterol:
- Protein:
- Total Fat:

322. Wicked Witch Cupcakes

Serving: about 1 dozen. | Prep: 01hours15mins | Cook: 20mins | Ready in:

Ingredients

- 1/2 cup butter, softened
- 1 cup sugar
- 2 eggs
- 1-1/2 cups all-purpose flour
- 1/2 cup baking cocoa
- 1 teaspoon baking soda
- 1/2 teaspoon baking powder
- 1/2 teaspoon salt
- 1-1/4 cups milk
- 1 can (16 ounces) vanilla frosting
- Green food coloring
- WITCH HATS:
- 1 can (16 ounces) vanilla frosting
- 2 teaspoons milk
- Assorted food coloring of your choice
- 12 to 16 ice cream sugar cones
- Fruit Roll-Ups, licorice and assorted candies of your choice

Direction

- Cream the sugar and butter in a large bowl until fluffy and light. Add the eggs, one at a time and whisking well after every addition. Combine the salt, baking soda, baking powder, flour and cocoa and add this mixture alternately with the milk to the creamed mixture. Whisk well until blended.
- Fill the foil or paper-lined muffin cups with the mixture, about 2/3 full. Bake it at 350° for 18 to 22 minutes until the toothpick will come out clean. Let them cool for 10 minutes. Remove them from the pan and place them on a wire rack. Let them cool completely.
- Tint the frosting with green and use it to frost the cupcakes. Combine the frosting with the milk for the hats. Tint the mixture with a food coloring and use it to frost the cones of ice cream. Cut out some shapes from the Fruit Roll-ups using the small cookie cutters. Arrange the shapes onto the hats. For the faces, add some candies. For the hair, add the licorice. Arrange the hat onto each witch.

Nutrition Information

- Calories:
- Cholesterol:
- Protein:
- Total Fat:
- Sodium:
- Fiber:
- Total Carbohydrate:

323. Wide Eyed Owl Cupcakes

Serving: 2 dozen. | Prep: 60mins | Cook: 20mins | Ready in:

Ingredients

- 1 package cake mix of your choice (regular size)
- 1 can (16 ounces) vanilla frosting
- 24 Nutter Butter cookies
- 1/2 cup Froot Loops
- 1/4 cup chocolate frosting
- Assorted candies: candy corn, butterscotch or chocolate chips
- 48 ginger thin cookies

Direction

- Follow the directions on the packaging to prepare and bake cake batter; let it fully cool. Frost vanilla frosting on top of the cupcakes.
- To make the eyes, attach two Froot Loops to each cookie and pipe chocolate frosting in the center. Remove the yellow part in the candy corn. Attach them for beaks using chocolate frosting and use butterscotch chips to make the ears.
- In each cupcake, make a slit and put the cookies owl into the slit carefully. Insert the rye chips into the white frosting to make the wings.

Nutrition Information

- Calories:
- Protein:
- Total Fat:
- Sodium:
- Fiber:
- Total Carbohydrate:
- Cholesterol:

324. Witch Cupcakes

Serving: 2 dozen. | Prep: 02hours00mins | Cook: 20mins | Ready in:

Ingredients

- 1 package cake mix of your choice (regular size)
- 1-1/2 cups semisweet chocolate chips

- 1 tablespoon shortening
- 24 Bugles
- 12 chocolate wafers, cut in half
- 1 cup chow mein noodles
- 2 teaspoons sugar
- 2 teaspoons baking cocoa
- 1 can (16 ounces) vanilla frosting
- Green paste food coloring
- 1/3 cup miniature marshmallows
- Assorted candies: miniature chocolate chips, black licorice twists, black shoestring licorice and purple Nerds

Direction

- Follow the package directions on how to prepare and bake the cake mix for cupcakes. Let it cool completely.
- For the witches' hats, melt the shortening and chocolate chips in a microwave-safe bowl; stir the mixture until smooth. Dip a Bugle in chocolate, letting the excess to drip off. Place it on a chocolate wafer half to form a witch's hat. Transfer it on a waxed paper and let it dry. Do the same with the remaining Bugles, chocolate, and wafers.
- For the hair, mix the cocoa, chow mein noodles, and sugar in a small bowl; put aside. Color the frosting green, and then frost the cupcakes. Place witch's hat into each cupcake.
- For the eyes, cut the miniature marshmallows in half. Pinch the marshmallows slightly. Attach the miniature chocolate chips using the frosting for the pupils. Place the eyes onto the cupcakes. For the noses, add the licorice twists pieces. For the mouths, add the shoestring licorice. For warts, add the Nerds. For their hairs, arrange the reserved chow mein noodles onto each cupcake.

Nutrition Information

- Calories:
- Sodium:
- Fiber:
- Total Carbohydrate:
- Cholesterol:
- Protein:
- Total Fat:

325. Yellow Cupcakes

Serving: about 2 dozen. | Prep: 20mins | Cook: 15mins | Ready in:

Ingredients

- 2/3 cup butter, softened
- 1-3/4 cups sugar
- 2 large eggs
- 1-1/2 teaspoons vanilla extract
- 2-1/2 cups all-purpose flour
- 2-1/2 teaspoons baking powder
- 1/2 teaspoon salt
- 1-1/4 cups 2% milk
- Frosting of your choice

Direction

- Set the oven to 350° for preheating. Use the paper liners to line 22 to 24 muffin cups.
- Cream the sugar and butter in a large bowl until fluffy and light. Add the eggs, one at a time, whisking well after every addition. Mix in the vanilla. In a separate bowl, mix the baking powder, flour, and salt. Add the mixture to the creamed mixture, alternating with the milk. Make sure to whisk the mixture after every addition.
- Pour the mixture into the prepared cups, filling them to 3/4 full. Bake them for 15 to 20 minutes until the inserted toothpick into the center will come out clean. Let them cool in the pans for 10 minutes. Remove and place them on wire racks. Let them cool completely before spreading with the frosting.

Nutrition Information

- Calories: 163 calories
- Sodium: 138mg sodium
- Fiber: 0 fiber)

- Total Carbohydrate: 25g carbohydrate (15g sugars
- Cholesterol: 32mg cholesterol
- Protein: 2g protein.
- Total Fat: 6g fat (4g saturated fat)

Chapter 8: Cupcake Frosting Recipes

***

326. Apple Spice Cupcakes

Serving: 2 dozen. | Prep: 25mins | Cook: 20mins | Ready in:

Ingredients

- 1 package spice cake mix (regular size)
- 1-1/4 cups water
- 3 eggs
- 1/3 cup applesauce
- FROSTING:
- 1 package (8 ounces) cream cheese, softened
- 1/4 cup butter, softened
- 1 teaspoon vanilla extract
- 4 cups confectioners' sugar
- Red paste or liquid food coloring
- 24 pieces black licorice (3/4 inch)
- 12 green spice gumdrops

Direction

- Beat together applesauce, eggs, water and cake mix in a big bowl on low speed for a half minute, then beat on medium speed about 2 minutes.
- Put into muffin cups lined with paper until 2/3 full. Bake at 350 degrees until a toothpick pricked in the center exits clean, about 18 to 22 minutes. Allow to cool about 10 minutes, then transfer from pans to wire racks to cool through.
- Beat together vanilla, butter and cream cheese in a small bowl until fluffy. Put in sugar slowly while beating until the mixture is smooth, then add food coloring and stir.
- Frost tops of cupcakes and stuck licorice into the centers to make apple stems. Halve the gumdrops, then flatten and pinch to make leaves. Position a leaf next to each stem.

Nutrition Information

- Calories: 241 calories
- Sodium: 222mg sodium
- Fiber: 0 fiber)
- Total Carbohydrate: 39g carbohydrate (31g sugars
- Cholesterol: 48mg cholesterol
- Protein: 3g protein.
- Total Fat: 8g fat (4g saturated fat)

327. Banana Cupcakes

Serving: 1-1/2 dozen. | Prep: 20mins | Cook: 15mins | Ready in:

Ingredients

- 1/2 cup shortening
- 1-1/2 cups sugar
- 2 large eggs
- 1 teaspoon vanilla extract
- 1 cup mashed ripe bananas (about 2 medium)
- 2 cups all-purpose flour
- 1 teaspoon baking powder
- 3/4 teaspoon baking soda
- 1/2 teaspoon salt
- 1/4 cup buttermilk
- FROSTING:
- 1/2 cup butter, softened
- 2-1/2 cups confectioners' sugar
- 3 to 4 tablespoons milk
- Colored sprinkles, optional

Direction

- Cream sugar and shortening till fluffy and light in a big bowl. One by one, add eggs; beat well after each. Beat in bananas and vanilla. Mix salt, baking soda, baking powder and flour. Alternately with buttermilk, add to banana mixture; beat well after each.
- Fill 18 paper-lined muffin cups to 2/3 full; bake it at 350° till inserted toothpick in middle exits clean for 15-20 minutes. Transfer to wire racks; fully cool.
- Cream confectioners' sugar and butter till fluffy and light in a small bowl; to get preferred spreading consistency, add enough milk. Frost cupcakes; if desired, garnish with sprinkles.

Nutrition Information

- Calories: 297 calories
- Cholesterol: 38mg cholesterol
- Protein: 3g protein.
- Total Fat: 11g fat (5g saturated fat)
- Sodium: 204mg sodium
- Fiber: 1g fiber)
- Total Carbohydrate: 47g carbohydrate (35g sugars

328. Bananas Foster Surprise Cupcakes

Serving: 2 dozen. | Prep: 50mins | Cook: 20mins | Ready in:

Ingredients

- 3/4 cup butter, softened
- 2 cups sugar
- 2 tablespoons dark brown sugar
- 3 eggs
- 1-3/4 cups mashed ripe bananas (about 4-5 medium)
- 1-1/2 cups buttermilk
- 2 teaspoons lemon juice
- 2 teaspoons vanilla extract
- 3 cups all-purpose flour
- 1-1/2 teaspoons baking soda
- 1 teaspoon ground cinnamon
- 1/4 teaspoon salt
- FILLING:
- 1 jar (12 ounces) hot caramel ice cream topping
- 1/2 teaspoon ground cinnamon
- 1/4 teaspoon rum extract
- FROSTING:
- 2-1/4 cups packed brown sugar
- 1 cup heavy whipping cream
- 1/2 teaspoon baking soda
- 1/2 cup butter, cubed
- 1/4 teaspoon rum extract
- Sliced bananas, whipped cream and turbinado (washed raw) sugar

Direction

- Cream brown sugar, sugar and butter till fluffy and light in a big bowl. One by one, add eggs; beat well after each. Beat in vanilla, lemon juice, buttermilk and bananas. Mix salt, cinnamon, baking soda and flour; add to creamed mixture till just moist.
- Fill paper-lined/greased muffin cups to 3/4 full; bake for 18-22 minutes at 375° till inserted toothpick in cupcake exits clean. Cool it for 10 minutes. Transfer from pans onto wire racks; fully cool.
- Mix filling ingredients in a small bowl. Cut small hole in corner of a plastic/pastry bag; insert very small tip. Use caramel filling to fill. Push tip through top to fill every cupcake.
- Frosting: Boil cream and brown sugar in a big saucepan on medium low heat. Mix in baking soda; mix and cook till smooth. Mix in extract and butter. Take off heat; slightly cool. Put into small bowl; refrigerate till chilled for a minimum of 30 minutes.
- Beat frosting at high for 15-20 minutes till thick. Put frosting, whipped cream and banana slices over cupcakes; sprinkle turbinado sugar.

Nutrition Information

- Calories: 389 calories
- Sodium: 284mg sodium
- Fiber: 1g fiber)
- Total Carbohydrate: 64g carbohydrate (41g sugars
- Cholesterol: 66mg cholesterol
- Protein: 4g protein.
- Total Fat: 14g fat (9g saturated fat)

---

329. Baseball Cupcakes

Serving: Makes 2 doz. or 24 servings, 1 cupcake each. | Prep: 15mins | Cook: | Ready in:

Ingredients

- 1 pkg. (2-layer size) white cake mix
- 10 OREO Cookies, crushed
- 2 cups thawed COOL WHIP Whipped Topping
- 3 Tbsp. red decorating gel

Direction

- Follow package directions to prep cake batter. Mix in cookie crumbs; evenly put into 24 paper-lined and medium muffin cups.
- Follow package directions to bake for cupcakes; fully cool.
- Use whipped topping to frost cupcakes. To draw stitching lines over each cupcake, use decorating gel to resemble a baseball. Keep refrigerated.

Nutrition Information

- Calories: 140
- Protein: 2 g
- Total Fat: 5 g
- Saturated Fat: 1.5 g
- Sodium: 180 mg
- Total Carbohydrate: 23 g
- Fiber: 0 g

- Sugar: 14 g
- Cholesterol: 0 mg

---

330. Berry Topped White Cupcakes

Serving: 22 cupcakes. | Prep: 30mins | Cook: 20mins | Ready in:

Ingredients

- 5 large egg whites
- 1/2 cup plus 2 tablespoons butter, softened
- 1 cup sugar, divided
- 3/4 teaspoon vanilla extract
- 2-1/4 cups cake flour
- 2-1/4 teaspoons baking powder
- 1/2 teaspoon salt
- 3/4 cup milk
- ICING:
- 4 ounces cream cheese, softened
- 1/3 cup butter, softened
- 2 cups confectioners' sugar
- 1/2 teaspoon lemon juice
- Assorted berries

Direction

- Put egg whites in a large bowl; allow to sit for 30 minutes at room temperature. Cream 3/4 cup of sugar and butter in another bowl, till fluffy and light. Beat in vanilla. Mix salt, baking powder and flour together; include alternately with milk into the creamed mixture, beating well after each addition.
- Whisk egg whites on medium speed, till it forms soft peaks. Slowly whisk in the remaining sugar, around 2 tablespoons per time, on high, till the sugar is completely dissolved and the mixture forms stiff glossy peaks. Fold 1/4 of the egg whites into the batter; bend in the remaining whites.
- Carefully fill a paper- or foil-lined muffin cups 2/3 full, using a spoon. Bake at 350° for 18-22 minutes. Allow to cool for 10 minutes; take

away from the pans and place on wire racks; cool completely.
- For icing, beat butter and cream cheese in a small bowl, till smooth. Slowly beat in lemon juice and confectioners' sugar. Frost the cupcakes. Arrange berries on top.

Nutrition Information

- Calories: 226 calories
- Fiber: 0 fiber)
- Total Carbohydrate: 31g carbohydrate (20g sugars
- Cholesterol: 28mg cholesterol
- Protein: 3g protein.
- Total Fat: 10g fat (6g saturated fat)
- Sodium: 207mg sodium

331. Box Of Chocolates Cupcakes

Serving: 2 dozen. | Prep: 60mins | Cook: 20mins | Ready in:

Ingredients

- 1 package devil's food cake mix (regular size)
- 1-1/3 cups strong brewed coffee
- 3 eggs
- 1/2 cup canola oil
- FILLING:
- 8 ounces bittersweet chocolate, chopped
- 3 tablespoons sugar
- 4 tablespoons strong brewed coffee, divided
- 3 egg yolks, beaten
- 2 tablespoons thawed orange juice concentrate
- 2 tablespoons Nutella
- 1 tablespoon heavy whipping cream
- 1-1/2 cups whipped topping
- GANACHE:
- 4 ounces bittersweet chocolate, chopped
- 2 ounces white baking chocolate, chopped
- 2/3 cup heavy whipping cream, divided
- 2-1/2 teaspoons corn syrup, divided
- Paste food coloring of your choice

Direction

- Set oven to 350 degrees and start preheating. Use paper liners to line 24 muffin cups. Mix together oil, eggs, coffee and cake mix in a big bowl; beat the mixture for half a minute on low speed. Increase speed to medium and beat for 2 minutes. Pour batter into muffin cups to 2/3 full.
- Bake until a toothpick is clean when coming out of the middle, 18 to 22 minutes. Keep in pans to cool for 10 minutes, then transfer to wire racks and finish cooling.
- In the meantime, heat 3 tablespoons coffee, sugar and chocolate in a metal bowl over simmering water or a double boiler's top until melted, whisking to dissolve sugar (mixture will become thick). Mix in egg yolks and cook, while stirring, until the mixture achieves 160 degrees, 4 to 5 minutes.
- Transfer evenly into 3 small bowls. In 1 bowl, mix orange juice concentrate. In another bowl, whisk cream and Nutella together; and in the last bowl, mix the rest of coffee. Fold in each bowl half a cup of whipped topping. Refrigerate for 10 minutes.
- In a food-safe plastic bag's corner or a pastry bag's tip, cut a small hole and fit in a very small pastry tip. Fill with one filling. Poke a hole through paper liner's bottom using a wooden or metal skewer. Put the tip through the hole and pipe filling into 8 cupcakes. Follow the same steps with the rest of cupcakes and filling.
- To make the ganache, put chocolates in different small bowls. Boil cream in a small saucepan. Transfer half a cup of cream to the bittersweet chocolate and pour the rest to white chocolate. Using a whisk, stir until forming smooth mixtures.
- In bittersweet ganache, mix 2 tsp corn syrup and in white ganache, mix 1/2 tsp corn syrup. Allow to cool until they become a little thicker, 10 minutes, stirring once in a while. Color

white ganache as preferred; cover and chill until thick.
- Using bittersweet ganache, dip in the cupcakes' tops. Pipe designs with tinted or white ganache on top. Chill to set. Keep refrigerated in airtight containers to store.

Nutrition Information

- Calories: 285 calories
- Cholesterol: 64mg cholesterol
- Protein: 4g protein.
- Total Fat: 18g fat (7g saturated fat)
- Sodium: 182mg sodium
- Fiber: 2g fiber)
- Total Carbohydrate: 31g carbohydrate (21g sugars

332. Carrot & Raisin Spice Cupcakes

Serving: 2 dozen. | Prep: 30mins | Cook: 20mins | Ready in:

Ingredients

- 4 large eggs
- 1 cup canola oil
- 1 cup sugar
- 1 cup packed brown sugar
- 1 teaspoon vanilla extract
- 2 cups all-purpose flour
- 2 teaspoons baking powder
- 2 teaspoons ground cinnamon
- 1 teaspoon baking soda
- 1 teaspoon salt
- 1/2 teaspoon ground cloves
- 1/2 teaspoon ground nutmeg
- 3 cups finely shredded carrots
- 1 cup raisins
- FILLING:
- 1 cup sugar
- 2 tablespoons plus 1-1/2 teaspoons cornstarch
- 1 can (20 ounces) crushed pineapple, drained and chopped
- FROSTING:
- 1 package (8 ounces) reduced-fat cream cheese
- 1/2 cup butter, softened
- 3-1/2 cups confectioners' sugar
- 1 teaspoon vanilla extract
- Additional ground cinnamon

Direction

- In a big bowl, beat the vanilla, sugars, oil, and eggs until properly blended. Combine the nutmeg, cloves, salt, baking soda, cinnamon, baking powder, and flour; slowly beat into egg mixture up to blended. Mix in raisins and carrots.
- Fill three-fourths full of paper-lined muffin cups. Bake at 350° for around 20-25 minutes or up to a toothpick pinned in the core comes out clean. Allow to cool for 10 minutes, then take away from pans and move to wire racks for complete cooling.
- Meanwhile, in a little saucepan, combine cornstarch and sugar together. Mix in pineapple up to blended. Let it boil over medium heat. Cook and combine for 2-3 minutes, or till thickened. Take away from the heat; leave aside to cool.
- In a big bowl, beat butter and cream cheese until fluffy. Fold in vanilla and confectioners' sugar; beat until smooth.
- Cut a big hole in the corner of a plastic bag or pastry; put in a round tip. Stuff with pineapple filling. Fill each cupcake by pushing the tip through the cupcake's top. Frost the tops then dust cinnamon atop. Reserve in the refrigerator to store.

Nutrition Information

- Calories: 403 calories
- Sodium: 277mg sodium
- Fiber: 1g fiber)
- Total Carbohydrate: 63g carbohydrate (51g sugars
- Cholesterol: 52mg cholesterol

- Protein: 4g protein.
- Total Fat: 16g fat (5g saturated fat)

333. Carrot Cake Cupcakes

Serving: 12 | Prep: 45mins | Cook: | Ready in:

Ingredients

- Cake
- 1 cup canned crushed pineapple
- 1 cup whole-wheat pastry flour
- 1 teaspoon ground cinnamon
- 1 teaspoon baking soda
- ¼ teaspoon salt
- 1 large egg
- ¾ cup granulated sugar
- ½ cup buttermilk
- ¼ cup canola oil
- 1 teaspoon vanilla extract
- 1 cup shredded carrots
- ¼ cup chopped toasted walnuts
- 2 tablespoons unsweetened flaked coconut
- Frosting
- 8 ounces reduced-fat cream cheese, softened
- ¼ cup low-fat plain Greek yogurt
- ⅓ cup confectioners' sugar
- 1 teaspoon vanilla extract
- 2 tablespoons unsweetened flaked coconut (optional)

Direction

- For the cupcakes: Start preheating the oven to 325°F. Use paper liners to line twelve 1/2-cup muffin cups.
- In a sieve set over a bowl, drain pineapple, pressing on the solids. (Dispose the juice or keep to use later).
- In a medium-sized bowl, combine salt, baking soda, cinnamon, and flour. In a big bowl, combine 1 teaspoon vanilla, oil, buttermilk, granulated sugar, and egg until mixed. Mix in the drained pineapple, 2 tablespoons coconut, walnuts, and carrots. Add the dry ingredients and use a rubber spatula to stir until barely combined. Distribute the batter between the prepared muffin cups.
- Bake the cupcakes for 25-30 minutes until a toothpick comes out clean when you insert one into the middle. Remove onto a wire rack to thoroughly cool.
- For the frosting and complete the cupcakes: In a mixing bowl, use an electric mixer to beat together vanilla, confectioners' sugar, yogurt, and cream cheese until creamy and smooth. Spread onto each cooled cupcake with a scant 2 tablespoons of the frosting and use coconut to garnish if you want.

Nutrition Information

- Calories: 238 calories;
- Total Fat: 12
- Total Carbohydrate: 29
- Sodium: 240
- Fiber: 2
- Cholesterol: 30
- Sugar: 20
- Protein: 5
- Saturated Fat: 4

334. Carrot Cupcakes With Cream Cheese Frosting

Serving: 15 | Prep: 30mins | Cook: | Ready in:

Ingredients

- Nonstick cooking spray
- 1 cup all-purpose flour
- 1 cup whole wheat flour
- ¾ cup packed brown sugar or brown sugar substitute blend equivalent to ¾ cup brown sugar (see Tip)
- 1 teaspoon baking powder
- 1 teaspoon baking soda
- ¾ teaspoon ground cinnamon
- ¼ teaspoon salt

- ¼ teaspoon ground ginger
- 2 eggs, lightly beaten
- 2 cups shredded carrots (4 medium)
- 1 cup unsweetened applesauce
- ⅓ cup canola oil
- 6 ounces reduced-fat cream cheese (Neufchâtel)
- 3 tablespoons agave nectar or honey
- 5 tablespoons finely shredded carrot or 15 wide, very thin carrot strips

Direction

- Set an oven to preheat to 350 degrees F. Line paper bake cups on fifteen muffin cups of 2 1/2-inch. Use cooking spray to coat the paper cups lightly, then put aside.
- Stir together the ginger, salt, cinnamon, baking soda, baking powder, brown sugar and flours in a big bowl, then put aside.
- Mix together the oil, applesauce, carrots and eggs in a medium bowl. Add the egg mixture to the flour mixture, then mix until blended. Scoop the batter into the prepped muffin cups, then fill each 3/4 full.
- Let it bake for 18-20 minutes or until an inserted toothpick near the middle exits clean. Allow it to cool for 5 minutes in the muffin cups on a wire rack. Take it out of the muffin cups, then let it fully cool on a wire rack.
- To make the frosting, beat the cream cheese in a small bowl on medium speed using an electric mixer, until it becomes smooth. Add the agave nectar, then beat it for another 1 minute. Spread the frosting on the cupcakes. Put 1 very thin carrot strip or 1 tsp of the finely shredded carrots on top of each cake cupcake.

Nutrition Information

- Calories: 254 calories;
- Total Fat: 11
- Sodium: 188
- Fiber: 3
- Saturated Fat: 2
- Cholesterol: 3
- Total Carbohydrate: 34
- Sugar: 19
- Protein: 5

335. Chai Cupcakes

Serving: 12 | Prep: 15mins | Cook: 20mins | Ready in:

Ingredients

- 1 cup milk
- 2 black tea bags
- 2 chai tea bags
- 1/2 cup plain yogurt
- 3/4 cup white sugar
- 1/4 cup canola oil
- 1 teaspoon vanilla extract
- 1 cup all-purpose flour
- 1/4 teaspoon baking soda
- 1/2 teaspoon baking powder
- 2 teaspoons ground cinnamon
- 1/2 teaspoon ground ginger
- 1/4 teaspoon ground cloves
- 1/2 teaspoon salt
- 1 pinch ground black pepper

Direction

- Preheat an oven to 175°C/350°F. Grease/line paper baking cups on 12-cup muffin pan.
- Heat milk till nearly boiling in a saucepan; take off heat. Add chai tea and black tea bags; cover. Stand for 10 minutes. Wring tea bags out into milk; discard bags. Whisk vanilla, oil, sugar, yogurt and tea-milk in a medium bowl. Mix pepper, salt, cloves, ginger, cinnamon, baking powder, baking soda and flour in a big bowl. Put wet ingredients into dry mixture; mix till blended. Put batter in prepped cups, evenly dividing.
- In preheated oven, bake for 20-25 minutes till tops spring back when pressed lightly; cool in pan above wire rack. Put cupcakes onto serving platter when cool. Frost using desired frosting.

Nutrition Information

- Calories: 147 calories;
- Cholesterol: 2
- Protein: 2.3
- Total Fat: 5.3
- Sodium: 159
- Total Carbohydrate: 22.8

336. Cherry Chocolate Coconut Cupcakes

Serving: 2 dozen. | Prep: 35mins | Cook: 20mins | Ready in:

Ingredients

- 1 package (10 to 12 ounces) vanilla or white chips
- 1/2 cup butter, cubed
- 1 cup heavy whipping cream
- 1 teaspoon coconut extract
- 1 can (21 ounces) cherry pie filling
- 1 cup buttermilk
- 2 large eggs
- 2 cups all-purpose flour
- 2 cups sugar
- 3/4 cup baking cocoa
- 2 teaspoons baking soda
- 1 teaspoon baking powder
- 1/2 teaspoon salt
- 6 packages (1.9 ounces each) chocolate-covered coconut candy bars
- 1/2 cup semisweet chocolate chips
- 1 teaspoon shortening
- 24 maraschino cherries, well drained
- 3-1/4 cups confectioners' sugar
- 2 tablespoons coarse sugar

Direction

- For making ganache, in a large bowl, place butter and vanilla chips. In a small saucepan, bring cream just to a boil. Pour over chip mixture; whisk until smooth. Blend in extract. Allow at least 4 hours to cool while covering in refrigerator, stirring occasionally.
- In a large bowl, beat the eggs, buttermilk and pie filling until well blended. Combine the sugar, flour, baking soda, cocoa, salt and baking powder; beat into pie filling mixture gradually until blended.
- Fill 24 paper-lined muffin cups to about one-third full. Break candy bars in half; in center of each cupcake, place half of a candy bar. Using 2 tablespoonful batter to cover each.
- Bake at 375° for nearly 16 to 20 minutes or until a toothpick inserted in the center comes out clean. Allow 10 minutes to cool before taking away from pans to wire racks for cooling completely.
- In the meantime, in a microwave, melt chocolate chips and shortening; stir until smooth. Dip cherries in chocolate mixture; allow excess to drip off. On a baking sheet with waxed paper-lined, place the mixture. Cool in refrigerator until set.
- Take away ganache from refrigerator; beat in confectioners' sugar gradually until frosting is fluffy and light. Pipe over cupcakes; use coarse sugar to sprinkle. Have chocolate-dipped cherries for garnishing.

Nutrition Information

- Calories: 426 calories
- Total Carbohydrate: 67g carbohydrate (54g sugars
- Cholesterol: 44mg cholesterol
- Protein: 4g protein.
- Total Fat: 16g fat (10g saturated fat)
- Sodium: 255mg sodium
- Fiber: 1g fiber)

337. Cherry Gingerbread Cupcakes

Serving: 2 dozen. | Prep: 30mins | Cook: 20mins | Ready in:

Ingredients

- 1/2 cup shortening
- 1 cup sugar
- 2 eggs
- 1 cup molasses
- 3 cups all-purpose flour
- 1 teaspoon baking soda
- 1 teaspoon ground ginger
- 1 teaspoon ground cinnamon
- 1 cup buttermilk
- 1/2 cup chopped walnuts
- 24 maraschino cherries, well drained
- LEMON CREAM CHEESE FROSTING:
- 4 ounces cream cheese, softened
- 1/4 cup butter, softened
- 1 teaspoon vanilla extract
- 1 teaspoon grated lemon peel
- 1-3/4 to 2 cups confectioners' sugar

Direction

- Cream sugar and shortening till fluffy and light in a big bowl. One by one, add eggs; beat well after each. Beat in molasses. Mix cinnamon, ginger, baking soda and flour. Alternately with buttermilk, add to creamed mixture slowly; beat well after each. Mix in walnuts.
- Fill the paper-lined muffin cups to 2/3 full; put cherry in middle of each. Bake it at 375° till inserted toothpick in middle exits clean for 20-24 minutes. Cool for 10 minutes. Transfer from pans onto wire racks; fully cool.
- Frosting: Beat butter and cream cheese till fluffy in a small bowl. Add lemon peel and vanilla. Beat in confectioners' sugar slowly till smooth; frost cupcakes.

Nutrition Information

- Calories: 266 calories
- Total Carbohydrate: 42g carbohydrate (28g sugars
- Cholesterol: 28mg cholesterol
- Protein: 3g protein.
- Total Fat: 10g fat (4g saturated fat)
- Sodium: 107mg sodium
- Fiber: 1g fiber)

338. Chip Lover's Cupcakes

Serving: 1-1/2 dozen. | Prep: 30mins | Cook: 20mins | Ready in:

Ingredients

- 1 package white cake mix (regular size)
- 1/4 cup butter, softened
- 1/4 cup packed brown sugar
- 2 tablespoons sugar
- 1/3 cup all-purpose flour
- 1/4 cup confectioners' sugar
- 1/4 cup miniature semisweet chocolate chips
- BUTTERCREAM FROSTING:
- 1/2 cup butter, softened
- 1/2 cup shortening
- 4-1/2 cups confectioners' sugar
- 4 tablespoons 2% milk, divided
- 1-1/2 teaspoons vanilla extract
- 1/4 cup baking cocoa
- 18 miniature chocolate chip cookies

Direction

- Follow package directions to prep cake batter; put aside. Filling: Cream sugars and butter till fluffy and light in small bowl; beat in confectioners' sugar and flour slowly till blended. Fold in the chocolate chips.
- Use cake batter to fill the paper-lined muffin cups to 1/2 full. By tablespoonfuls, drop filling in middle of each; cover with leftover batter.
- Bake at 350° till inserted toothpick in cake exits clean for 20-22 minutes. Cool for 10 minutes. Transfer from pans onto wire racks; fully cool.

- Frosting: Cream confectioners' sugar, shortening and butter till smooth in a big bowl; beat in vanilla and 3 tbsp. milk till creamy. Put 1 cup frosting aside; use leftover frosting to frost cupcakes.
- Mix leftover milk and baking cocoa into reserved frosting. Cut small hole in corner of plastic/pastry bag; insert the star tip. Use chocolate frosting to fill bag. Pipe rosette over each cupcake; use a cookie to garnish.

Nutrition Information

- Calories:
- Total Fat:
- Sodium:
- Fiber:
- Total Carbohydrate:
- Cholesterol:
- Protein:

339. Chocolate Angel Cupcakes With Coconut Cream Frosting

Serving: 2 dozen. | Prep: 15mins | Cook: 15mins | Ready in:

Ingredients

- 1 package (16 ounces) angel food cake mix
- 3/4 cup baking cocoa
- 1 cup (8 ounces) reduced-fat sour cream
- 1 cup confectioners' sugar
- 1/8 teaspoon coconut extract
- 2-1/2 cups reduced-fat whipped topping
- 3/4 cup sweetened shredded coconut, toasted

Direction

- Follow the package directions to prepare cake mix for cupcakes and put in cocoa when mixing.
- Line muffin cups with foil or paper, then fill in the cake mix to 2/3 full. Bake at 375° until cake springs back when slightly touched and cracks feel dry, about 11 to 15 minutes. Allow to cool about 10 minutes before transferring from pans to wire racks to cool thoroughly.
- For frosting, mix together extract, confectioners' sugar and sour cream in a big bowl until smooth. Fold in whipped topping and frost cupcakes. Sprinkle over with coconut and chill the leftovers.
- ,

Nutrition Information

- Calories: 142 calories
- Protein: 3g protein. Diabetic Exchanges: 1-1/2 starch
- Total Fat: 3g fat (2g saturated fat)
- Sodium: 154mg sodium
- Fiber: 1g fiber)
- Total Carbohydrate: 27g carbohydrate (16g sugars
- Cholesterol: 3mg cholesterol

340. Chocolate Banana Split Cupcakes

Serving: 1 dozen. | Prep: 20mins | Cook: 20mins | Ready in:

Ingredients

- 1-1/4 cups all-purpose flour
- 1/2 cup sugar
- 1/4 teaspoon baking soda
- 1/4 teaspoon salt
- 1/2 cup mashed banana (about 1 medium)
- 1/2 cup butter, melted
- 1/4 cup buttermilk
- 1 egg, lightly beaten
- 1/2 teaspoon vanilla extract
- 1/2 cup chopped walnuts

- 2 milk chocolate bars (1.55 ounces each), broken into squares, divided
- FROSTING:
- 1-1/2 cups confectioners' sugar
- 1 tablespoon butter, melted
- 1/2 teaspoon vanilla extract
- 1 to 2 tablespoons milk
- 12 maraschino cherries with stems

Direction

- Mix in a large bowl the salt, baking soda, sugar and flour. Mix in a separate bowl the vanilla, egg, buttermilk, butter and banana. Then add to the dry ingredients; whisk just until blended. Add in walnuts then fold. Put 1 tablespoon of batter in each of 12 paper-lined muffin cups. Put one candy bar square on top of each. Then fill cups two-thirds full with batter.
- Put in the oven and bake for 20-25 minutes at 350°F or until a toothpick pricked in the cupcake comes out clean. Let it cool for 10 minutes before taking out from the pan to a wire rack to fully cool.
- Mix in a large bowl the vanilla, butter, confectioner's sugar and enough milk to reach a spreading consistency, then frost cupcakes. Melt the remaining candy bar squares in a microwave; drizzle over frosting. Put a cherry on top of each cupcake.

Nutrition Information

- Calories: 292 calories
- Protein: 4g protein.
- Total Fat: 13g fat (6g saturated fat)
- Sodium: 177mg sodium
- Fiber: 1g fiber)
- Total Carbohydrate: 42g carbohydrate (29g sugars
- Cholesterol: 42mg cholesterol

341. Chocolate Cream Cheese Cupcakes

Serving: Makes 12 cupcakes | Prep: | Cook: | Ready in:

Ingredients

- 1 8-ounce package cream cheese
- 1 large egg
- 2 tablespoons sugar
- 1/2 teaspoon salt
- 1/2 teaspoon vanilla extract
- 1/4 cup mini semisweet chocolate chips
- 1 cup all purpose flour
- 3 tablespoons sifted unsweetened cocoa powder
- 3/4 teaspoon baking powder
- 1/2 teaspoon coarse kosher salt
- 1/8 teaspoon baking soda
- 3/4 cup plus 2 tablespoons sugar
- 1/2 cup (1 stick) unsalted butter, room temperature
- 2 large eggs
- 1 teaspoon vanilla extract
- 3 ounces bittersweet chocolate, chopped, melted, warm
- 1/2 cup whole milk

Direction

- Beat cream cheese in a medium bowl with an electric mixer. Put in vanilla, salt, sugar and egg, and beat until almost smooth. Fold chocolate chips into the mixture.
- Cupcakes: Set oven to 350 degrees F and start preheating. Line 12 paper liners on standard muffin pan. Combine the first 5 ingredients in a small bowl. Cream butter and sugar with an electric mixer until fluffy. Whip in eggs. Whisk in chocolate and vanilla; beat for 5 seconds on high speed. Alternately whip in flour mixture along with milk. Beat for 5 seconds over high speed to incorporate. Distribute batter between cups until 1/3 full. Scoop out the middle of each cupcake with a tablespoon. Fill each middle part with 1 heaping tablespoonful of cream cheese filling.

- Bake cupcakes for about 20 minutes until toothpick slid into the middle (without poking through cream cheese filling) comes out with no batter streaks. Let cool in pan for 10 minutes. Take out of the pan, then place on a rack to cool through.

Nutrition Information

- Calories: 315
- Sodium: 212 mg(9%)
- Fiber: 1 g(6%)
- Total Carbohydrate: 34 g(11%)
- Cholesterol: 89 mg(30%)
- Protein: 5 g(10%)
- Total Fat: 19 g(29%)
- Saturated Fat: 11 g(56%)

342. Chocolate Cream Cupcakes

Serving: 20 cupcakes. | Prep: 30mins | Cook: 20mins | Ready in:

Ingredients

- 1 package yellow cake mix (regular size)
- 1 package (3.4 ounces) cook-and-serve chocolate pudding mix
- GLAZE:
- 2/3 cup semisweet chocolate chips
- 2-1/2 tablespoons butter
- 1-1/4 cups confectioners' sugar
- 3 tablespoons hot water
- White decorating icing, optional

Direction

- Following directions on cupcakes package, prepare and bake cake mix in 20 muffin cups lined with paper. Allow to fully cool.
- In the meantime, make pudding mix in a small bowl following directions on package. Cover the pudding with plastic wrap, pressing down the surface; put in the refrigerator to cool.
- In a food-safe plastic bag's corner or a pastry bag's tip, cut out a small hole; fit in a small pastry tip. Fill in the pudding. Poke a hole through the cupcake liners' bottom with a metal or wooden skewer. Insert tip through hole and pipe filling into the cupcakes.
- Microwave butter and chocolate chips until melted; stir until the mixture is smooth. Mix in water and confectioners' sugar. Dip the cupcakes' tops into glaze mixture. Decorate by piping designs onto cupcakes (optional).

Nutrition Information

- Calories: 239 calories
- Fiber: 1g fiber)
- Total Carbohydrate: 35g carbohydrate (24g sugars
- Cholesterol: 37mg cholesterol
- Protein: 3g protein.
- Total Fat: 11g fat (3g saturated fat)
- Sodium: 210mg sodium

343. Chocolate Cupcake Cones

Serving: about 3 dozen. | Prep: 25mins | Cook: 25mins | Ready in:

Ingredients

- 1 package chocolate cake mix (regular size)
- 1 package (8 ounces) cream cheese, softened
- 1/3 cup sugar
- 1 egg
- 1/2 teaspoon vanilla extract
- 1 cup miniature semisweet chocolate chips
- 36 ice-cream cake cones (about 3 inches tall)
- FROSTING:
- 1/2 cup shortening
- 3-3/4 cups confectioners' sugar
- 1 teaspoon vanilla extract

- 4 to 5 tablespoons milk
- Sprinkles

Direction

- Ready cake mix based on the package directions; reserve. Mix in a large bowl the vanilla, egg, sugar and cream cheese until it turns smooth; mix in chocolate chips.
- Put ice-cream cones in muffin cups. Then spoon about 1 tablespoon of cake batter into each cone; put a rounded teaspoon of cream cheese mixture on top. Then fill with remaining batter to within 3/4-inch of top.
- Place in the oven and bake for 25-30 minutes at 350°F or until a toothpick comes out clean.
- Mix in a small bowl the vanilla, confectioner's sugar and shortening until smooth. Mix in enough milk to reach the spreading consistency, then frost tops of cooled cones and put sprinkles on top.

Nutrition Information

- Calories: 223 calories
- Protein: 2g protein.
- Total Fat: 10g fat (4g saturated fat)
- Sodium: 146mg sodium
- Fiber: 1g fiber)
- Total Carbohydrate: 33g carbohydrate (24g sugars
- Cholesterol: 27mg cholesterol

344. Chocolate Frosted Peanut Butter Cupcakes

Serving: 2 dozen. | Prep: 30mins | Cook: 20mins | Ready in:

Ingredients

- 1 package yellow cake mix (regular size)
- 3/4 cup creamy peanut butter
- 3 large eggs
- 1-1/4 cups water
- 1/4 cup canola oil
- FROSTING:
- 1-2/3 cups semisweet chocolate chips
- 1/2 cup heavy whipping cream
- 1/2 cup butter, softened
- 1 cup confectioners' sugar

Direction

- Mix the oil, water, eggs, peanut butter and cake mix in a big bowl; whip on low speed for half a minute. Whip on medium for 2 minutes.
- Put batter in paper-lined muffin tins 2/3 full. Bake for 18 to 22 mins at 350° or until a toothpick inserted in the middle exits clean. Let cool for 10 minutes before taking out from pans to wire racks to cool entirely.
- In a big bowl, put chocolate chips. Heat up cream in a small saucepan just to a boil. Put over chocolate; mix until smooth. Let cool to room temperature, mixing once in a while. Put in confectioners' sugar and butter; whip until smooth. Put on cupcakes to frost.

Nutrition Information

- Calories: 289 calories
- Fiber: 1g fiber)
- Total Carbohydrate: 32g carbohydrate (22g sugars
- Cholesterol: 43mg cholesterol
- Protein: 4g protein.
- Total Fat: 18g fat (8g saturated fat)
- Sodium: 217mg sodium

345. Chocolate Peanut Butter Cupcakes

Serving: 2 dozen. | Prep: 20mins | Cook: 15mins | Ready in:

Ingredients

- 2-1/2 cups all-purpose flour
- 2/3 cup baking cocoa
- 2 teaspoons baking soda
- 1/3 cup reduced-fat creamy peanut butter
- 1/4 cup canola oil
- 1 cup sugar
- 1/2 cup sugar blend
- 2 cups fat-free milk
- 2 tablespoons white vinegar
- 1 teaspoon vanilla extract
- FROSTING:
- 1/3 cup reduced-fat creamy peanut butter
- 1/4 cup reduced-fat butter
- 3 cups confectioners' sugar
- 3/4 cup baking cocoa
- 1/4 cup fat-free milk
- 2 teaspoons vanilla extract
- 1/4 teaspoon salt
- 1/2 cup jimmies or sprinkles, optional

Direction

- Into a big bowl, sift the baking soda, cocoa and flour; put aside. Cook oil and peanut butter for 2-3 minutes in a small saucepan over low heat or until melted. Take it off the heat; mix in sugar and sugar blend until smooth. Mix in the vanilla, vinegar and milk. Add into flour mixture; mix until combined.
- Fill paper-lined muffin tins 1/2 full. Bake for 15 to 20 mins at 350° or until a toothpick inserted in the middle exits clean. Let cool for 10 minutes before taking out from pans to wire racks to cool completely.
- To make frosting, whip butter and peanut butter in a big bowl until light and fluffy. Whip in salt, vanilla, milk, cocoa and confectioners' sugar. Spread on cupcakes to frost. Garnish with jimmies (optional).

Nutrition Information

- Calories: 246 calories
- Cholesterol: 4mg cholesterol
- Protein: 5g protein.
- Total Fat: 7g fat (1g saturated fat)
- Sodium: 197mg sodium
- Fiber: 2g fiber)
- Total Carbohydrate: 44g carbohydrate (28g sugars

346. Chocolate Toffee Cupcakes

Serving: about 1-1/2 dozen. | Prep: 20mins | Cook: 20mins | Ready in:

Ingredients

- 1-1/2 cups all-purpose flour
- 1 cup sugar
- 1/4 cup baking cocoa
- 1 teaspoon baking soda
- 1 cup water
- 1/4 cup vegetable oil
- 1 tablespoon white vinegar
- 1 teaspoon vanilla extract
- 1/2 cup milk chocolate toffee bits
- FROSTING:
- 1-1/2 cups confectioners' sugar
- 1/3 cup baking cocoa
- 1/3 cup butter, softened
- 2 tablespoons milk
- 3/4 teaspoon vanilla extract
- 3/4 cup English toffee bits or almond brickle chips

Direction

- Mix in a large bowl the baking soda, cocoa, sugar and flour. Combine the vanilla, vinegar, oil and water until smooth. Gently add to dry ingredients just until mixed. Mix in toffee bits.
- Put into paper-lined muffin cups and fill two-thirds full. Put in the oven and bake for 20-25 minutes at 350°F or until a toothpick comes out clean. Let it cool for 10 minutes prior to taking out from pans to wire racks to fully cool.
- To make frosting, mix cocoa and confectioner's sugar; reserve. Beat 1/2 cup cocoa mixture and

butter in a large bowl until smooth. Put in remaining cocoa mixture, vanilla and milk; whisk until desired spreading consistency is achieved. Mix in 1/2 cup toffee bits.
- Frost cupcakes. Put in the refrigerator, covered until serving time. Put remaining toffee bits on top prior to serving.

Nutrition Information

- Calories: 275 calories
- Protein: 2g protein.
- Total Fat: 12g fat (5g saturated fat)
- Sodium: 192mg sodium
- Fiber: 1g fiber)
- Total Carbohydrate: 40g carbohydrate (30g sugars
- Cholesterol: 18mg cholesterol

347. Chocolate Glazed Cupcakes

Serving: 16 cupcakes. | Prep: 25mins | Cook: 15mins | Ready in:

Ingredients

- 1-1/2 cups all-purpose flour
- 3/4 cup sugar
- 1/3 cup baking cocoa
- 1 teaspoon baking soda
- 3/4 teaspoon salt
- 1 cup water
- 1/4 cup unsweetened applesauce
- 1/4 cup canola oil
- 1 tablespoon white vinegar
- 1 teaspoon vanilla extract
- 2/3 cup semisweet chocolate chips, optional
- GLAZE:
- 1/2 cup semisweet chocolate chips
- 1/4 cup half-and-half cream
- White nonpareils, optional

Direction

- Preheat oven to 350°. Use foil liners to line sixteen muffin cups.
- Whisk the first 5 ingredients together in a big bowl. Whisk together vanilla, vinegar, oil, applesauce and water in another bowl, until combined. Put into the flour mixture and stir just until moistened. Stir in chocolate chips, if wanted.
- Fill prepared muffin cups until 3/4 full. Bake until a toothpick comes out clean after inserting into the center, about 14 to 16 minutes. Allow to cool about 5 minutes before turning from pans to wire racks to cool thoroughly.
- To make glaze, mix cream and chocolate chips together in a small saucepan, then cook and stir on low heat until smooth, about 3 to 5 minutes. Take away from the heat. Allow to cool at room temperature while stirring sometimes for a half hour, or until glaze is thickened a bit. Dip tops of cupcakes into glaze, then sprinkle with nonpareils, if wanted.

Nutrition Information

- Calories: 148 calories
- Cholesterol: 2mg cholesterol
- Protein: 2g protein. Diabetic Exchanges: 1-1/2 starch
- Total Fat: 6g fat (1g saturated fat)
- Sodium: 192mg sodium
- Fiber: 1g fiber)
- Total Carbohydrate: 23g carbohydrate (13g sugars

348. Chocolate Mint Shamrock Cupcakes

Serving: 2 dozen. | Prep: 02hours00mins | Cook: 20mins | Ready in:

Ingredients

- 1 package chocolate cake mix (regular size)
- Pencil, paper, scissors and waxed paper
- 1 cup light green candy coating disks
- 24 chocolate wafers
- 2 tablespoons corn syrup, warmed
- Gold pearl dust
- 2 packages (4.67 ounces each) mint Andes candies, chopped
- 1/2 cup heavy whipping cream

Direction

- Follow package directions to prepare and bake cake batter for cupcakes; chill thoroughly.
- In the meantime, draw shamrock design using a pencil and paper. Cut out pattern. In a microwave-safe bowl, heat candy coating until melted; whisk until no lumps remain. Pour into a resealable plastic bag and cut a small hole in corner of the bag. Set waxed paper onto the pattern, then pipe a shamrock design. Do the same thing for 23 times. Leave in the fridge until set.
- Brush a thin layer of corn syrup onto wafers, then brush using pearl dust. Careful lift candy shamrocks out of waxed paper. Brush a thin layer of corn syrup onto the bottoms, then attach to the wafers. Put aside.
- Arrange Andes candies to a small bowl. Lightly boil cream in a small saucepan. Drizzle onto the candies, then stir until no lumps remain. Lightly chill and stir every now and then. Dip cupcakes into melted mints, then allow to rest till set. Lay and press on each cupcake a shamrock-topped wafer.

Nutrition Information

- Calories:
- Sodium:
- Fiber:
- Total Carbohydrate:
- Cholesterol:
- Protein:
- Total Fat:

349. Cinnamon Cupcakes

Serving: 1-1/2 dozen. | Prep: 25mins | Cook: 20mins | Ready in:

Ingredients

- 3/4 cup butter, softened
- 1-1/4 cups sugar
- 4 large egg whites
- 1 teaspoon vanilla extract
- 2-1/4 cups cake flour
- 2 teaspoons baking powder
- 1/2 teaspoon salt
- 3/4 cup 2% milk
- TOPPING:
- 2 tablespoons sugar
- 1/2 teaspoon ground cinnamon
- CINNAMON FROSTING:
- 1/4 cup butter, softened
- 1 teaspoon clear vanilla extract
- 1/4 teaspoon ground cinnamon
- 2-1/4 cups confectioners' sugar
- 3 tablespoons 2% milk
- Additional ground cinnamon

Direction

- Cream sugar and butter till fluffy and light in a small bowl; beat in vanilla and egg whites. Mix salt, flour and baking powder; alternately with milk, add to creamed mixture slowly, beating well after each.
- Fill the paper-lined muffin cups to 2/3 full. Mix cinnamon and sugar; sprinkle 1/4 tsp. on each cupcake.
- Bake for 16-18 minutes at 375° till inserted toothpick in middle exits clean; cool it for 10 minutes. Transfer from pans onto wire racks; fully cool.
- Frosting: Cream cinnamon, vanilla and butter in a small bowl; beat in confectioners' sugar slowly. Add milk; beat till fluffy and light. Frost cupcakes; sprinkle extra cinnamon.

Nutrition Information

- Calories: 280 calories
- Cholesterol: 28mg cholesterol
- Protein: 3g protein.
- Total Fat: 11g fat (7g saturated fat)
- Sodium: 201mg sodium
- Fiber: 0 fiber)
- Total Carbohydrate: 44g carbohydrate (30g sugars

350. Coconut Cupcakes

Serving: 12 | Prep: 20mins | Cook: 20mins | Ready in:

Ingredients

- 1 cup white sugar
- 1/2 cup applesauce
- 1/4 cup butter, softened
- 2 eggs, separated
- 1 tablespoon vanilla extract
- 1 1/2 cups all-purpose flour
- 1 3/4 teaspoons baking powder
- 1/2 teaspoon salt
- 1/2 (13.5 ounce) can coconut milk
- 1 1/4 cups unsweetened shredded coconut

Direction

- Set oven to 350 0 F (175 0 C) and preheat. Coat 12 muffin cups with grease or use paper liners to line.
- In a bowl, mix together butter, applesauce and sugar.
- In a glass or metal bowl, beat egg whites until medium peaks form. When you lift your whisk or beater straight up, the tip of the peak formed by the egg whites should curl over slightly.
- Mix vanilla extract and egg yolks into applesauce mixture; fold in egg whites. Mix in salt, baking powder and flour until just combined. Blend coconut milk into batter for about 1 minute until smooth. Blend in shredded coconut for about 30 seconds. Pour the batter into the greased muffin cups.
- Put into the prepared oven and bake for about 20 minutes until when you insert a toothpick in the center of a cupcake, it should come out clean.

Nutrition Information

- Calories: 271 calories;
- Total Carbohydrate: 32.9
- Cholesterol: 41
- Protein: 3.7
- Total Fat: 14.5
- Sodium: 213

351. Coconut Pecan Cupcakes

Serving: 2 dozen. | Prep: 50mins | Cook: 20mins | Ready in:

Ingredients

- 5 eggs, separated
- 1/2 cup butter, softened
- 1/2 cup shortening
- 2 cups sugar
- 3/4 teaspoon vanilla extract
- 1/4 teaspoon almond extract
- 1-1/2 cups all-purpose flour
- 1/4 cup cornstarch
- 1/2 teaspoon baking soda
- 1/2 teaspoon salt
- 1 cup buttermilk
- 2 cups sweetened shredded coconut
- 1 cup finely chopped pecans
- FROSTING:
- 1 package (8 ounces) cream cheese, softened
- 1/4 cup butter, softened
- 1/2 teaspoon vanilla extract
- 1/4 teaspoon almond extract
- 3-3/4 cups confectioners' sugar
- 3/4 cup chopped pecans

Direction

- Stand eggs for 30 minutes at room temperature. Cream sugar, shortening and butter till fluffy and light in a big bowl. One by one, add egg yolks; beat well after each. Mix in extracts. Mix salt, baking soda, cornstarch and flour. Alternately with buttermilk, add to creamed mixture, beating well after each.
- Beat egg whites at high speed till stiff peaks form in a small bowl; fold into batter. Mix in pecans and coconut.
- Fill the paper-lined muffin cups to 3/4 full; bake for 20-25 minutes at 350° till inserted toothpick in middle exits clean. Cool for 10 minutes. Transfer from pans onto wire racks; fully cool.
- Mix frosting ingredients till smooth in a big bowl; frost cupcakes. Keep in the fridge.

Nutrition Information

- Calories: 410 calories
- Protein: 4g protein.
- Total Fat: 23g fat (10g saturated fat)
- Sodium: 206mg sodium
- Fiber: 1g fiber)
- Total Carbohydrate: 48g carbohydrate (38g sugars
- Cholesterol: 70mg cholesterol

352. Coconut Filled Chocolate Cupcakes

Serving: 26 cupcakes. | Prep: 45mins | Cook: 20mins | Ready in:

Ingredients

- 1 egg white
- Dash salt
- 1 cup sweetened shredded coconut
- 1 tablespoon all-purpose flour
- 2 tablespoons sugar
- BATTER:
- 2/3 cup shortening
- 1-1/2 cups sugar
- 2 eggs
- 1 teaspoon vanilla extract
- 2-1/2 cups all-purpose flour
- 1/2 cup baking cocoa
- 1 teaspoon salt
- 3/4 teaspoon baking soda
- 1 cup buttermilk
- 1/2 cup water
- GLAZE:
- 2 cups sugar
- 1/2 cup milk
- 1/2 cup shortening
- 1 cup (6 ounces) semisweet chocolate chips
- Toasted unsweetened coconut flakes and chocolate curls

Direction

- Put salt and egg white into a small bowl to make filling; allow to sit for half an hour at room temperature. Mix flour and coconut; put aside. Beat egg white over medium speed until it forms soft peaks. Slowly add in sugar, beating over high speed until it forms sheeny peaks and no sugar lumps remain. Slowly fold in coconut mixture, approximately a quarter cup each time; put aside.
- Beat sugar and shortening in a big bowl until fluffy and light. Put in vanilla and eggs; combine thoroughly. Mix together baking soda, salt, cocoa and flour; alternately put into the creamed mixture with water and buttermilk. Pour mixture into muffin cups lined with paper until 1/2 full. Dollop teaspoonfuls of filling into the middle of each cupcake. Put 2 tablespoons of batter on top to cover.
- Bake at 350 degrees until a toothpick slid inside the cake comes out without any batter streaks, 18 to 22 minutes. Let cool in pans for 10 minutes, then transferring to wire racks to cool through.
- Mix together milk and sugar to make glaze in a small saucepan. Boil, while stirring

continuously. Turn off the heat; whisk in chocolate chips and shortening until melted. Beat to achieve a thick consistency. Glaze the cupcakes and decorate with chocolate curls and toasted coconut.

Nutrition Information

- Calories: 298 calories
- Sodium: 162mg sodium
- Fiber: 1g fiber)
- Total Carbohydrate: 45g carbohydrate (34g sugars
- Cholesterol: 17mg cholesterol
- Protein: 3g protein.
- Total Fat: 13g fat (5g saturated fat)

353. Coconut Frosted Chocolate Cupcakes

Serving: 1 dozen. | Prep: 30mins | Cook: 15mins | Ready in:

Ingredients

- 2 tablespoons butter, softened
- 3/4 cup sugar
- 1 large egg
- 1 large egg white
- 1/3 cup buttermilk
- 1/3 cup water
- 1 teaspoon vanilla extract
- 1-1/2 cups all-purpose flour
- 1/3 cup baking cocoa
- 3/4 teaspoon baking soda
- 1/2 teaspoon salt
- FROSTING:
- 1/2 cup fat-free evaporated milk
- 1/2 cup sugar
- 1/4 cup marshmallow creme
- 1 large egg yolk, lightly beaten
- 1/2 teaspoon vanilla extract
- 1/2 cup sweetened shredded coconut
- 1/4 cup chopped pecans

Direction

- Whip sugar and butter in a big bowl until crumbly. Whip in egg white and egg. Whip in the vanilla, water and buttermilk. Mix the salt, baking soda, cocoa and flour; add to the batter just until moistened.
- Put batter into foil- or paper-lined muffin tins 2/3 full. Bake for 13 to 15 mins at 375° or until a toothpick inserted in the middle exits clean. Let cool for 5 minutes before taking out from pan to a wire rack.
- To make frosting, mix the egg yolk, marshmallow crème, sugar and milk in a small saucepan. Cook and mix over medium heat for about 15 minutes until thickened (don't boil). Take it off the heat; mix in vanilla. Fold in pecans and coconut. Let cool completely at room temperature. Put on cupcakes to frost.

Nutrition Information

- Calories: 229 calories
- Sodium: 238mg sodium
- Fiber: 1g fiber)
- Total Carbohydrate: 40g carbohydrate (25g sugars
- Cholesterol: 41mg cholesterol
- Protein: 4g protein.
- Total Fat: 6g fat (3g saturated fat)

354. Conversation Cupcakes

Serving: 28 cupcakes. | Prep: 45mins | Cook: 20mins | Ready in:

Ingredients

- 1 package white cake mix (regular size)
- 4 cups confectioners' sugar
- 1/2 cup butter, softened
- 1/2 cup shortening
- 1 teaspoon vanilla extract
- 1/8 teaspoon butter flavoring, optional

- 2 tablespoons milk
- 1 to 2 drops red food coloring, optional
- 1 to 2 drops yellow food coloring, optional
- 1 to 2 drops blue food coloring, optional

Direction

- Follow the package directions on how to prepare the cake mix batter for the cupcakes.
- Place foil or paper liners in a standard or heart-shaped muffin tin. Distribute batter among the cups, filling them half full. Bake them according to the package instructions for cupcakes. Let them cool for 10 minutes. Transfer them from the pans onto the wire racks; cool completely.
- For the frosting, mix the shortening, confectioners' sugar, vanilla, milk, butter, and butter flavoring, if desired in a big bowl until smooth.
- If desired, divide the frosting into fourths. Place the frosting into four separate bowls. Leaving 1 bowl untinted, fill each of the three bowls with one color of food coloring, and then mix them until well-blended. Frost the cupcakes. Pipe the edges of the cupcakes with the untinted frosting. Decorate the tops of the cupcakes with the Valentine phrases.

Nutrition Information

- Calories:
- Total Carbohydrate:
- Cholesterol:
- Protein:
- Total Fat:
- Sodium:
- Fiber:

355. Cookie Dough Cupcakes With Ganache Frosting

Serving: 2 dozen. | Prep: 25mins | Cook: 20mins | Ready in:

Ingredients

- 1 package yellow cake mix (regular size)
- 1 cup milk
- 3 eggs
- 1/2 cup butter, melted
- 1 teaspoon vanilla extract
- 1 tube (16-1/2 ounces) refrigerated chocolate chip cookie dough
- FROSTING:
- 2 cups (12 ounces) semisweet chocolate chips
- 1 cup heavy whipping cream
- 1/2 cup miniature semisweet chocolate chips

Direction

- Beat vanilla, butter, eggs, milk and cake mix for 30 seconds on low speed in a big bowl; beat for 2 minutes on medium.
- Fill the paper-lined muffin cups to 1/3 full. Roll cookie dough by tablespoonfuls to balls. Drop in middle of every cupcake; put leftover batter over.
- Bake at 350° till toothpick exits clean for 15-20 minutes. Cool for 10 minutes. Transfer from pans onto wire racks; fully cool.
- Frosting: Melt cream and chocolate chips in a small saucepan on low heat; mix till blended. Take off heat. Put into small bowl; cover. Refrigerate, mixing every 15 minutes, till it gets spreading consistency for 45-60 minutes.
- Cut small hole in corner of plastic/pastry bag; insert the #20 star pastry tip. Use chocolate mixture to fill bag; pipe cupcakes. Sprinkle miniature chocolate chips.

Nutrition Information

- Calories: 339 calories
- Sodium: 227mg sodium
- Fiber: 1g fiber
- Total Carbohydrate: 41g carbohydrate (20g sugars
- Cholesterol: 56mg cholesterol
- Protein: 3g protein.
- Total Fat: 19g fat (10g saturated fat)

356. Cream Filled Banana Cupcakes

Serving: 1-1/2 dozen. | Prep: 30mins | Cook: 20mins | Ready in:

Ingredients

- 1/2 cup shortening
- 1-1/3 cups sugar
- 2 eggs
- 1 teaspoon vanilla extract
- 2 cups all-purpose flour
- 3/4 teaspoon salt
- 1/2 teaspoon baking soda
- 1/4 teaspoon baking powder
- 1 cup mashed ripe bananas
- 1/3 cup buttermilk
- FILLING:
- 3 tablespoons all-purpose flour
- 1/2 cup milk
- 1/3 cup butter, softened
- 1/4 cup shortening
- 1 teaspoon vanilla extract
- 2 cups confectioners' sugar
- Additional confectioners' sugar, optional

Direction

- Cream the sugar and shortening in a large bowl until fluffy and light. Add the eggs, one at a time and whisking well after every addition. Mix in vanilla. Combine the baking powder, flour, salt, and baking soda and add the mixture alternately with bananas and buttermilk to the creamed mixture, whisking well after every addition. Fill the paper-lined muffin cups with 2/3 full of the mixture.
- Bake them at 350° for 20 to 25 minutes until the inserted toothpick into the center will come out clean. Let them cool for 10 minutes. Remove them from the pans and let them cool on wire racks completely.
- In the meantime, combine milk and flour in a small saucepan for the filling until smooth. Bring the mixture to a boil. Cook for 2 minutes, stirring, until thickened. You will have a very thick mixture. Let it cool to room temperature.
- Cream the shortening and butter in a small bowl until fluffy and light. Whisk in the cooled milk mixture and vanilla until smooth. Whisk in the confectioners' sugar.
- Cut a 1-inch circle with 1-inch deep on top of each cupcake using the sharp knife. Remove the tops carefully; put aside. Fill the cupcakes with the filling and replace the tops. If desired, sprinkle the cupcakes with more confectioners' sugar.

Nutrition Information

- Calories: 294 calories
- Sodium: 179mg sodium
- Fiber: 1g fiber)
- Total Carbohydrate: 43g carbohydrate (30g sugars
- Cholesterol: 33mg cholesterol
- Protein: 3g protein.
- Total Fat: 12g fat (4g saturated fat)

357. Creepy Cupcakes

Serving: 9 cupcakes. | Prep: 30mins | Cook: 25mins | Ready in:

Ingredients

- 1 package devil's food cake mix (regular size)
- 1/4 cup butter, softened
- 3 ounces cream cheese, softened
- 3 cups confectioners' sugar
- 2 tablespoons plus 1 teaspoon milk, divided
- 1/2 teaspoon vanilla extract
- Red and yellow liquid food coloring or orange paste food coloring
- 1 tablespoon baking cocoa
- Round pastry tip #3
- 9 chocolate kisses

- 9 semisweet chocolate chips
- Black shoestring licorice, cut into 3/4-inch pieces
- 18 white nonpareils

Direction

- Ready the cake mix based on package directions. Put 1/2 cup batter in a greased jumbo muffin cups. Place in the oven and bake for 25-30 minutes at 350°F or until a toothpick pricked in the middle comes out clean. Let cool for 5 minutes before taking from pans to wire racks to fully cool. Slice a thin slice off the top of the each cupcake. Beat vanilla, 2 tablespoons milk, confectioner's sugar, cream cheese and butter in a large bowl; combine well. Take out 1 cup;color with orange and frost cupcakes. Add baking cocoa and remaining milk to the remaining frosting. Slice a small hole in the corner of a plastic bag or pastry; insert round tip. Pack with chocolate frosting. Pipe a web on each cupcake; reserve left frosting. To make spider, insert chocolate kiss, point side down, next to edge of cupcake. Next to kiss, insert chocolate chip, point side down. Put four licorice pieces on each side of kiss. To make eyes, put 2 small circles of chocolate frosting on chocolate chip; then insert nonpareils.

Nutrition Information

- Calories:
- Sodium:
- Fiber:
- Total Carbohydrate:
- Cholesterol:
- Protein:
- Total Fat:

358. Cupcake Easter Baskets

Serving: 1-1/2 dozen. | Prep: 20mins | Cook: 20mins | Ready in:

Ingredients

- 1/2 cup butter, softened
- 1 cup sugar
- 1 large egg
- 1 teaspoon grated orange zest
- 2 cups cake flour
- 3/4 teaspoon baking soda
- 1/2 teaspoon baking powder
- 1/4 teaspoon salt
- 2/3 cup buttermilk
- FROSTING:
- 3/4 cup butter, softened
- 6 ounces cream cheese, softened
- 1 teaspoon vanilla extract
- 3 cups confectioners' sugar
- 1 teaspoon water
- 4 drops green food coloring
- 1-1/2 cups sweetened shredded coconut
- Red shoestring licorice
- Jelly beans

Direction

- Cream sugar and butter in a large bowl, then beat in orange zest and egg. Mix salt, baking powder, baking soda and flour. Transfer into the creamed mixture alternating with the buttermilk.
- Fill muffin cups that are lined with paper until two-thirds full, then bake for 20 to 25 minutes at 350° or until a toothpick comes out clean when inserted in the middle. Let it cool for ten minutes prior to transferring from the pans onto wire racks to completely cool.
- Beat vanilla, cream cheese and butter in a small bowl until smooth. Slowly beat in the confectioners' sugar and then spread atop cupcakes. In a large resealable plastic bag, mix food coloring and water. Place in coconut. Seal the bag and then shake to tint. Sprinkle atop cupcakes.

- Poke a hole at the top on the opposite sides of every cupcake using a wooden or metal skewer. For handles, cut licorice into 6-inch strips and then insert every end into a hole. Stud with the jelly beans.

Nutrition Information

- Calories: 351 calories
- Protein: 3g protein.
- Total Fat: 18g fat (11g saturated fat)
- Sodium: 273mg sodium
- Fiber: 1g fiber)
- Total Carbohydrate: 47g carbohydrate (33g sugars
- Cholesterol: 51mg cholesterol

359. Elvis Cupcakes

Serving: 1-1/2 dozen. | Prep: 30mins | Cook: 20mins | Ready in:

Ingredients

- 1-1/3 cups mashed ripe bananas (about 3 medium)
- 1 cup mayonnaise
- 1 teaspoon vanilla extract
- 2 cups all-purpose flour
- 3/4 cup sugar
- 1 teaspoon baking soda
- 1/2 teaspoon salt
- 18 milk chocolate kisses
- PEANUT BUTTER FROSTING:
- 1/3 cup creamy peanut butter
- 2 cups confectioners' sugar
- 1 teaspoon vanilla extract
- 3 to 4 tablespoons milk
- Milk chocolate chips, optional

Direction

- Mix vanilla, mayonnaise and bananas till well blended in a small bowl. Mix salt, baking soda, sugar and flour in a big bowl; beat into banana mixture slowly till blended.
- In each paper-lined muffin cup, put 1 tbsp. batter. Put a chocolate kiss on each, pointed side down; use leftover batter to fill cups to 2/3 full.
- Bake at 350° till inserted toothpick in middle exits clean for 20-25 minutes. Cool for 10 minutes. Transfer from pans onto wire racks; fully cool.
- Mix vanilla, confectioners' sugar, peanut butter with enough milk to get spreading consistency in a big bowl; frost cupcakes. If desired, garnish with chocolate chips.

Nutrition Information

- Calories: 294 calories
- Cholesterol: 6mg cholesterol
- Protein: 3g protein.
- Total Fat: 14g fat (3g saturated fat)
- Sodium: 230mg sodium
- Fiber: 1g fiber)
- Total Carbohydrate: 40g carbohydrate (27g sugars

360. Famous Chocolate Cupcakes

Serving: 2 dozen. | Prep: 30mins | Cook: 20mins | Ready in:

Ingredients

- 4 ounces milk chocolate,chopped
- 1/4 cup hot water
- 1/2 cup butter, softened
- 1 cup sugar
- 2 eggs
- 1-1/2 teaspoons vanilla extract
- 1-1/4 cups all-purpose flour
- 1/4 cup baking cocoa
- 3/4 teaspoon baking soda
- 1/2 teaspoon salt

- 1/2 cup buttermilk
- PEANUT BUTTER FROSTING:
- 1-1/2 cups creamy peanut butter
- 1/2 cup butter, softened
- 2-1/4 cups confectioners' sugar
- 24 miniature peanut butter cups

Direction

- Mix together hot water and chocolate in a small bowl. Stir to form a smooth mixture. Let cool slightly.
- Beat sugar and butter in a big bowl until fluffy and light. Put in eggs, one by one, beating thoroughly between additions. Beat vanilla into the mixture.
- Mix together salt, baking soda, cocoa and flour. Mix buttermilk in chocolate mixture. Alternate between chocolate mixture and dry ingredients to add in the beaten mixture, beating well between additions. Pour mixture to 1/2 full of muffin cups lined with paper.
- Bake in 350-degree oven until a toothpick comes out clean when pierced into the middle, 20 to 22 minutes. Allow to cool for 10 minutes in pans, then transfer to wire racks and cool entirely.
- To make frosting, mix together confectioners' sugar, butter and peanut butter; beat to form a smooth mixture. Spread onto cupcakes. Sprinkle peanut butter cups on top to garnish.

Nutrition Information

- Calories: 332 calories
- Protein: 7g protein.
- Total Fat: 20g fat (8g saturated fat)
- Sodium: 250mg sodium
- Fiber: 2g fiber)
- Total Carbohydrate: 35g carbohydrate (26g sugars
- Cholesterol: 39mg cholesterol

361. Gin & Tonic Cupcakes

Serving: 16 cupcakes. | Prep: 30mins | Cook: 20mins | Ready in:

Ingredients

- 3 large eggs, separated
- 3/4 cup all-purpose flour
- 3/4 cup sugar
- 1-1/2 teaspoons baking powder
- 1/4 teaspoon salt
- 1/4 cup tonic water
- 1/4 cup canola oil
- 2 tablespoons lime juice
- 2 teaspoons grated lime zest
- 1/2 teaspoon vanilla extract
- 1/4 teaspoon cream of tartar
- FROSTING:
- 2 cartons (8 ounces each) Mascarpone cheese
- 2/3 cup heavy whipping cream
- 1/2 cup confectioners' sugar
- 1/3 cup gin
- 6 to 8 drops green food coloring
- Lime slices

Direction

- Stand egg whites for 30 minutes in a big bowl at room temperature. Mix salt, baking powder, sugar and flour in a big bowl. Whisk vanilla, zest, lime juice, oil, water and egg yolks in another bowl. Add to dry ingredients and beat till blended well.
- Put cream of tartar in egg whites; beat using clean beaters till stiff peaks form. Fold into the batter.
- Fill the paper-lined muffin cups to 3/4 full; bake for 18-22 minutes at 325° till inserted toothpick in middle exits clean. Cool it for 10 minutes. Transfer from pans onto wire racks; fully cool.
- Beat food coloring, gin, confectioners' sugar, cream and cheese till stiff peaks form in a big bowl; pipe on cupcakes. Use lime slices to garnish; refrigerate leftovers.

Nutrition Information

- Calories: 285 calories
- Sodium: 107mg sodium
- Fiber: 0 fiber)
- Total Carbohydrate: 19g carbohydrate (13g sugars
- Cholesterol: 89mg cholesterol
- Protein: 4g protein.
- Total Fat: 21g fat (10g saturated fat)

---

362.   Heavenly Surprise Cupcakes

Serving: 1-1/2 dozen. | Prep: 20mins | Cook: 20mins | Ready in:

Ingredients

- 2 large eggs
- 1-1/4 cups sugar
- 1 cup buttermilk
- 2/3 cup canola oil
- 1 teaspoon vanilla extract
- 1-1/2 cups all-purpose flour
- 1/2 cup baking cocoa
- 1-1/4 teaspoons baking soda
- 1 teaspoon salt
- FROSTING:
- 2/3 cup butter-flavored shortening
- 2/3 cup butter, softened
- 1 cup sugar
- 1 can (5 ounces) evaporated milk
- 1 tablespoon water
- 1/2 teaspoon vanilla extract
- 2 cups confectioners' sugar

Direction

- Mix vanilla, oil, buttermilk, sugar and eggs in a large bowl until combined. Mix the salt, baking soda, cocoa and flour; gently add to egg mixture until combined. Then put into paper-lined muffin cups and fill two-thirds full. Place in the oven and bake for 20-22 minutes at 350°F or until a toothpick pricked in the middle comes out clean. Let cool for 10 minutes before taking from pans to wire racks to fully cool. To make frosting, cream the sugar, butter and shortening in a large bowl until fluffy and light. Mix in the vanilla, water and milk. Gently mix in confectioner's sugar until become smooth. Slice a small hole in the corner of a resealable plastic bag or pastry; insert a small star tip. Then fill bag with frosting. Push tip 1-inch into middle of cupcake and fill with frosting just until top of cake starts to crack. Pipe frosting over the tops.

Nutrition Information

- Calories: 415 calories
- Fiber: 1g fiber)
- Total Carbohydrate: 49g carbohydrate (39g sugars
- Cholesterol: 44mg cholesterol
- Protein: 3g protein.
- Total Fat: 24g fat (7g saturated fat)
- Sodium: 296mg sodium

---

363.   Heavenly Surprise Mini Cupcakes

Serving: 6 dozen. | Prep: 35mins | Cook: 15mins | Ready in:

Ingredients

- FILLING:
- 1 package (8 ounces) cream cheese, softened
- 1/3 cup sugar
- 1 egg
- 1/8 teaspoon salt
- 1 cup sweetened shredded coconut
- 1 cup finely chopped walnuts
- 1 cup (6 ounces) miniature semisweet chocolate chips
- BATTER:
- 2 cups sugar

- 1-1/2 cups water
- 3/4 cup canola oil
- 2 eggs
- 2 teaspoons vanilla extract
- 1 teaspoon white vinegar
- 3 cups all-purpose flour
- 1/2 cup baking cocoa
- 1 teaspoon baking soda
- 1 teaspoon salt
- FROSTING:
- 1/2 cup heavy whipping cream
- 1-1/3 cups semisweet chocolate chips

Direction

- Filling: Beat sugar and cream cheese till fluffy and light in a small bowl. Add salt and egg; stir well. Mix in chocolate chips, walnuts and coconut; put aside.
- Batter: Beat vinegar, vanilla, eggs, oil, water and sugar till well blended in a big bowl. Mix salt, baking soda, cocoa and flour; beat into oil mixture slowly till blended.
- Fill the paper-lined mini muffin cups to 1/3 full using batter. By teaspoonfuls, drop filling in middle of each; put extra batter over, filling muffin cups to 3/4 full.
- Bake for 12-15 minutes at 350° till inserted toothpick in cake portion of cupcake exits clean. Cool it for 10 minutes. Transfer from pans onto wire racks; fully cool.
- Frosting: Melt cream and chocolate in a small saucepan on low heat; mix till blended. Take off heat. Cool it to room temperature. Frost the cupcakes. Refrigerate leftovers.

Nutrition Information

- Calories: 130 calories
- Protein: 2g protein. Diabetic Exchanges: 1 starch
- Total Fat: 7g fat (3g saturated fat)
- Sodium: 71mg sodium
- Fiber: 1g fiber)
- Total Carbohydrate: 15g carbohydrate (10g sugars
- Cholesterol: 15mg cholesterol

364. Jalapeno Popper Corn Cupcakes

Serving: 1 dozen. | Prep: 40mins | Cook: 25mins | Ready in:

Ingredients

- 1-1/4 cups all-purpose flour
- 1 cup sugar
- 1/2 cup cornmeal
- 2 teaspoons baking powder
- 1/4 teaspoon salt
- 2 large eggs
- 1/2 cup 2% milk
- 1/2 cup olive oil
- 1/2 teaspoon vanilla extract
- 3/4 cup frozen corn, thawed
- 2 tablespoons finely chopped seeded jalapeno pepper
- FROSTING:
- 1/4 cup panko (Japanese) bread crumbs
- 4 ounces cream cheese, softened
- 1/4 cup butter, softened
- 1-3/4 cups confectioners' sugar
- 1 teaspoon vanilla extract
- Sliced jalapeno peppers

Direction

- Mix salt, baking powder, cornmeal, sugar and flour in a big bowl. Mix vanilla, oil, milk and eggs in another bowl; mix into dry ingredients till just moist. Fold in jalapeno and corn.
- Fill paper-lined/greased muffin cups to 3/4 full; bake at 350° till inserted toothpick in cupcake exits clean for 24-28 minutes. Cool for 5 minutes. Transfer from pan onto wire rack; fully cool.
- On ungreased baking sheet, put breadcrumbs; bake at 400° till toasted for 2-3 minutes. Cool. Beat butter and cream cheese till fluffy in a big bowl. Add vanilla and confectioners' sugar;

beat till smooth. Frost cupcakes. Use jalapeno slices and toasted breadcrumbs to garnish; keep refrigerated.

Nutrition Information

- Calories: 380 calories
- Sodium: 192mg sodium
- Fiber: 1g fiber)
- Total Carbohydrate: 52g carbohydrate (34g sugars
- Cholesterol: 56mg cholesterol
- Protein: 4g protein.
- Total Fat: 17g fat (6g saturated fat)

365. Key Lime Pie Cupcakes

Serving: 32 cupcakes. | Prep: 45mins | Cook: 20mins | Ready in:

Ingredients

- 2 packages (14.1 ounces each) refrigerated pie pastry
- 1 cup butter, softened
- 2-1/2 cups sugar
- 4 large eggs
- 1/2 cup Key lime juice
- 2 cups all-purpose flour
- 1-1/2 cups self-rising flour
- 1-1/2 cups buttermilk
- FROSTING:
- 12 ounces cream cheese, softened
- 1-1/2 cups butter, softened
- 1-1/2 teaspoons vanilla extract
- 2-3/4 to 3 cups confectioners' sugar
- 6 tablespoons Key lime juice
- Fresh raspberries

Direction

- Preheat an oven to 350°. Line foil liners on 32 muffin cups. Unroll pastry sheets on lightly floured work surface. Use floured 2 1/4-inch round cookie cutter to cut 32 circles; discard/keep leftover pastry for another time. In each liner, press 1 pastry circle; bake till light brown for 10-12 minutes. On wire racks, cool.
- Beat sugar and butter till crumbly in a big bowl. One by one, add eggs; beat well after each. Beat in lime juice. Whisk flours in another bowl. Alternately with buttermilk, add to butter mixture; beat well after each.
- Put in prepped cups; bake till inserted toothpick in middle exits clean for 20-22 minutes. Cool for 10 minutes in pans. Transfer onto wire racks; fully cool.
- Beat vanilla, butter and cream cheese till blended in a big bowl; alternately with lime juice, beat in enough of confectioners' sugar to get preferred consistency. Frost cupcakes; put raspberries over. Refrigerate leftovers.

Nutrition Information

- Calories: 368 calories
- Protein: 4g protein.
- Total Fat: 21g fat (13g saturated fat)
- Sodium: 256mg sodium
- Fiber: 0 fiber)
- Total Carbohydrate: 42g carbohydrate (27g sugars
- Cholesterol: 78mg cholesterol

366. Kitty Cat Cupcakes

Serving: about 1-1/2 dozen. | Prep: 30mins | Cook: 15mins | Ready in:

Ingredients

- 2/3 cup shortening
- 1-3/4 cups sugar, divided
- 4 eggs, separated
- 2-1/2 cups all-purpose flour
- 2-1/2 teaspoons baking powder
- 1/2 teaspoon salt

- 1 cup orange juice
- 1 cup sweetened shredded coconut
- FROSTING:
- 1-1/4 cups sugar
- 1/4 cup water
- 1/4 cup light corn syrup
- 1/8 teaspoon salt
- 1 egg white
- 1/2 cup miniature marshmallows (about 50)
- 1/2 teaspoons vanilla extract
- Assorted M&M's
- 1 piece red shoestring licorice, cut into 3/4-inch pieces
- Chocolate sprinkles
- About 9 vanilla wafers
- 2 cups sweetened shredded coconut, toasted

Direction

- Allow eggs to stand for a half hour at room temperature. Cream together 1 1/2 cups sugar and shortening in a big bowl until fluffy and light. Beat in egg yolk until well combined. Mix together salt, baking powder and flour, then alternately put into the cream mixture together with orange juice, while beating well after each addition.
- Use clean beaters to beat egg whites in a small bowl until create soft peaks. One tablespoon at a time, add in the leftover sugar gradually on high until create stiff peaks. Fold into the batter gradually along with coconut.
- Fill paper-lined muffin cups until 2/3 full. Bake at 350° until a toothpick inserted into the center comes out clean, about 15 minutes. Allow to cool for 10 minutes before turning from pans to wire racks to cool thoroughly.
- For frosting, mix together salt, egg white, corn syrup, water and sugar in a heavy saucepan. Beat the mixture on low speed about a minute, using a portable mixer. Keep in beating on low for 12 to 18 minutes, until frosting reaches 160°, over low heat. Turn into the bowl of a heavy-duty stand mixer, then put in vanilla and marshmallow. Beat on high for 5 minutes, until create stiff peaks. Frost cupcakes.
- Place M&M's for nose and eyes, sprinkles for whiskers and licorice for mouth. To make ears, use a serrated knife to quarter wafers and put two on each cupcake with rounded side down. Sprinkle over with coconut and chill until ready to serve.

Nutrition Information

- Calories: 387 calories
- Sodium: 209mg sodium
- Fiber: 1g fiber)
- Total Carbohydrate: 62g carbohydrate (43g sugars
- Cholesterol: 47mg cholesterol
- Protein: 4g protein.
- Total Fat: 14g fat (7g saturated fat)

367. Lemon Coconut Cupcakes

Serving: 12 | Prep: 20mins | Cook: 20mins | Ready in:

Ingredients

- Cupcakes:
- 1 1/4 cups all-purpose flour
- 3/4 teaspoon baking soda
- 1 pinch salt
- 5 tablespoons butter, cut into chunks
- 2/3 cup milk
- 1 cup white sugar
- 2 eggs
- 1 egg yolk
- 1 teaspoon vanilla extract
- 1/2 cup shredded coconut
- Frosting:
- 1/4 cup butter, softened
- 4 ounces cream cheese, softened
- 1 cup confectioners' sugar
- 1/2 teaspoon vanilla extract
- 1 teaspoon grated lemon zest
- 1/4 cup shredded coconut, or to taste

Direction

- Preheat an oven to 175°C/350°F; line paper liners on 12-cup muffin tin.
- Mix salt, baking soda and flour in a bowl.
- Heat milk and 5 tbsp. butter in a saucepan on low heat for 3-5 minutes till butter melts; take off heat.
- Beat 1 tsp. vanilla extract, egg yolk, eggs and white sugar using electric hand mixer at low till thick and smooth in a bowl. Put flour mixture in sugar-egg mixture slowly, mixing with electric mixer just till incorporated. Add butter-milk mixture slowly; beat just till combined. Fold in 1/2 cup of shredded coconut; use batter to fill muffin cups.
- In preheated oven, bake for 20 minutes till inserted toothpick in middle of cupcake exits clean; cool for 10 minutes in pans. Transfer onto wire rack; fully cool.
- Beat cream cheese and softened butter using an electric mixer at medium in a bowl. Beat confectioners' sugar slowly into creamed butter mixture at low till incorporated. Beat in lemon zest and 1/2 tsp. vanilla extract till creamy and smooth. Spread frosting on cooled cupcakes; sprinkle each cupcake with 1 tsp. shredded coconut.

Nutrition Information

- Calories: 308 calories;
- Total Fat: 14.8
- Sodium: 199
- Total Carbohydrate: 40.5
- Cholesterol: 82
- Protein: 4

368. Lemon Cupcakes

Serving: 30 | Prep: 48mins | Cook: 17mins | Ready in:

Ingredients

- 3 cups self-rising flour
- 1/2 teaspoon salt
- 1 cup unsalted butter, at room temperature
- 2 cups white sugar
- 4 eggs, at room temperature
- 1 teaspoon vanilla extract
- 2 tablespoons lemon zest
- 1 cup whole milk, divided
- 2 1/2 tablespoons fresh lemon juice, divided
- Lemon Cream Icing
- 2 cups chilled heavy cream
- 3/4 cup confectioners' sugar
- 1 1/2 tablespoons fresh lemon juice

Direction

- Preheat an oven to 190°C/375°F; line paper liners on 30 cupcake pan cups.
- Sift together salt and self-rising flour in a bowl. Beat sugar and unsalted butter using electric mixer till fluffy and light in another bowl. One by one, beat in eggs; beat each egg till incorporated prior to adding next. Mix in lemon zest and vanilla extract.
- Beat flour mixture, 1/3 at a time, into butter mixture gently, alternating with 1/2 lemon juice and 1/2 milk after each of initial 2 flour additions; beat till just combined, don't overmix.
- Fill prepped cupcake liners to 3/4 full with batter; in preheated oven, bake for 17 minutes till inserted toothpick in middle exits clean. Cool them for 10 minutes in pans. Transfer onto rack; finish cooling.
- Icing: Beat cream using an electric mixer on low till cream starts to thicken in a chilled bowl. Little by little, add lemon juice and confectioners' sugar; beat after every addition till incorporated fully. Put mixer speed on high; beat for 5 minutes till icing makes soft peaks. Spread on cooled cupcakes; refrigerate the leftovers.

Nutrition Information

- Calories: 232 calories;
- Total Fat: 13.1

- Sodium: 260
- Total Carbohydrate: 26.7
- Cholesterol: 64
- Protein: 2.7

369. Lemon Curd Cupcakes

Serving: 1 dozen. | Prep: 40mins | Cook: 20mins |Ready in:

Ingredients

- 3 tablespoons plus 1-1/2 teaspoons sugar
- 3 tablespoons lemon juice
- 4-1/2 teaspoons butter
- 1 egg, lightly beaten
- 1 teaspoon grated lemon peel
- BATTER:
- 3/4 cup butter, softened
- 1 cup sugar
- 2 eggs
- 1 teaspoon vanilla extract
- 1 teaspoon grated lemon peel
- 1-1/2 cups cake flour
- 1/2 teaspoon baking powder
- 1/4 teaspoon baking soda
- 1/4 teaspoon salt
- 2/3 cup buttermilk
- FROSTING:
- 2 tablespoons butter, softened
- 1/2 teaspoon vanilla extract
- Pinch salt
- 2 cups confectioners' sugar
- 2 to 4 tablespoons milk
- Edible flowers or additional grated lemon peel, optional

Direction

- Cook and stir the butter and lemon juice in a heavy saucepan for the lemon curd until smooth. Mix a small amount of the hot mixture into the egg. Pour the mixture back into the pan. Bring the mixture to a gentle boil while constantly stirring it. Allow it to cook for 2 minutes until thickened. Mix in the lemon peel and let the mixture cool for 10 minutes. Cover the mixture and let it chill for 1 1/2 hours until thickened.
- Cream the sugar and butter in a large bowl until fluffy and light. Add the eggs, one at a time and whisking well after every addition. Add the lemon peel and vanilla. Combine the salt, flour, baking soda, and baking powder and add the mixture to the creamed mixture, adding it alternately with the buttermilk.
- Pour the mixture into the paper-lined muffin cups, filling them up to 3/4 full. Bake them at 350° for 20 to 25 minutes until the toothpick will come out clean. Allow them to cool for 10 minutes. Remove them from the pan and let them cool on a wire rack completely.
- Make a small hole in the plastic or pastry bag's corner. Fill the hole with a small round pastry tip. Pour the lemon curd into the bag. Insert 1 inch into the center of each cupcake with the tip. Fill the cupcake with the curd until the tops of each of the cupcakes start to crack.
- Combine the salt, butter, confectioners' sugar, vanilla, and enough amount of milk in a small bowl until the desired frosting consistency was reached. Use the mixture to frost the cupcakes. Let them store inside the fridge. If desired, garnish them with lemon peel or flowers.

Nutrition Information

- Calories: 376 calories
- Fiber: 0 fiber)
- Total Carbohydrate: 55g carbohydrate (40g sugars
- Cholesterol: 94mg cholesterol
- Protein: 4g protein.
- Total Fat: 16g fat (10g saturated fat)
- Sodium: 286mg sodium

370. Maple Carrot Cupcakes

Serving: 1-1/2 dozen. | Prep: 15mins | Cook: 20mins | Ready in:

Ingredients

- 2 cups all-purpose flour
- 1 cup sugar
- 1 teaspoon baking powder
- 1 teaspoon baking soda
- 1 teaspoon ground cinnamon
- 1/2 teaspoon salt
- 4 large eggs
- 1 cup canola oil
- 1/2 cup maple syrup
- 3 cups grated carrots (about 6 medium)
- FROSTING:
- 1 package (8 ounces) cream cheese, softened
- 1/4 cup butter, softened
- 1/4 cup maple syrup
- 1 teaspoon vanilla extract
- Walnuts, optional

Direction

- Combine the first six ingredients in a large bowl. In another bowl, beat syrup, oil and eggs. Blend mixture into dry ingredients just until moistened. Fold in carrots.
- Fill about two-thirds full to 18 paper-lined or greased muffin cups. Bake at 350° for nearly 20 to 25 minutes or until a toothpick inserted in the center comes out clean. Allow 5 minutes for cooling before taking away from pans to wire racks.
- For frosting, in a bowl, combine the butter, cream cheese, vanilla and syrup; beat until smooth. Frost cooled cupcakes. Add nuts if you want. Place in the refrigerator for storing.

Nutrition Information

- Calories: 327 calories
- Protein: 4g protein.
- Total Fat: 20g fat (6g saturated fat)
- Sodium: 243mg sodium
- Fiber: 1g fiber)
- Total Carbohydrate: 33g carbohydrate (21g sugars
- Cholesterol: 68mg cholesterol

371. Mocha Cupcakes

Serving: about 1-1/2 dozen. | Prep: 15mins | Cook: 20mins | Ready in:

Ingredients

- 1 cup boiling water
- 1 cup mayonnaise
- 1 teaspoon vanilla extract
- 2 cups all-purpose flour
- 1 cup sugar
- 1/2 cup baking cocoa
- 2 teaspoons baking soda
- MOCHA FROSTING:
- 3/4 cup confectioners' sugar
- 1/4 cup baking cocoa
- 1/2 to 1 teaspoon instant coffee granules
- Pinch salt
- 1-1/2 cups heavy whipping cream

Direction

- Mix vanilla, mayonnaise and water in a large bowl. Mix the baking soda, cocoa, sugar and flour; put into the mayonnaise mixture and whisk until well combined. Then put into a greased or paper-lined muffin cups and fill two-thirds full. Place in the oven and bake for 20-25 minutes at 350°F or until a toothpick comes out clean. Let cool for 10 minutes before taking to wire racks to fully cool. To make frosting, mix salt, coffee granules, cocoa and confectioner's sugar in a large bowl. Mix in cream. Put mixer beaters in bowl; then cover and chill for 30 minutes. Whip frosting until form a stiff peaks. Frost the cupcakes. Keep leftovers in the refrigerator.

Nutrition Information

- Calories: 421 calories
- Total Fat: 26g fat (9g saturated fat)
- Sodium: 334mg sodium
- Fiber: 2g fiber)
- Total Carbohydrate: 44g carbohydrate (24g sugars
- Cholesterol: 47mg cholesterol
- Protein: 4g protein.

372. Moist Carrot Cupcakes

Serving: 12 | Prep: 20mins | Cook: 25mins | Ready in:

Ingredients

- 2 eggs, room temperature
- 1 cup white sugar
- 2 tablespoons white sugar
- 1/3 cup brown sugar
- 1/2 cup olive oil
- 1 teaspoon vanilla extract
- 2 cups shredded carrots
- 1/2 cup drained crushed pineapple
- 1/2 cup shredded coconut
- 1 1/2 cups all-purpose flour
- 1 1/4 teaspoons baking soda
- 1/2 teaspoon salt
- 1 1/2 teaspoons ground cinnamon
- 1/2 teaspoon ground nutmeg
- 1/4 teaspoon ground ginger

Direction

- Preheat the oven to 350°F (175 °C). Line a 12-cup muffin tin with paper liners or grease it.
- In a bowl, beat brown sugar, 1 cup plus 2 tablespoons white sugar and eggs together; mixing in the vanilla extract and oil. Fold coconut, pineapple and carrots into mixture.
- In a separate bowl, mix ginger, salt, nutmeg, baking soda, flour and cinnamon together; then add it to the carrot mixture and mix until thoroughly moistened. Move the batter to the prepped muffin tin and divide evenly.
- Put it into the oven and bake for 25 minutes or until a toothpick poked in a cupcake comes out spotless.

Nutrition Information

- Calories: 274 calories;
- Sodium: 263
- Total Carbohydrate: 42
- Cholesterol: 31
- Protein: 3
- Total Fat: 10.9

373. Orange Applesauce Cupcakes

Serving: 1 dozen. | Prep: 20mins | Cook: 20mins | Ready in:

Ingredients

- 6 tablespoons butter, softened
- 1 cup packed brown sugar
- 1 large egg
- 1/2 cup unsweetened applesauce
- 1 teaspoon vanilla extract
- 1 teaspoon grated orange zest
- 1 cup all-purpose flour
- 1 teaspoon baking powder
- 1/2 teaspoon salt
- 1/4 teaspoon baking soda
- 1/2 cup chopped pecans
- FROSTING:
- 1/4 cup butter, softened
- 2 cups confectioners' sugar
- 1-1/2 teaspoons grated orange zest
- 2 to 4 teaspoons orange juice

Direction

- Cream the brown sugar and butter in a large bowl until fluffy and light. Whisk in the egg.

Stir in the orange zest, applesauce, and vanilla. Combine the baking soda, flour, salt, and baking powder and add the mixture to the creamed mixture gradually. Whisk the mixture well before stirring in the pecans.
- Pour the mixture into the paper-lined muffin cups, filling them half-full. Bake them at 350° for 20 to 25 minutes until the toothpick comes out very clean. Let them cool for 10 minutes. Remove them from the pan and place them on a wire rack to cool completely.
- Cream the confectioners' sugar and butter in a small bowl for the frosting until fluffy and light. Add the orange zest and enough amount of orange juice until the spreading consistency is achieved. Use it to frost the cupcakes.

Nutrition Information

- Calories: 315 calories
- Sodium: 267mg sodium
- Fiber: 1g fiber)
- Total Carbohydrate: 48g carbohydrate (38g sugars
- Cholesterol: 43mg cholesterol
- Protein: 2g protein.
- Total Fat: 14g fat (6g saturated fat)

374. Orange Cream Filled Cupcakes

Serving: 20 cupcakes. | Prep: 20mins | Cook: 20mins | Ready in:

Ingredients

- 3 large eggs
- 1-1/2 cups sugar
- 1 cup canola oil
- 1/2 cup buttermilk
- 1/3 cup orange juice
- 2 teaspoons grated orange zest
- 1 teaspoon orange extract
- 1 teaspoon vanilla extract
- 3 cups all-purpose flour
- 2 teaspoons baking powder
- 1 teaspoon baking soda
- 3/4 teaspoon salt
- FROSTING:
- 3/4 cup butter, softened
- 1 cup confectioners' sugar
- 1/4 teaspoon vanilla extract
- 1/4 teaspoon orange extract
- 1 jar (7 ounces) marshmallow creme
- 2 cups vanilla ice cream
- Orange peel strips

Direction

- Mix the first 8 ingredients in a large bowl until well combined. Add in the salt, baking soda, baking powder and flour' slowly mix into egg mixture until combined well. Fill three-fourths full the paper-lined muffin cups.
- Place inside the oven at 350 degrees F for 18-22 minutes or until used toothpick to insert in the middle comes out clean. Let it cool for 10 minutes then get from pan and put on wire racks to fully cool. Beat butter until fluffy in a large bowl; add in extracts and confectioner's sugar until turns smooth. Stir in marshmallow crème; whip until fluffy and light in weight.
- Use a melon scoop to remove a small amount of cake from tops of cupcakes. Then replace removed tops with a little scoop of ice cream. Garnish with orange peel strips and frosting. Present right away.

Nutrition Information

- Calories: 386 calories
- Sodium: 276mg sodium
- Fiber: 1g fiber)
- Total Carbohydrate: 48g carbohydrate (31g sugars
- Cholesterol: 56mg cholesterol
- Protein: 4g protein.
- Total Fat: 20g fat (6g saturated fat)

375. Orange Date Cupcakes

Serving: 1-1/2 dozen. | Prep: 20mins | Cook: 15mins | Ready in:

Ingredients

- 1/2 cup butter-flavored shortening
- 1 cup sugar
- 2 large eggs
- 1 tablespoon orange extract
- 2 cups cake flour
- 1 teaspoon baking powder
- 1/2 teaspoon baking soda
- 1/2 teaspoon salt
- 1 cup whole milk
- 1 cup chopped dates
- 4 teaspoons grated orange zest
- FROSTING:
- 3 ounces cream cheese, softened
- 3/4 cup confectioners' sugar
- 1 teaspoon orange extract
- 2 to 3 teaspoons whole milk

Direction

- Cream sugar and shortening till fluffy and light in a big bowl. One by one, add eggs; beat well after each. Mix in extract. Mix salt, baking soda, baking powder and flour. Alternately with milk, add to creamed mixture; beat well after each. Mix in orange zest and dates.
- Fill the paper-lined muffin cups to 2/3 full; bake it at 350° till toothpick exits clean for 15-20 minutes. Cool for 10 minutes. Transfer from pans onto wire racks; fully cool.
- Frosting: Beat cream cheese till fluffy in a small bowl. Add extract and confectioners' sugar; beat till smooth. To get desired consistency, add enough milk. Frost cupcakes and refrigerate leftovers.

Nutrition Information

- Calories: 233 calories
- Cholesterol: 30mg cholesterol
- Protein: 3g protein.
- Total Fat: 8g fat (3g saturated fat)
- Sodium: 151mg sodium
- Fiber: 1g fiber)
- Total Carbohydrate: 36g carbohydrate (23g sugars

376. Orange Dream Mini Cupcakes

Serving: 4 dozen. | Prep: 60mins | Cook: 15mins | Ready in:

Ingredients

- 1/2 cup butter, softened
- 1 cup sugar
- 2 large eggs
- 1 tablespoon grated orange zest
- 1 tablespoon orange juice
- 1/2 teaspoon vanilla extract
- 1-1/2 cups all-purpose flour
- 1-1/2 teaspoons baking powder
- 1/4 teaspoon salt
- 1/2 cup buttermilk
- BUTTERCREAM:
- 1/2 cup butter, softened
- 1/4 teaspoon salt
- 2 cups confectioners' sugar
- 2 tablespoons 2% milk
- 1-1/2 teaspoons vanilla extract
- 1/2 cup orange marmalade

Direction

- Set the oven at 325° to preheat. Use paper liners to line 48 mini-muffin cups. Cream sugar and butter in a large bowl until fluffy and light. Put in the eggs, 1 at a time, beat well after each addition. Then continue to beat in vanilla, orange juice, and orange zest. Whisk flour, salt, and baking powder in another bowl; add to the creamed mixture alternately

with buttermilk, keep beating well after each addition.
- Fill 2/3 full into the prepared cups. Bake for 11-13 minutes, until inserting a toothpick in the center and it comes out clean. Let cool in the pans for 5 minutes before moving to wire racks to completely cool.
- To make the buttercream: Beat salt and butter in a large bowl until creamy. Beat in vanilla, milk, and confectioners' sugar slowly until smooth.
- From the top of each cupcake, cut a 1-in.-wide cone-shaped piece using a paring knife; discard the removed part. Fill with marmalade into the cavity. Spread or pipe the buttercream over tops.

Nutrition Information

- Calories: 96 calories
- Protein: 1g protein.
- Total Fat: 4g fat (2g saturated fat)
- Sodium: 72mg sodium
- Fiber: 0 fiber)
- Total Carbohydrate: 15g carbohydrate (11g sugars
- Cholesterol: 19mg cholesterol

377. Pad Thai Cupcakes

Serving: 1-1/2 dozen. | Prep: 25mins | Cook: 25mins | Ready in:

Ingredients

- 3/4 cup creamy peanut butter
- 1/2 cup butter, softened
- 1-1/2 cups sugar
- 4 eggs
- 2 teaspoons vanilla extract
- 2 cups all-purpose flour
- 1 teaspoon baking powder
- 1/2 teaspoon salt
- 1/4 teaspoon baking soda
- 1/4 teaspoon cayenne pepper
- 3/4 cup sour cream
- FROSTING:
- 1 cup creamy peanut butter
- 6 ounces cream cheese, softened
- 1/2 cup heavy whipping cream
- 1/3 cup confectioners' sugar
- 1/4 teaspoon salt
- Chopped salted peanuts, minced fresh cilantro and crushed red pepper flakes

Direction

- Cream sugar, butter and peanut butter till fluffy and light in a big bowl; beat in vanilla and eggs. Mix cayenne, baking soda, salt, baking powder and flour. Alternately with sour cream, add to creamed mixture; beat well after each.
- Fill the paper-lined muffin cups to 2/3 full; bake at 350° till inserted toothpick in middle exits clean for 22-26 minutes. Cool for 10 minutes. Transfer from pans onto wire racks; fully cool.
- Cream the cream cheese and peanut butter till fluffy and light in a small bowl; beat in salt, confectioners' sugar and cream slowly. Frost cupcakes. Sprinkle pepper flakes, cilantro and peanuts.

Nutrition Information

- Calories: 409 calories
- Sodium: 340mg sodium
- Fiber: 2g fiber)
- Total Carbohydrate: 35g carbohydrate (21g sugars
- Cholesterol: 86mg cholesterol
- Protein: 10g protein.
- Total Fat: 26g fat (11g saturated fat)

378. Peanut Butter Chocolate Cupcakes

Serving: 1 dozen. | Prep: 30mins | Cook: 25mins | Ready in:

Ingredients

- 3 ounces cream cheese, softened
- 1/4 cup creamy peanut butter
- 2 tablespoons sugar
- 1 tablespoon 2% milk
- BATTER:
- 2 cups sugar
- 1-3/4 cups all-purpose flour
- 1/2 cup baking cocoa
- 1-1/2 teaspoons baking powder
- 1 teaspoon salt
- 1/4 teaspoon baking soda
- 2 large eggs
- 1 cup water
- 1 cup 2% milk
- 1/2 cup canola oil
- 2 teaspoons vanilla extract
- FROSTING:
- 1/3 cup butter, softened
- 2 cups confectioners' sugar
- 6 tablespoons baking cocoa
- 3 to 4 tablespoons 2% milk

Direction

- Beat milk, sugar, peanut butter and cream cheese in a small bowl to form a smooth mixture and put aside.
- Mix together baking soda, salt, baking powder, cocoa, flour and sugar in a big bowl. In a separate bowl, mix together vanilla, oil, milk, water and eggs. Mix into the dry mixture just until moist. (The mixture will have a thin consistency).
- In jumbo muffin cups lined with paper liners, add batter to 1/2 full. Dollop peanut butter mixture by a scant tablespoonful to each cup's center; fill with the rest of batter.
- Bake in 350-degree oven until a toothpick is clean when pierced into the middle, 25 to 30 minutes. Allow to cool for 10 minutes, then transfer from pans to wire racks. Allow to fully cool.
- Mix together frosting ingredients in a big bowl until smooth; frost the cupcakes. Keep in the refrigerator to store.

Nutrition Information

- Calories: 509 calories
- Cholesterol: 60mg cholesterol
- Protein: 7g protein.
- Total Fat: 22g fat (7g saturated fat)
- Sodium: 394mg sodium
- Fiber: 2g fiber)
- Total Carbohydrate: 75g carbohydrate (55g sugars

379. Peanut Butter Cup Chocolate Cupcakes

Serving: 2 dozen. | Prep: 30mins | Cook: 20mins | Ready in:

Ingredients

- 1 package chocolate cake mix (regular size)
- 1-1/4 cups water
- 1/2 cup peanut butter
- 1/3 cup canola oil
- 3 eggs
- 24 miniature peanut butter cups
- FROSTING:
- 6 ounces semisweet chocolate, chopped
- 2/3 cup heavy whipping cream
- 1/3 cup peanut butter
- Additional miniature peanut butter cups, chopped

Direction

- Mix together eggs, oil, peanut butter, water and cake mix in a big bowl; beat for half a

minute over low speed. Beat for 2 minutes over medium until smooth.
- Pour creamed mixture into paper-lined muffin cups until 1/2 full. Arrange a peanut butter cup in the middle of each cupcake. Top with 1 tablespoonful of batter to cover.
- Bake at 350 degrees until a toothpick slid into the middle of the cupcake comes out with no batter streaks, 18 to 22 minutes. Let cool down on the pans for 10 minutes, then move onto wire racks to cool fully.
- Put chocolate into a small bowl. Let cream come just to a boil in a small saucepan. Add onto the chocolate; stir until no lumps remain. Mix in peanut butter. Cool for about 10 minutes, while stirring every now and then, to room temperature until mixture is spreadable.
- Lather onto the cupcakes; sprinkle more peanut butter cups over at once. Allow to stand until set.

Nutrition Information

- Calories: 269 calories
- Protein: 5g protein.
- Total Fat: 17g fat (6g saturated fat)
- Sodium: 220mg sodium
- Fiber: 2g fiber)
- Total Carbohydrate: 27g carbohydrate (18g sugars
- Cholesterol: 36mg cholesterol

380. Peanut Butter Cupcakes

Serving: 24 | Prep: 10mins | Cook: 12mins | Ready in:

Ingredients

- 2 cups brown sugar
- 1/2 cup shortening
- 1 cup peanut butter
- 2 eggs
- 1 1/2 cups milk
- 1 teaspoon vanilla extract
- 2 1/2 cups all-purpose flour
- 1 teaspoon baking soda
- 2 teaspoons cream of tartar
- 1 pinch salt

Direction

- Preheat an oven to 175°C/350°F. Grease then flour/line paper liners on a cupcake pan.
- Mix peanut butter, shortening and brown sugar till fluffy and light in a big bowl. One by one, beat in eggs; mix in vanilla. Mix salt, baking soda, cream of tartar and flour; alternately with milk, mix into batter. Put into prepped muffin cups.
- In the preheated oven, bake till cupcake's tops spring back when pressed lightly for 15-20 minutes; cool for a minimum of 10 minutes in pan. Transfer to a wire rack; fully cool.

Nutrition Information

- Calories: 209 calories;
- Total Fat: 10.5
- Sodium: 118
- Total Carbohydrate: 24.8
- Cholesterol: 17
- Protein: 5.1

381. Peanut Butter Cupcakes With Creamy Chocolate Frosting

Serving: 22 cupcakes. | Prep: 30mins | Cook: 25mins | Ready in:

Ingredients

- 3/4 cup creamy peanut butter
- 1/2 cup butter, softened
- 1 cup sugar
- 1/2 cup packed brown sugar
- 4 eggs
- 2 teaspoons vanilla extract

- 2 cups all-purpose flour
- 3/4 teaspoon baking soda
- 1/2 teaspoon baking powder
- 1/4 teaspoon salt
- 3/4 cup buttermilk
- CREAMY CHOCOLATE FROSTING:
- 1/4 cup butter, softened
- 3-1/2 cups confectioners' sugar
- 1/2 cup baking cocoa
- 6 tablespoons milk
- 1-1/2 teaspoons vanilla extract
- 1/4 teaspoon salt

Direction

- Cream together sugars, butter and peanut butter in a big bowl until fluffy and light. Beat in vanilla and eggs. Mix together salt, baking powder, baking soda and flour, then add into the creamed mixture together with buttermilk, alternately while beating well after each addition. Fill paper-lined cups until 2/3 full.
- Bake at 350° until a toothpick tucked in the center comes out clean, for about 24 to 26 minutes. Allow to cool for 10 minutes before turning from pans to wire racks to cool thoroughly.
- For frosting, cream butter in a small bowl until fluffy and light. Beat in salt, vanilla, milk, baking cocoa and sugar gradually, then frost cupcakes.

Nutrition Information

- Calories: 302 calories
- Sodium: 216mg sodium
- Fiber: 1g fiber)
- Total Carbohydrate: 45g carbohydrate (33g sugars
- Cholesterol: 56mg cholesterol
- Protein: 5g protein.
- Total Fat: 12g fat (5g saturated fat)

382. Peanut Butter Truffle Cupcakes

Serving: 1 dozen. | Prep: 40mins | Cook: 15mins | Ready in:

Ingredients

- 6 ounces white baking chocolate, coarsely chopped
- 1/4 cup creamy peanut butter
- 2 tablespoons baking cocoa
- BATTER:
- 1/2 cup butter, softened
- 3/4 cup sugar
- 2 large eggs
- 1 teaspoon vanilla extract
- 3/4 cup all-purpose flour
- 1/2 cup baking cocoa
- 1/2 teaspoon baking soda
- 1/4 teaspoon salt
- 1/2 cup buttermilk
- 1/2 cup strong brewed coffee
- FROSTING:
- 3 ounces semisweet chocolate, chopped
- 1/3 cup heavy whipping cream
- 3 tablespoons creamy peanut butter

Direction

- Truffles: Melt chocolate for 1 minute at 70% power in microwave-safe bowl; mix. Microwave in extra 10-20-sec intervals, mixing till smooth; mix in peanut butter. Cover; refrigerate till firm enough to shape to balls for 15-20 minutes. Form to 12 1-in. balls then roll in cocoa; put aside.
- Cream sugar and butter till fluffy and light in a big bowl. One by one, add eggs; beat well after each. Beat in vanilla. Mix salt, baking soda, cocoa and flour. Alternately with coffee and buttermilk, add to creamed mixture slowly; stir well.
- Fill the paper-lined muffin cups to 2/3 full. Put a truffle over each; don't press down.
- Bake at 350° till inserted toothpick in cake portion exits clean for 15-20 minutes. Cool for

10 minutes. Transfer from pan onto wire rack; fully cool.
- Melt cream and chocolate in a heavy saucepan on low heat, constantly mixing; take off heat. Mix in peanut butter till smooth. Put into small bowl; chill till it gets spreading consistency. Frost cupcakes. Keep refrigerated.

Nutrition Information

- Calories: 277 calories
- Protein: 6g protein.
- Total Fat: 18g fat (8g saturated fat)
- Sodium: 249mg sodium
- Fiber: 2g fiber)
- Total Carbohydrate: 26g carbohydrate (16g sugars
- Cholesterol: 66mg cholesterol

383. Peanut Filled Devil's Food Cupcakes

Serving: 2 dozen. | Prep: 30mins | Cook: 15mins | Ready in:

Ingredients

- 1/2 cup plus 2 tablespoons butter, softened
- 1-1/2 cups sugar
- 1 teaspoon vanilla extract
- 3 large eggs
- 1-1/4 cups cake flour
- 1/2 cup baking cocoa
- 1 teaspoon baking soda
- 1/2 teaspoon salt
- 1/4 teaspoon baking powder
- 1/2 cup buttermilk
- 1/2 cup strong brewed coffee, cooled
- FILLING:
- 1 cup creamy peanut butter
- 1/2 cup butter, softened
- 1-1/4 cups confectioners' sugar
- GANACHE:
- 4 ounces semisweet chocolate, chopped
- 1/2 cup heavy whipping cream
- 1/2 cup dry roasted peanuts

Direction

- Preheat the oven to 325 degrees. Put paper liners in 24 muffin cups.
- Mix sugar and butter in a bowl until texture is crumbly. Put in vanilla; beat eggs in one at a time, mix after each addition. Whisk cocoa, flour, salt, baking soda and baking powder in another bowl. Mix into creamed mixture alternating with coffee and buttermilk until combined.
- Pour into cups until half full. Bake for 15-20 minutes or until a toothpick poked in middle is clean. Let cool for 10 minutes. Take out of pans onto wire racks and let cool thoroughly.
- Scoop 1 in. deep the center of every cupcake out with a melon baller. For filling, mix butter and peanut butter until fluffy. Slowly add in the confectioner's sugar. Spoon or pipe 1 tablespoon of filling into each cupcake center.
- For ganache, put chocolate in a bowl. Bring the cream just to a boil in a saucepan. Pour the cream on the chocolate and mix until smooth. Let cool for 10 minutes or until mixture has thickened. Spread a scant tablespoon of ganache on each cupcake. Top with peanuts. Chill about 20 minutes or until set. Chill remaining cupcakes.

Nutrition Information

- Calories: 294 calories
- Sodium: 282mg sodium
- Fiber: 1g fiber)
- Total Carbohydrate: 29g carbohydrate (20g sugars
- Cholesterol: 57mg cholesterol
- Protein: 6g protein.
- Total Fat: 19g fat (8g saturated fat)

384. Peppermint Red Velvet Cupcakes

Serving: 2 dozen. | Prep: 25mins | Cook: 20mins | Ready in:

Ingredients

- 1 package German chocolate cake mix (regular size)
- 1 cup (8 ounces) sour cream
- 3 large eggs
- 1/4 cup water
- 1/3 cup canola oil
- 1 bottle (1 ounce) red food coloring
- 1 cup (6 ounces) miniature semisweet chocolate chips
- FROSTING:
- 1/2 cup butter, softened
- 1 package (8 ounces) reduced-fat cream cheese
- 12 ounces white baking chocolate, melted
- 2 teaspoons peppermint extract
- 7 cups confectioners' sugar
- White chocolate curls and crushed peppermint candies, optional

Direction

- Beat the cake mix, water, food coloring, oil, sour cream, and eggs in a large bowl on low speed for 30 seconds. Whisk the mixture at medium speed for 2 more minutes and then fold in the chocolate chips.
- Pour the mixture into the paper-lined muffin cups, filling them up to 2/3 full. Bake it inside the 350° oven for 18 to 22 minutes until the inserted toothpick into the center will come out clean. Let them cool for 10 minutes and then transfer them onto wire racks to fully cool.
- Mix the cream cheese and butter in a large bowl until fluffy for the frosting. Mix in the extract and melted white chocolate. Mix in the confectioners' sugar until smooth.
- Frost the cupcakes and sprinkle them with peppermint candies and chocolate curls if desired. Store them inside the fridge.

Nutrition Information

- Calories: 450 calories
- Protein: 4g protein.
- Total Fat: 20g fat (10g saturated fat)
- Sodium: 255mg sodium
- Fiber: 0 fiber)
- Total Carbohydrate: 66g carbohydrate (56g sugars
- Cholesterol: 52mg cholesterol

385. Pink Velvet Cupcakes

Serving: 2 dozen. | Prep: 30mins | Cook: 25mins | Ready in:

Ingredients

- 1 cup butter, softened
- 1-1/4 cups sugar
- 1/8 teaspoon pink paste food coloring
- 3 eggs
- 1 teaspoon vanilla extract
- 2-1/2 cups all-purpose flour
- 1-1/2 teaspoons baking powder
- 1/4 teaspoon baking soda
- 1/4 teaspoon salt
- 1 cup buttermilk
- WHITE CHOCOLATE GANACHE:
- 2 cups white baking chips
- 1/2 cup heavy whipping cream
- 1 tablespoon butter
- Pink coarse sugar and sugar pearls

Direction

- Cream food coloring, sugar and butter till fluffy and light in a big bowl. One by one, add eggs; beat well after each. Beat in vanilla. Mix salt, baking soda, baking powder and flour. Alternately with buttermilk, add to creamed mixture; beat well after each.

- Fill the paper-lined muffin cups to 2/3 full; bake it at 350° till inserted toothpick in middle exits clean for 23-27 minutes. Cool for 10 minutes. Transfer from pans onto wire racks; fully cool.
- Meanwhile, in a small bowl, put in white chips. Boil cream in a small saucepan. Put on chips; whisk till smooth. Mix in butter; put into big bowl. Chill, mixing once, for 30 minutes.
- Beat at high speed till frosting is fluffy and light and soft peaks form for 2-3 minutes. Frost cupcakes. Roll cupcake's edges with coarse sugar; use sugar pearls to decorate. Keep refrigerated.

Nutrition Information

- Calories: 266 calories
- Cholesterol: 57mg cholesterol
- Protein: 3g protein.
- Total Fat: 15g fat (9g saturated fat)
- Sodium: 154mg sodium
- Fiber: 0 fiber)
- Total Carbohydrate: 29g carbohydrate (20g sugars

386. Pumpkin Pecan Bites

Serving: about 6 dozen. | Prep: 20mins | Cook: 20mins | Ready in:

Ingredients

- 1 package spice cake mix (regular size)
- 1 can (15 ounces) solid-pack pumpkin
- 3 large eggs
- 1/2 cup canola oil
- 1 tablespoon ground cinnamon
- 1 teaspoon baking soda
- 1/4 teaspoon ground cloves
- 36 pecan halves, cut in half
- CREAM CHEESE FROSTING:
- 1/2 cup butter, softened
- 4 ounces cream cheese, softened
- 1 teaspoon vanilla extract
- 3-3/4 cups confectioners' sugar
- 2 to 3 tablespoons whole milk
- Ground cinnamon

Direction

- Combine the cake mix, cloves, baking soda, cinnamon, oil, eggs, and pumpkin in a large bowl; beat for 30 seconds on low speed. Then continue to beat for 2 minutes on medium.
- Fill 2/3 full into the paper-lined mini muffin cups. Next, press into each with a pecan piece. Bake for 17-20 minutes at 350°, or until inserting in the center with a toothpick and it comes out clean. Then let it cool for around 5 minutes before transferring from pans to wire racks to completely cool.
- Cream the cream cheese, butter, and vanilla in a small bowl until fluffy and light. Add confectioners' sugar gradually and mix well. Next, add enough milk to get the spreading consistency. Then frost the cupcakes and scatter with cinnamon.

Nutrition Information

- Calories: 191 calories
- Total Fat: 10g fat (3g saturated fat)
- Sodium: 186mg sodium
- Fiber: 1g fiber)
- Total Carbohydrate: 25g carbohydrate (19g sugars
- Cholesterol: 32mg cholesterol
- Protein: 2g protein.

387. Pumpkin Spice Cupcakes

Serving: 24 | Prep: 25mins | Cook: 25mins | Ready in:

Ingredients

- 2 1/4 cups all-purpose flour

- 1 teaspoon ground cinnamon
- 1/2 teaspoon ground nutmeg
- 1/2 teaspoon ground ginger
- 1/2 teaspoon ground cloves
- 1/2 teaspoon ground allspice
- 1/2 teaspoon salt
- 1 tablespoon baking powder
- 1/2 teaspoon baking soda
- 1/2 cup butter, softened
- 1 cup white sugar
- 1/3 cup brown sugar
- 2 eggs, room temperature
- 3/4 cup milk
- 1 cup pumpkin puree
- Cinnamon Cream Cheese Frosting
- 1 (8 ounce) package cream cheese, softened
- 1/4 cup butter, softened
- 3 cups confectioners' sugar
- 1 teaspoon vanilla extract
- 1 teaspoon ground cinnamon

Direction

- Set the oven at 190° C (375° F) to preheat. Coat 24 muffin cups with cooking spray or line them with paper muffin liners. Sift baking soda, baking powder, salt, allspice, clove, ginger, nutmeg, 1 teaspoon of cinnamon and flour together; put aside.
- In a big bowl, beat brown sugar, white sugar and 1/2 cup of butter using an electric mixer until fluffy and light. The color of the mixture should be visibly lighter. Put in room-temperature eggs, 1 egg at a time, let egg blend into the butter mixture after each addition. Stir in pumpkin puree and milk after adding the last egg. Stir in the flour mixture and mix until just incorporated. Fill prepared muffin cups with the batter.
- Bake in the preheated oven for 25 minutes until the cupcakes turn golden and when you press it lightly, the tops spring back. Let it cool in the pans for 5 minutes before transferring to a wire rack to cool completely.
- As the cupcakes cool, prepare the frosting by beating 1/4 butter and cream cheese in a bowl using an electric mixer until smooth. Beat in a little confectioners' sugar at a time until incorporated. Put in 1 teaspoon ground cinnamon and vanilla extract; beat until the mixture is fluffy. Frost the cupcake with cream cheese icing when the cupcakes are already cool.

Nutrition Information

- Calories: 244 calories;
- Total Fat: 9.8
- Sodium: 220
- Total Carbohydrate: 37.2
- Cholesterol: 42
- Protein: 2.9

388. Pumpkin Spice Cupcakes With Cream Cheese Frosting

Serving: 2 dozen. | Prep: 25mins | Cook: 20mins | Ready in:

Ingredients

- 3/4 cup butter, softened
- 2-1/2 cups sugar
- 3 large eggs
- 1 can (15 ounces) solid-pack pumpkin
- 2-1/3 cups all-purpose flour
- 1 tablespoon pumpkin pie spice
- 1 teaspoon baking powder
- 1 teaspoon ground cinnamon
- 3/4 teaspoon salt
- 1/2 teaspoon baking soda
- 1/2 teaspoon ground ginger
- 1 cup buttermilk
- FROSTING:
- 1 package (8 ounces) cream cheese, softened
- 1/2 cup butter, softened
- 4 cups confectioners' sugar
- 1 teaspoon vanilla extract
- 2 teaspoons ground cinnamon

Direction

- Preheat oven to 350°. In a big bowl, cream sugar and butter until fluffy and light. Put in one egg at a time, beating properly after each addition. Put in pumpkin. Blend ginger, baking soda, salt, cinnamon, baking powder, pie spice and flour together; move to the creamed mixture alternately with buttermilk, properly beating after each addition.
- Fill three-fourths full of each 24 paper-lined muffin cups. Bake for 20-25 minutes, or till a toothpick pinned into the middle comes out clean. Let cool for 10 minutes before shifting from pans to wire racks for totally cooling.
- For frosting, in a big bowl, beat butter and cream cheese until fluffy. Put in cinnamon, vanilla and confectioners' sugar; beat till smooth. Frost the cupcakes. Chill the leftovers.

Nutrition Information

- Calories: 340 calories
- Sodium: 233mg sodium
- Fiber: 1g fiber)
- Total Carbohydrate: 53g carbohydrate (41g sugars
- Cholesterol: 62mg cholesterol
- Protein: 4g protein.
- Total Fat: 14g fat (8g saturated fat)

389. Raisin Zucchini Spice Cupcakes

Serving: 2 dozen. | Prep: 30mins | Cook: 20mins | Ready in:

Ingredients

- 1 package spice cake mix (regular size)
- 1-1/3 cups water
- 1/4 cup canola oil
- 3 large eggs
- 2 cups shredded zucchini
- 1/2 cup raisins
- CINNAMON FROSTING:
- 1/4 cup butter, softened
- 1-3/4 cups confectioners' sugar
- 1 teaspoon vanilla extract
- 1/2 teaspoon ground cinnamon
- 1/8 teaspoon ground nutmeg
- 1 to 2 tablespoons 2% milk

Direction

- Mix eggs, oil, water, and cake mix in a large bowl; whisk for half a minute at low speed. Whisk for 2 minutes at medium speed. Stir in raisins and zucchini. Pour in paper-lined muffin cups to 2/3 full.
- Bake at 350 degrees until a toothpick comes out clean when inserted into the center, for 18-22 minutes. Let cool for 10 minutes, then transfer onto wire racks and cool entirely.
- To make the frosting: Whisk butter until it is fluffy and light in a small bowl. Whisk in enough milk, nutmeg, cinnamon, vanilla, and confectioners' sugar to reach spreading consistency. Then frost the cupcakes.

Nutrition Information

- Calories: 183 calories
- Total Carbohydrate: 28g carbohydrate (20g sugars
- Cholesterol: 37mg cholesterol
- Protein: 2g protein. Diabetic Exchanges: 2 starch
- Total Fat: 7g fat (3g saturated fat)
- Sodium: 188mg sodium
- Fiber: 0 fiber)

390. Raspberry Peach Cupcakes

Serving: 2 dozen. | Prep: 25mins | Cook: 15mins | Ready in:

Ingredients

- 1 cup white baking chips
- 6 tablespoons butter, cubed
- 1 package white cake mix (regular size)
- 1 cup 2% milk
- 3 eggs
- 1 teaspoon vanilla extract
- 1 cup fresh raspberries
- 1/2 cup chopped peeled fresh peaches or frozen unsweetened peach slices, thawed and chopped
- LEMON FROSTING:
- 1/2 cup butter, softened
- 3 cups confectioners' sugar
- 2 tablespoons lemon juice
- Fresh raspberries and peach pieces, optional

Direction

- Melt butter and chips in a microwave; stir until smooth.
- Combine the melted chips, vanilla, eggs, milk and cake mix in a large bowl; beat on low speed for half a minute. Continue beating on medium for 2 minutes more. Fold in peaches and raspberries.
- Fill into muffin cups lined with paper until it reaches three-fourths full. Bake for 15-20 minutes at 350°, or until a toothpick put into the middle comes out clean. Allow to cool for 10 minutes before transferring from pans to wire racks to cool entirely.
- To make frosting, beat the lemon juice, confectioners' sugar and butter in a small bowl until smooth. Frost the cupcakes. If preferred, put fruit on top.

Nutrition Information

- Calories: 267 calories
- Protein: 3g protein.
- Total Fat: 12g fat (7g saturated fat)
- Sodium: 224mg sodium
- Fiber: 1g fiber)
- Total Carbohydrate: 38g carbohydrate (24g sugars
- Cholesterol: 47mg cholesterol

391. Raspberry Swirl Cupcakes

Serving: 2 dozen. | Prep: 20mins | Cook: 20mins | Ready in:

Ingredients

- 1 package white cake mix (regular size)
- 1/4 cup raspberry pie filling
- 1/2 cup shortening
- 1/3 cup 2% milk
- 1 teaspoon vanilla extract
- 1/4 teaspoon salt
- 3 cups confectioners' sugar
- Fresh raspberries and decorative sprinkles, optional

Direction

- For cake batter mix, prepare following to package instructions for cupcakes. Fill into paper-lined muffin cups until two-thirds full. Drop 1/2 teaspoon of pie filling in the middle of each; using a knife, cut through batter to swirl.
- Bake for 20-25 minutes at 350°, or until a toothpick put into the middle comes out clean. Let them cool for 10 minutes before transferring from pans to wire racks to completely cool.
- Beat shortening in a large bowl until fluffy. Add the salt, vanilla and milk; slowly add confectioners' sugar; continue beating until it gets smooth. Frost cupcakes. If preferred, garnish with sprinkles and raspberries.

Nutrition Information

- Calories: 230 calories
- Total Carbohydrate: 34g carbohydrate (25g sugars
- Cholesterol: 27mg cholesterol
- Protein: 2g protein.
- Total Fat: 10g fat (2g saturated fat)

- Sodium: 183mg sodium
- Fiber: 0 fiber)

392. Red Velvet Cupcakes With Coconut Frosting

Serving: 2 dozen. | Prep: 25mins | Cook: 20mins | Ready in:

Ingredients

- 3/4 cup butter, softened
- 1-1/2 cups sugar
- 2 eggs
- 1 tablespoon red food coloring
- 1 teaspoon vanilla extract
- 1-3/4 cups all-purpose flour
- 1/4 cup baking cocoa
- 3/4 teaspoon baking soda
- 3/4 teaspoon salt
- 1 cup buttermilk
- 1 teaspoon white vinegar
- FROSTING:
- 2 packages (8 ounces each) cream cheese, softened
- 1/4 cup butter, softened
- 1-1/2 cups confectioners' sugar
- 1 teaspoon vanilla extract
- 2 cups sweetened shredded coconut, divided

Direction

- Set the oven to 350° for preheating. Cream the sugar and butter in a large bowl until fluffy and light. Add the eggs, one at a time and whisking well every after addition. Mix in the vanilla and food coloring. Mix the salt, flour, baking soda, and cocoa. Mix vinegar and buttermilk. Add the dry ingredients to the creamed mixture, adding it alternately with the buttermilk mixture and whisking well every after addition.
- Fill the paper or foil-lined muffin cups with the mixture, about 2/3 full. Bake them for 18-22 minutes or until the inserted toothpick into the center comes out clean. Let them cool for 10 minutes. Remove them from the pans and place them onto a wire rack. Let them cool totally.
- Beat the butter and cream cheese in a large bowl for the frosting until fluffy. Add the vanilla and confectioners' sugar. Whisk the mixture until smooth. Mix in a cup of coconut. Use this to frost the cupcakes.
- Toast the remaining coconut, and then sprinkle it all over the cupcakes. Store them inside the fridge.

Nutrition Information

- Calories: 296 calories
- Cholesterol: 59mg cholesterol
- Protein: 4g protein.
- Total Fat: 18g fat (12g saturated fat)
- Sodium: 260mg sodium
- Fiber: 1g fiber)
- Total Carbohydrate: 32g carbohydrate (23g sugars

393. Red Wine And Chocolate Cupcakes

Serving: 2 dozen. | Prep: 15mins | Cook: 20mins | Ready in:

Ingredients

- 1/2 cup baking cocoa
- 4 ounces bittersweet chocolate, chopped
- 1/2 cup boiling water
- 1 cup butter, softened
- 1-1/2 cups sugar
- 4 large eggs
- 1-3/4 cups all-purpose flour
- 1-1/2 teaspoons baking powder
- 1 teaspoon salt
- 1/2 cup dry red wine
- MASCARPONE ICING:
- 2 cartons (8 ounces each) mascarpone cheese

- 2 cups confectioners' sugar
- 1/2 teaspoon vanilla extract

Direction

- Combine chocolate and cocoa in a small bowl. Add boiling water and whisk until chocolate is melted and mixture is well blended.
- Meanwhile, in a large bowl, cream butter and sugar until light and fluffy. Drop in eggs, one at a time, beating the mixture well after each addition. Combine the flour, salt and baking powder. Add into the creamed mixture alternately with wine and chocolate mixture, beating well after every addition. Arrange the paper-lined muffin cups and fill each with the batter to three-fourths full.
- Bake at 350 degrees for 18-22 minutes or until an inserted toothpick in the center comes out clean. Let the muffin cups cool for 10 minutes then transfer to wire racks and let it cool completely.
- Beat confectioner's sugar, mascarpone cheese and vanilla extract in a small bowl. Beat all ingredients together until creamy. Frost individual cupcakes then store in the refrigerator to chill.

Nutrition Information

- Calories: 318 calories
- Protein: 4g protein.
- Total Fat: 19g fat (11g saturated fat)
- Sodium: 212mg sodium
- Fiber: 1g fiber)
- Total Carbohydrate: 31g carbohydrate (23g sugars
- Cholesterol: 75mg cholesterol

394. Rich Chocolate Cupcakes

Serving: 14 cupcakes. | Prep: 30mins | Cook: 25mins | Ready in:

Ingredients

- 1/2 cup butter, softened
- 1 cup sugar
- 1 egg
- 1 teaspoon vanilla extract
- 1-1/2 cups all-purpose flour
- 1/2 cup baking cocoa
- 1 teaspoon baking soda
- 1/4 teaspoon salt
- 1/2 cup buttermilk
- 1/2 cup strong brewed coffee
- CHOCOLATE GANACHE:
- 4 ounces semisweet chocolate, coarsely chopped
- 1/2 cup heavy whipping cream
- 1/2 teaspoon vanilla extract

Direction

- Beat sugar and butter in a small bowl until light and fluffy. Whip in vanilla and egg. Mix the salt, baking soda, cocoa and flour; slowly put to creamed mixture alternately with buttermilk and coffee, whipping thoroughly after each time.
- Scoop into paper-lined muffin tins, about 2/3 full. Bake for 25 to 30 mins at 350° or until a toothpick inserted in the middle comes out clean. Let cool for 10 minutes before taking out from pans to wire racks to cool completely.
- Melt chocolate with cream in a small saucepan over low heat; mix until combined. Take off from the heat. Mix in vanilla. Put to a bowl; cover and chill until mixture has a spreading consistency, mixing from time to time. Put on cupcakes to frost.

Nutrition Information

- Calories: 219 calories
- Total Carbohydrate: 28g carbohydrate (16g sugars
- Cholesterol: 45mg cholesterol
- Protein: 3g protein.
- Total Fat: 11g fat (7g saturated fat)
- Sodium: 216mg sodium

- Fiber: 1g fiber)

395. Simply Decorated Cupcakes

Serving: 2 dozen (3 cups frosting). | Prep: 30mins | Cook: 20mins | Ready in:

Ingredients

- 1 package chocolate cake mix (regular size)
- BUTTERCREAM FROSTING:
- 1/2 cup butter, softened
- 4-1/2 cups confectioners' sugar
- 1-1/2 teaspoons vanilla extract
- 5 to 6 tablespoons milk
- Halved large marshmallows and gumdrops

Direction

- Follow package directions to prep cake batter. Fill the paper-lined muffin cups to 2/3 full; bake at 350° till toothpick exits clean for 20-22 minutes. Cool for 10 minutes. Transfer from pans onto wire racks; fully cool.
- Frosting: Cream butter till fluffy and light in a big bowl; beat in vanilla and confectioners' sugar. To get spreading consistency, add enough milk.
- In corner of pastry bag, cut a small hole; insert a #20 star pastry tip. Use frosting to fill bag 1/2 full. Pipe frosting into thin, concentric circles, 1/2-in. apart, starting with outer edge of every cupcake. If desired, tie a ribbon around every cupcake.

Nutrition Information

- Calories:
- Sodium:
- Fiber:
- Total Carbohydrate:
- Cholesterol:
- Protein:

- Total Fat:

396. Sour Cream Chocolate Cupcakes

Serving: 2 dozen. | Prep: 30mins | Cook: 20mins | Ready in:

Ingredients

- 1/4 cup butter, cubed
- 4 ounces unsweetened chocolate, chopped
- 2 eggs
- 2 cups sugar
- 1 cup water
- 3/4 cup sour cream
- 1 teaspoon vanilla extract
- 2 cups all-purpose flour
- 1 teaspoon baking soda
- FROSTING:
- 1/2 cup butter, cubed
- 4 ounces unsweetened chocolate, chopped
- 4 cups confectioners' sugar
- 1/2 cup sour cream
- 2 teaspoons vanilla extract

Direction

- Microwave chocolate and butter until melted and mix to smoothen. Allow to cool for 10 minutes. Beat vanilla, sour cream, water, sugar and eggs in a big bowl. Mix together baking soda and flour; pour into egg mixture and stir thoroughly. Put in chocolate mixture; on high speed, beat the mixture for 2 to 3 minutes.
- In muffins cup lined with paper liners, pour in batter to 2/3 full. Bake in 350-degree oven until a toothpick is clean when coming out of the middle, 18 to 20 minutes. Allow to cool for 10 minutes in pans, then transfer to wire racks and finish cooling.
- To make the frosting, microwave chocolate and butter in a microwaveable bowl until melted and whisk until smooth. Allow to cool for 10 minutes. Using a portable mixer on low,

beat in vanilla, sour cream and confectioners' sugar until smooth. Frost onto cupcakes. Keep in the refrigerator to store.

Nutrition Information

- Calories: 275 calories
- Total Fat: 10g fat (6g saturated fat)
- Sodium: 123mg sodium
- Fiber: 1g fiber)
- Total Carbohydrate: 46g carbohydrate (35g sugars
- Cholesterol: 41mg cholesterol
- Protein: 2g protein.

397. Special Mocha Cupcakes

Serving: 1 dozen. | Prep: 25mins | Cook: 20mins | Ready in:

Ingredients

- 1 cup sugar
- 1/2 cup cold brewed coffee
- 1/2 cup canola oil
- 2 large eggs
- 3 teaspoons cider vinegar
- 3 teaspoons vanilla extract
- 1-1/2 cups all-purpose flour
- 1/3 cup baking cocoa
- 1 teaspoon baking soda
- 1/2 teaspoon salt
- MOCHA FROSTING:
- 3 tablespoons milk chocolate chips
- 3 tablespoons semisweet chocolate chips
- 1/3 cup butter, softened
- 2 cups confectioners' sugar
- 1 to 2 tablespoons brewed coffee
- 1/2 cup chocolate sprinkles

Direction

- Preheat oven to 350°. Beat coffee, sugar, eggs, oil, vanilla and vinegar in a large bowl until blended well. Combine baking soda, flour, salt and cocoa in a small bowl; beat into coffee mixture gradually until blended.
- Fill about three-fourths full of paper-lined muffin cups. Bake for around 20 to 25 minutes or until a toothpick inserted in center comes out clean. Allow 10 minutes to cool before taking away from pan to a wire rack for cooling.
- For frosting, in a microwave, melt butter and chips; stir until smooth. Remove to a large bowl. Beat in enough coffee and confectioners' sugar gradually to achieve the level of desired consistency. On cupcakes, pipe frosting. Place sprinkles on top; press down gently.

Nutrition Information

- Calories: 412 calories
- Total Carbohydrate: 59g carbohydrate (42g sugars
- Cholesterol: 49mg cholesterol
- Protein: 4g protein.
- Total Fat: 19g fat (5g saturated fat)
- Sodium: 255mg sodium
- Fiber: 1g fiber)

398. Spice Cupcakes

Serving: 15 | Prep: 20mins | Cook: 15mins | Ready in:

Ingredients

- 1 1/2 cups all-purpose flour
- 1/2 cup cornstarch
- 2 teaspoons baking powder
- 1 teaspoon ground cinnamon
- 4 pinches ground nutmeg
- 4 pinches salt
- 12 tablespoons butter
- 1 1/3 cups sugar
- 4 eggs
- 1 teaspoon vanilla extract
- 1/2 cup milk

Direction

- Set the oven to 350°F or 175°C for preheating. Use the paper muffin liners to line 15 muffin cups.
- In a bowl, sift the baking powder, salt, nutmeg, flour, cinnamon, and cornstarch.
- In a large bowl, beat the sugar and butter using the electric mixer until fluffy and light. Add eggs to the mixture, one at a time and let each egg blend into the butter mixture before adding the next one. Mix in the vanilla together with the last egg. Whisk in the flour mixture, adding it alternately with the milk. Spread the batter into the prepared cups.
- Let them bake inside the preheated oven for 15-20 minutes until golden and their tops will spring back once pressed lightly.

Nutrition Information

- Calories: 238 calories;
- Cholesterol: 75
- Protein: 3.4
- Total Fat: 10.9
- Sodium: 136
- Total Carbohydrate: 32.1

399. Spice Cupcakes With Mocha Frosting

Serving: 15 cupcakes. | Prep: 30mins | Cook: 20mins | Ready in:

Ingredients

- 1/2 cup butter, softened
- 1/2 cup sugar
- 1 large egg
- 1/2 cup molasses
- 1-1/2 cups all-purpose flour
- 1/2 teaspoon baking soda
- 1/4 teaspoon salt
- 1/4 teaspoon each ground cinnamon, cloves and nutmeg
- 1/2 cup buttermilk
- FROSTING:
- 1-3/4 cups confectioners' sugar
- 1 tablespoon baking cocoa
- 2 tablespoons strong brewed coffee
- 1 tablespoon butter, softened
- 1/4 teaspoon vanilla extract
- Chocolate-covered coffee beans and assorted candies, optional

Direction

- Beat sugar and butter in a big bowl until fluffy and light. Mix in molasses and egg. Combine the nutmeg, cloves, cinnamon, salt, baking soda, and flour; put in creamed mixture alternately with the buttermilk.
- Fill muffin cups lined with paper; two-thirds full. Place in the oven and bake for 20-25 minutes at 350°F or until a toothpick pricked in the middle exits clean. Let cool for 10 minutes before taking out of pans to wire racks to fully cool. In a small bowl, mix the cocoa and confectioner's sugar. Mix in the vanilla, butter, and coffee until it turns smooth. Frost the cupcakes. Decorate with candies and coffee beans if you want.

Nutrition Information

- Calories: 227 calories
- Sodium: 147mg sodium
- Fiber: 0 fiber)
- Total Carbohydrate: 39g carbohydrate (26g sugars
- Cholesterol: 32mg cholesterol
- Protein: 2g protein.
- Total Fat: 7g fat (4g saturated fat)

400. Spiced Apple Cupcakes

Serving: 2 dozen. | Prep: 25mins | Cook: 20mins | Ready in:

Ingredients

- 1 medium apple, peeled and finely chopped
- 1/2 teaspoon ground coriander
- 1/2 cup butter, softened
- 3/4 cup packed brown sugar
- 1/2 cup sugar
- 4 eggs
- 1 cup unsweetened applesauce
- 2 cups all-purpose flour
- 1 teaspoon baking soda
- 1/2 teaspoon salt
- 1/2 teaspoon ground cinnamon
- 1/4 teaspoon ground nutmeg
- 1/4 teaspoon ground allspice
- 1/4 teaspoon cayenne pepper
- MAPLE CREAM CHEESE FROSTING:
- 1 package (8 ounces) cream cheese, softened
- 1/2 cup butter, softened
- 4 cups confectioners' sugar
- 2 tablespoons maple syrup
- Ground allspice

Direction

- Sauté coriander and apple till tender in a small skillet. Take off heat; put aside.
- Cream sugars and butter till fluffy and light in a big bowl. One by one, add eggs; beat well after each. Beat in applesauce; it'll look curdled. Mix cayenne, allspice, nutmeg, cinnamon, salt, baking soda and flour; add to creamed mixture slowly till combined. Fold in the apple mixture; fill the paper-lined muffin cups to 2/3 full.
- Bake for 18-22 minutes at 350° till inserted toothpick in middle exits clean. Cool it for 10 minutes. Transfer from pans onto wire racks; fully cool.
- Beat butter and cream cheese till fluffy and light in a small bowl. Add maple syrup and confectioners' sugar; beat till smooth. Pipe frosting on cupcakes; sprinkle allspice. Keep refrigerated.

Nutrition Information

- Calories: 282 calories
- Total Carbohydrate: 42g carbohydrate (32g sugars
- Cholesterol: 66mg cholesterol
- Protein: 3g protein.
- Total Fat: 12g fat (7g saturated fat)
- Sodium: 198mg sodium
- Fiber: 1g fiber)

401. Spiced Carrot Cupcakes

Serving: 1 dozen. | Prep: 30mins | Cook: 25mins | Ready in:

Ingredients

- 1-1/2 cups all-purpose flour
- 1 cup plus 2 tablespoons sugar
- 1/3 cup packed brown sugar
- 1-1/2 teaspoons ground cinnamon
- 1 teaspoon baking soda
- 1/2 teaspoon salt
- 1/2 teaspoon ground nutmeg
- 1/4 teaspoon ground ginger
- 2 eggs
- 1/2 cup canola oil
- 1 teaspoon vanilla extract
- 2 cups finely shredded carrots
- 1/2 cup crushed pineapple, drained
- 1/2 cup chopped walnuts
- WHITE CHOCOLATE CREAM CHEESE FROSTING:
- 4 ounces cream cheese, softened
- 1/4 cup butter, softened
- 1 ounce white baking chocolate, melted and cooled
- 1 tablespoon heavy whipping cream
- 1/2 teaspoon vanilla extract
- 1/4 teaspoon orange extract

- 2 cups confectioners' sugar
- Chopped walnuts, optional

Direction

- Mix together the first eight ingredients in a large bowl. Beat vanilla, oil and eggs in another bowl. Mix into the dry ingredients just till moisten. Fold in walnuts, pineapple and carrots.
- Fill paper-lined muffin cup three-fourths full. Bake at 350° till a toothpick comes out clean when inserted into the center, 25-28 minutes. Allow to cool for 10 minutes; take out of pan and place on a wire rack.
- For frosting, beat butter and cream cheese in a small bowl, till smooth. Beat in extracts, cream and chocolate. Slowly beat in confectioners' sugar till smooth. Spread or pipe over the cupcakes; use walnuts for garnish if you want. Keep in a refrigerator.

Nutrition Information

- Calories: 458 calories
- Protein: 5g protein.
- Total Fat: 21g fat (7g saturated fat)
- Sodium: 188mg sodium
- Fiber: 1g fiber)
- Total Carbohydrate: 63g carbohydrate (48g sugars
- Cholesterol: 58mg cholesterol

402. Spooky Spider Cupcakes

Serving: 1 dozen. | Prep: 20mins | Cook: 20mins | Ready in:

Ingredients

- 6 tablespoons butter, softened
- 1 cup packed brown sugar
- 1 large egg
- 1/2 cup unsweetened applesauce
- 1 teaspoon vanilla extract
- 1 teaspoon grated orange zest
- 1 cup all-purpose flour
- 1 teaspoon baking powder
- 1/2 teaspoon salt
- 1/4 teaspoon baking soda
- 1/2 cup chopped pecans
- FROSTING:
- 1/4 cup butter, softened
- 2 cups confectioners' sugar
- 1-1/2 teaspoons grated orange zest
- Orange paste food coloring
- 2 to 4 teaspoons orange juice
- 1/2 cup chocolate frosting
- Black shoestring licorice
- 12 black gumdrops

Direction

- Cream brown sugar and butter till fluffy and light in a small bowl; beat in egg then beat in orange zest, vanilla and applesauce. Mix baking soda, salt, baking powder and flour. Add to creamed mixture slowly till combined well; mix in pecans.
- Fill the paper-lined muffin cups to 1/2 full; bake it at 350° till inserted toothpick in middle exits clean for 20-25 minutes. Cool for 10 minutes. Transfer from pan onto wire rack; fully cool.
- Frosting: Cream confectioners' sugar and butter till fluffy and light in a small bowl. Add enough orange juice, food coloring and orange zest to get spreading consistency; put 1/4 cup orange frosting aside. Frost cupcakes.
- Put chocolate frosting into heavy-duty resealable bag; in corner of bag, cut a small hole. Pipe chocolate circle in middle of every cupcake; pipe thin, evenly spaced concentric circles, 1/4-in. apart. Pull toothpick through circles toward the outer edge gently starting with the center circle. Wipe the toothpick clean. To complete web pattern, repeat.
- Cut licorice to 2-inch pieces; in every gumdrop for legs, press 8 pieces. Put reserved orange frosting into heavy-duty resealable bag; in corner of bag, cut a small hole. On every

spider gumdrop, pipe eyes; position onto cupcakes.

Nutrition Information

- Calories: 361 calories
- Sodium: 294mg sodium
- Fiber: 1g fiber)
- Total Carbohydrate: 55g carbohydrate (44g sugars
- Cholesterol: 43mg cholesterol
- Protein: 2g protein.
- Total Fat: 16g fat (7g saturated fat)

403. Strawberry Cheesecake Cupcakes

Serving: 24 servings | Prep: 15mins | Cook: | Ready in:

Ingredients

- 2 cups graham cracker crumbs
- 1 cup sugar, divided
- 6 Tbsp. butter, melted
- 2 cups fresh strawberries, divided
- 2 Tbsp. strawberry jam
- 3 pkg. (8 oz. each) PHILADELPHIA Cream Cheese, softened
- 1 pkg. (3 oz.) JELL-O Lemon Flavor Gelatin
- 1 tub (8 oz.) COOL WHIP Whipped Topping, thawed
- 1 Tbsp. lemon zest

Direction

- 1. Combine together in a bowl the butter, 1/4 cup sugar and graham crumbs and mix well; place onto a 24 paper-lined muffin cups and compress onto bottoms. Place inside the refrigerator until prepared.
- 2. Slice strawberries enough to measure 1-1/2 cups; put in a medium bowl. Add in jam; lightly stir. Set aside left berries for garnishing later.
- 3. Whip in a bowl together the left sugar and cream cheese until well combined. Mix in gelatin mix; combine well. Mix in COOL WHIP. Scoop about 1 tbsp. cream cheese mixture on top of every crust. Put chopped strawberry mixture and left cream cheese mixture on top.
- 4. Place inside the refrigerator for 4 hours or until solid. Use set aside lemon zest and berries to garnish.

Nutrition Information

- Calories: 240
- Sugar: 18 g
- Total Carbohydrate: 24 g
- Cholesterol: 45 mg
- Protein: 3 g
- Total Fat: 15 g
- Fiber: 1 g
- Saturated Fat: 9 g
- Sodium: 200 mg

404. Sugar Ghost Cupcakes

Serving: 2 dozen. | Prep: 03hours00mins | Cook: 20mins | Ready in:

Ingredients

- 1 package chocolate cake mix (regular size)
- FONDANT:
- 1 package (16 ounces) miniature marshmallows
- 4 to 5 tablespoons water
- 1 package (2 pounds) confectioners' sugar
- 1/2 cup shortening
- DECORATING:
- 1 can (16 ounces) vanilla frosting
- Blue, orange and green paste food coloring
- Miniature peanut butter cups
- Malted milk balls
- Clear vanilla extract

Direction

- Follow the package directions to prepare and bake the cake mix for the cupcakes. Let them cool completely on wire racks.
- Combine 2 tbsp. of water and marshmallows in a large and microwave-safe bowl. Microwave the mixture while uncovered on high setting for 1 1/2-2 minutes, stirring every 30 seconds until melted. Mix in 3/4 of the sugar. Coat the work surface with 3 tbsp. of shortening and lay the mixture on it.
- Knead the mixture until pliable and smooth, adding leftover shortening and sugar gradually. If needed, moisten the mixture with additional water. To keep it from drying out, wrap it with a plastic wrap.
- Reserve 1/4 cup of the frosting for decorating. Tint the remaining frosting with blue and use it to frost the cupcakes.
- For the ghosts, invert two of the peanut butter cups and stack them, making sure they are secured with a small amount of the reserved frosting. Top the cups with a malted milk ball, attaching it using the frosting. Repeat the same procedures until you have a total of 24 stacks.
- Sprinkle the work surface with confectioners' sugar lightly. Roll 1 1/4-inches of fondant ball onto the work surface until it forms a 4-inches circle. Drape the circle over the stack. Cut out some shapes for the mouth and eyes using the pastry tips. Do the same process for leftover ghosts.
- For the tendrils, stems, and pumpkins, tint enough amount of fondant with orange. Wrap the fondant around the malted milk balls and shape them into pumpkins. Use a toothpick or veining tool to imprint lines on it.
- For the tendrils and stems, tint enough amount of fondant with green. Shape it into stems and attach it into pumpkins using the vanilla. For the tendrils, roll the remaining green fondant out and cut it into thin strips using the pizza cutter. Wrap the strips around the toothpicks gently and put them aside until dry. (You can wrap the remaining fondant in a plastic wrap tightly and store it inside the resealable plastic bag for future use.) To finalize the cupcakes, top each cupcake with a small amount of the reserved frosting. Place the prepared ghost on top of the cupcake. Remove the tendrils from the toothpick carefully. Use the vanilla to attach the tendrils to the pumpkins. As desired, attach the pumpkins into the cupcakes.

Nutrition Information

- Calories: 441 calories
- Total Carbohydrate: 84g carbohydrate (68g sugars
- Cholesterol: 23mg cholesterol
- Protein: 2g protein.
- Total Fat: 11g fat (3g saturated fat)
- Sodium: 225mg sodium
- Fiber: 1g fiber)

405. Sugar Plum Fairy Cupcakes

Serving: 18 cupcakes. | Prep: 40mins | Cook: 20mins | Ready in:

Ingredients

- 1/2 cup butter, softened
- 1-1/2 cups sugar
- 4 egg whites
- 2 teaspoons vanilla extract
- 2 cups all-purpose flour
- 1 teaspoon baking powder
- 1/2 teaspoon baking soda
- 1/4 teaspoon salt
- 1-1/3 cups buttermilk
- 1 cup plum jam
- FROSTING:
- 1 cup sugar
- 2 egg whites
- 1/4 cup water
- 1/4 teaspoon cream of tartar
- 1 teaspoon vanilla extract

- Edible glitter and coarse sugar

Direction

- Cream the sugar and butter in a large bowl until fluffy and light. Add the egg whites, one at a time and whisking well every after addition. Whisk in the vanilla. Mix the baking powder, salt, baking soda, and flour, and then add the mixture into the creamed mixture, adding it alternately with buttermilk. Make sure to whisk the mixture every after addition.
- Distribute the mixture among the paper-lined muffin cups, filling them 2/3 full. Bake them inside the 350° oven for 18 to 22 minutes or until the inserted toothpick into the center will come out clean. Let them cool for 10 minutes. Remove them from the pan and place them onto a wire rack. Let them cool completely.
- Slice a small hole into the plastic or pastry bag's corner. Insert a very small tip into the hole. Fill the bag with jam. Fill each cupcake by pushing the tip through the top.
- For the frosting, mix the cream of tartar, egg whites, sugar, and water in a large heavy saucepan over low heat. Using the hand mixer, whisk the mixture at low speed for a minute. Whisk for 8-10 minutes at low speed over low heat until the frosting reaches 160°. Transfer the mixture into a large bowl, and then add the vanilla. Whisk the mixture on high speed for 7 minutes until it forms stiff peaks.
- Pipe the frosting over each cupcake and sprinkle each with coarse sugar and glitter.

Nutrition Information

- Calories: 262 calories
- Sodium: 164mg sodium
- Fiber: 0 fiber)
- Total Carbohydrate: 51g carbohydrate (40g sugars
- Cholesterol: 14mg cholesterol
- Protein: 3g protein.
- Total Fat: 5g fat (3g saturated fat)

406. Surprise Red Cupcakes

Serving: 2 dozen. | Prep: 60mins | Cook: 20mins | Ready in:

Ingredients

- 2 cups sugar, divided
- 3 tablespoons plus 2 cups all-purpose flour, divided
- 1/2 cup milk
- 1/2 cup plus 1/3 cup shortening, divided
- 2 eggs
- 1 bottle (1 ounce) red food coloring
- 1 tablespoon white vinegar
- 2 teaspoons vanilla extract, divided
- 3 tablespoons baking cocoa
- 1 teaspoon baking soda
- 1 cup buttermilk
- 1/2 cup butter, softened
- 3 tablespoons confectioners' sugar
- FROSTING:
- 1 cup (6 ounces) semisweet chocolate chips
- 1/3 cup plus 1 to 3 teaspoons evaporated milk, divided
- 1-1/2 cups confectioners' sugar

Direction

- Boil milk, 3 tbsp. flour and 1/2 cup sugar in a heavy saucepan till smooth; mix and cook till thick for 1-2 minutes. Take off heat; cool.
- Cream leftover sugar and 1/2 cup shortening till fluffy and light in a big bowl. One by one, add eggs; beat well after each. Beat in 1 tsp. vanilla, vinegar and food coloring. Mix leftover flour, baking soda and cocoa. Alternately with buttermilk, add to creamed mixture slowly; beat well after each.
- Fill the paper-lined muffin cups to 2/3 full; bake it at 350° till inserted toothpick in middle exits clean for 20-25 minutes. Cool for 10 minutes. Transfer from pans onto wire racks; fully cool.
- Beat leftover shortening and butter till smooth in a small bowl; beat in leftover vanilla, cooled

sugar mixture and confectioners' sugar for 3 minutes till fluffy and light. Insert big round tip in plastic/pastry bag; use filling to fill. Insert tip halfway into middle of every cupcake; fill using small filling amount.
- Frosting: Melt 1/3 cup evaporated milk and chips in a heavy saucepan on low heat; mix till smooth. Take off heat. Beat in the confectioners' sugar. To get spreading consistency, add enough leftover milk; frost cupcakes.

Nutrition Information

- Calories: 288 calories
- Fiber: 1g fiber)
- Total Carbohydrate: 40g carbohydrate (29g sugars
- Cholesterol: 30mg cholesterol
- Protein: 3g protein.
- Total Fat: 14g fat (6g saturated fat)
- Sodium: 114mg sodium

407. Sweet Potato Cupcakes

Serving: Makes 16 cupcakes | Prep: | Cook: | Ready in:

Ingredients

- 1/2 cup oat flour
- 6 tablespoons all-purpose flour
- 1/2 teaspoon baking soda
- 6 tablespoons granulated sugar
- 2 tablespoons unsalted butter, at room temperature
- 1 egg white
- 1/4 cup cooked or canned sweet potato
- 1/4 teaspoon vanilla extract
- 2 tablespoons skim milk
- 1/4 cup confectioners' sugar
- 3 tablespoons reduced-fat cream cheese, at room temperature
- 1/4 teaspoon cinnamon
- 1/8 teaspoon ground cardamom
- 1/8 teaspoon ground cloves
- 2 tablespoons dried cranberries, chopped

Direction

- Heat an oven to 350°F. Use mini-muffin papers to line 16 cups of 2 12-cup mini-muffin pans. Mix baking soda and flours in a bowl. Cream butter and sugar together with electric mixer at medium in another bowl. Add vanilla, sweet potato and egg white; beat till well combined on low. Add milk and flour mixture; beat till just combined on low. Don't overmix then fill muffin cups to 2/3 full. Bake for 15-18 minutes till toothpick exits clean; cool in pans for 10 minutes. Remove from pans; fully cool. Beat spices, cream cheese and confectioners' sugar till smooth in a 3rd bowl. Frost cupcakes; use cranberries as garnish.

Nutrition Information

408. Texas Chocolate Cupcakes

Serving: 2 dozen. | Prep: 30mins | Cook: 15mins | Ready in:

Ingredients

- 2 cups all-purpose flour
- 2 cups sugar
- 1 teaspoon salt
- 1/2 teaspoon baking soda
- 1/4 cup baking cocoa
- 1 cup water
- 1 cup canola oil
- 1/2 cup butter, cubed
- 2 eggs
- 1/3 cup buttermilk
- 1 teaspoon vanilla extract
- CARAMEL ICING:
- 1 cup packed brown sugar

- 1/2 cup butter, cubed
- 1/4 cup milk
- 2 to 2-1/4 cups confectioners' sugar

Direction

- Mix the baking soda, salt, sugar and flour in a big bowl. Heat up the butter, oil, water and cocoa to a boil in a big saucepan over medium heat. Put to dry ingredients gradually and blend thoroughly. Mix the vanilla, buttermilk and eggs; put to batter gradually and stir well (batter will be very thin).
- Put batter in paper-lined muffin tins, about 3/4 full. Bake for 15 to 20 mins at 350° or until a toothpick inserted in the middle comes out clean. Let cool for 10 minutes before taking out from pans to wire racks to cool entirely.
- To make the icing, mix the milk, butter and brown sugar in a heavy saucepan. Cook and mix on low heat until sugar dissolved. Turn the heat up to medium. Don't mix. Cook for 3 to 6 minutes or until bubbles form in the middle of mixture and syrup turns into an amber color. Take off from the heat; put to a small bowl. Let cool to room temperature. Whip in confectioners' sugar gradually until smooth. Put on cupcakes to frost.

Nutrition Information

- Calories: 335 calories
- Fiber: 0 fiber)
- Total Carbohydrate: 44g carbohydrate (35g sugars
- Cholesterol: 39mg cholesterol
- Protein: 2g protein.
- Total Fat: 17g fat (6g saturated fat)
- Sodium: 216mg sodium

409. Walnut Banana Cupcakes

Serving: 1 dozen. | Prep: 25mins | Cook: 20mins | Ready in:

Ingredients

- 1/4 cup butter, softened
- 3/4 cup sugar
- 2 eggs
- 1/2 cup mashed ripe banana
- 1 teaspoon vanilla extract
- 1 cup all-purpose flour
- 1/2 teaspoon baking soda
- 1/2 teaspoon ground nutmeg
- 1/4 teaspoon salt
- 1/4 cup sour cream
- CREAM CHEESE FROSTING:
- 4 ounces cream cheese, softened
- 1/2 teaspoon vanilla extract
- 1-3/4 cups confectioners' sugar
- 3 tablespoons chopped walnuts

Direction

- Cream sugar and butter till fluffy and light in a big bowl. One by one, add eggs; beat well after each. Beat in vanilla and banana. Mix salt, nutmeg, baking soda and flour. Alternately with sour cream, add to creamed mixture slowly; mix well after each.
- Fill the paper-lined muffin cups to 1/2 full; bake at 350° till inserted toothpick in middle exits clean for 18-22 minutes. Cool for 10 minutes. Transfer from pan onto wire rack; fully cool.
- Frosting: Beat vanilla and cream cheese till smooth in a small bowl; beat in confectioners' sugar slowly. Frost cupcakes; sprinkle walnuts. Keep refrigerated.

Nutrition Information

- Calories: 265 calories
- Protein: 4g protein.
- Total Fat: 10g fat (5g saturated fat)
- Sodium: 182mg sodium
- Fiber: 1g fiber)
- Total Carbohydrate: 41g carbohydrate (31g sugars
- Cholesterol: 59mg cholesterol

Chapter 9: Awesome Cupcake Recipes

***

410. Apple Banana Cupcakes

Serving: 24 | Prep: 20mins | Cook: 25mins | Ready in:

Ingredients

- 2 cups all-purpose flour
- 1 teaspoon baking soda
- 1 teaspoon salt
- 1/2 teaspoon ground cinnamon
- 1/2 teaspoon ground nutmeg
- 2/3 cup shortening
- 1 1/4 cups white sugar
- 2 eggs
- 1 teaspoon vanilla extract
- 1/4 cup buttermilk
- 1 cup ripe bananas, mashed
- 2 apples - peeled, cored and shredded

Direction

- Preheat the oven to 190 degrees C/375 degrees F. Grease then flour or put paper liners on 24 muffin cups. Sift nutmeg, cinnamon, salt, baking soda and flour together. Put aside.
- Cream sugar and shortening in a big bowl until fluffy and light. One at a time, beat eggs in. Mix in buttermilk and vanilla. Beat flour mixture in, mixing until just incorporated. Fold in shredded apples and mashed bananas. Fill every muffin cup to half full.
- Bake for 20-25 minutes in preheated oven until an inserted toothpick in the middle exits clean. Cool.

Nutrition Information

- Calories: 151 calories;
- Sodium: 158
- Total Carbohydrate: 22.3
- Cholesterol: 16
- Protein: 1.8
- Total Fat: 6.3

411. Apple Pie Cupcakes

Serving: 24 | Prep: 20mins | Cook: 12mins | Ready in:

Ingredients

- 1 sweet red apple, peeled and roughly chopped
- 1 Granny Smith apple, peeled and roughly chopped
- 1 (15.25 ounce) package yellow cake mix (such as Betty Crocker®)
- 1 cup water
- 1/2 cup vegetable oil
- 3 eggs
- 2 cups graham cracker crumbs
- 1 teaspoon ground cinnamon
- 1/2 teaspoon nutmeg
- 1/4 cup melted butter

Direction

- Preheat an oven to 165°C/325°F; grease or line paper liners on 24 muffin cups.
- Process red apple till minced through a food processor; put in a bowl. Process Granny Smith apple till minced through a food processor; put in another bowl.
- By hand or with electric mixer, mix together eggs, vegetable oil, water and cake mix till smooth in bowl; fold 1/2 cup of Granny Smith apples and 1/2 cup of sweet apple into batter.
- Spread the graham cracker crumbs onto a waxed paper piece; add nutmeg and cinnamon. Transfer butter on top of crumbs; mix till crumbs are moist with hands. Add 1

tsp. crumb mixture to fill each muffin cup; fill the leftover with batter. Sprinkle all the leftover crumb mixture on top of batter.
- In preheated oven, bake for 12-17 minutes till an inserted toothpick in the middle exits clean; cool cupcakes for 5-10 minutes in tin. Transfer to a wire rack; cool.

Nutrition Information

- Calories: 179 calories;
- Sodium: 183
- Total Carbohydrate: 21.1
- Cholesterol: 29
- Protein: 2.1
- Total Fat: 9.9

412. Apple And Coconut Milk Cupcakes

Serving: 10 | Prep: 15mins | Cook: 30mins | Ready in:

Ingredients

- 1 cup all-purpose flour
- 1/3 cup white sugar
- 1/4 cup coconut flour
- 1 teaspoon baking powder
- 1/2 teaspoon ground cinnamon
- 1/4 teaspoon salt
- 1/4 teaspoon ground nutmeg
- 1 egg
- 3/4 cup applesauce
- 1/2 cup coconut milk
- 1/4 cup vegetable oil
- 1 tablespoon honey
- 1/2 teaspoon vanilla extract

Direction

- Preheat an oven to 175°C/350°F. Grease/line paper muffin liners on 10-cup muffin tin.
- Mix nutmeg, salt, cinnamon, baking powder, coconut flour, sugar and all-purpose flour in bowl.
- Lightly whisk egg in big bowl. Add vanilla extract, honey, vegetable oil, coconut milk and applesauce. Mix in flour mixture till batter just combined. Put into prepped muffin pan.
- In preheated oven, bake for 30 minutes till an inserted toothpick in middle exits clean and lightly pressing tops makes them spring back.

Nutrition Information

- Calories: 165 calories;
- Total Carbohydrate: 20.6
- Cholesterol: 19
- Protein: 2.2
- Total Fat: 8.5
- Sodium: 116

413. Banana Cupcakes With Ganache Frosting

Serving: about 1-1/2 dozen. | Prep: 45mins | Cook: 20mins | Ready in:

Ingredients

- 2 cups all-purpose flour
- 1-1/2 cups sugar
- 3/4 teaspoon baking soda
- 1/2 teaspoon baking powder
- 1/2 teaspoon salt
- 2 eggs
- 1/2 cup canola oil
- 1/4 cup buttermilk
- 1 teaspoon vanilla extract
- 1-1/3 cups mashed ripe bananas (2 to 3 medium)
- 3/4 cup chopped pecans
- FROSTING:
- 7 ounces semisweet chocolate, chopped
- 1/2 cup heavy whipping cream
- 6 tablespoons shortening

- 1/3 cup confectioners' sugar
- 1/2 cup marshmallow creme
- 1/2 teaspoon vanilla extract

Direction

- Combine the baking powder, flour, sugar, salt, and baking soda in a large bowl. In a separate bowl, combine the vanilla, oil, eggs, and buttermilk. Whisk the mixture into the dry ingredients until just moistened. Fold in the pecans and bananas.
- Pour the mixture into the paper-lined muffin cups, filling them 2/3 full. Bake them at 350° for 20 to 24 minutes until the inserted toothpick into the center comes out clean. Let them cool for 5 minutes, and then remove them from the pans. Let them cool on wire racks completely.
- In a small saucepan, melt the cream and chocolate over low heat for the frosting. Whisk the mixture until blended. Remove it from the heat and pour it into a small bowl. Allow the mixture to cool until it reaches room temperature.
- Cream the confectioners' sugar and shortening in a large bowl until fluffy and light. Whisk in the vanilla and marshmallow crème. Add the chocolate mixture and whisk it until fluffy and light. Use this mixture to frost the cupcakes.

Nutrition Information

- Calories: 310 calories
- Protein: 3g protein.
- Total Fat: 18g fat (5g saturated fat)
- Sodium: 125mg sodium
- Fiber: 2g fiber)
- Total Carbohydrate: 37g carbohydrate (25g sugars
- Cholesterol: 28mg cholesterol

414. Banana Nut Cupcakes

Serving: 15 cupcakes. | Prep: 15mins | Cook: 20mins | Ready in:

Ingredients

- 1/3 cup butter-flavored shortening
- 2/3 cup sugar
- 2 eggs
- 1 cup mashed ripe bananas (about 3 medium)
- 2 tablespoons 2% milk
- 1 tablespoon vanilla extract
- 1-1/3 cups all-purpose flour
- 2 teaspoons baking powder
- 1/2 teaspoon baking soda
- 1/4 teaspoon salt
- 1/4 cup chopped nuts

Direction

- Set the oven to 350° for preheating. Cream the sugar and shortening in a large bowl until fluffy and light. Whisk in the eggs. Mix in vanilla, bananas, and milk. Combine the salt, baking powder, flour, and baking soda and add the mixture gradually into the creamed mixture. Whisk the mixture well before mixing in the nuts.
- Pour the mixture into the paper-lined muffin cups, filling them up to 2/3 full. Bake them for 18-20 minutes until the inserted toothpick into the center will come out clean. Allow them to cool for 5 minutes. Transfer them from the pans onto the wire racks.

Nutrition Information

- Calories: 153 calories
- Fiber: 1g fiber)
- Total Carbohydrate: 21g carbohydrate (12g sugars
- Cholesterol: 29mg cholesterol
- Protein: 3g protein.
- Total Fat: 6g fat (1g saturated fat)
- Sodium: 145mg sodium

415. Banana And Vanilla Cupcakes With Buttercream Frosting

Serving: 12 | Prep: 30mins | Cook: 20mins | Ready in:

Ingredients

- Banana Cupcakes:
- 1 3/4 cups all-purpose flour
- 2 teaspoons baking powder
- 1/2 teaspoon salt
- 1/2 cup butter, at room temperature
- 1/2 cup white sugar
- 3 eggs, room temperature
- 1 teaspoon vanilla extract
- 1/4 cup milk
- 2 large bananas, chopped
- Buttercream Frosting:
- 2/3 cup butter, at room temperature
- 1/2 teaspoon vanilla extract
- 2 1/4 cups confectioners' sugar
- 2 tablespoons heavy cream
- 4 drops yellow food coloring, or as desired

Direction

- Preheat oven to 175°C/350°F; line paper muffin liners or grease 12 muffin cups.
- Whisk salt, baking powder and flour in a bowl; put aside. Beat white sugar and 1/2 cup butter with an electric mixer till fluffy and light in a big bowl. Put in eggs, one by one, blending each into butter mixture before adding next. Beat in the last egg and vanilla. Alternating with milk, add flour mixture, mixing till just incorporated. Fold in chopped bananas, stirring just enough to combine evenly; put batter in lined/greased cups.
- In preheated oven, bake for about 20 minutes till an inserted toothpick in middle exits clean. Cool for 10 minutes in pans. Transfer onto wire rack; fully cool.
- As cupcakes cool, make buttercream: Beat 2/3 cup butter till glossy and smooth in a bowl; beat in vanilla, then confectioners' sugar. Add food coloring and cream when there are no dry sugar lumps left; whip on high speed till fluffy and light. Use buttercream frosting to frost cooled cupcakes.

Nutrition Information

- Calories: 395 calories;
- Total Fat: 20.4
- Sodium: 327
- Total Carbohydrate: 50.5
- Cholesterol: 98
- Protein: 4.1

416. Black Bottom Cupcakes

Serving: 24 servings | Prep: 15mins | Cook: | Ready in:

Ingredients

- 1 pkg. (8 oz.) PHILADELPHIA Cream Cheese, softened
- 1 egg
- 1/3 cup granulated sugar
- 1 cup BAKER'S Semi-Sweet Chocolate Chunks
- 1 pkg. (2-layer size) chocolate cake mix
- 1/4 cup finely chopped PLANTERS Walnuts
- 1/4 cup packed brown sugar

Direction

- Beat granulated sugar, egg and cream cheese together till fluffy and light. Mix in chocolate chunks; set aside.
- Following the package directions, prepare cake batter properly.
- Spoon into 24 muffin cups lined with parchment paper; place a heaping teaspoonful of the cream cheese mixture on top of each. Mix nuts and sugar; sprinkle over the cupcakes.

- Bake for 20 minutes. Allow to cool for 10 minutes in the pans. Take away and cool completely on wire racks.

Nutrition Information

- Calories: 220
- Total Fat: 14 g
- Fiber: 1 g
- Saturated Fat: 4.5 g
- Sodium: 200 mg
- Sugar: 16 g
- Total Carbohydrate: 23 g
- Cholesterol: 45 mg
- Protein: 3 g

417. Black Sesame Cupcakes

Serving: 24 | Prep: 15mins | Cook: 20mins | Ready in:

Ingredients

- 1/4 cup black sesame seeds, crushed
- 1 1/2 sticks salted butter
- 1 1/2 cups white sugar
- 2 eggs
- 3 tablespoons black sesame paste
- 1 teaspoon vanilla extract
- 2 1/2 cups sifted all-purpose flour
- 2 1/2 teaspoons baking powder
- 1/4 teaspoon salt
- 1 1/4 cups milk

Direction

- Prepare the oven by preheating to 375°F (190°C). Use cupcake liners to line 2 muffin tins.
- Place sesame seeds in a dry frying pan and toast over medium heat for about 2 minutes, stirring and tossing constantly, until scented. Exclude this step if the seeds are already toasted.
- Use an electric mixer to whisk sugar and butter in a large bowl until creamy. Add vanilla extract, sesame paste, eggs, and toasted seeds. Whisk until blended. Slowly whisk in salt, baking powder, and flour. Add milk and whisk for a few more minutes until blended.
- Fill batter into cupcake liners.
- Place in the preheated oven and bake for 16-18 minutes until a toothpick poked into a cupcake comes out clean.

Nutrition Information

- Calories: 180 calories;
- Total Fat: 8.4
- Protein: 3
- Sodium: 127
- Total Carbohydrate: 24
- Cholesterol: 32

418. Blueberry Angel Cupcakes

Serving: 2-1/2 dozen. | Prep: 25mins | Cook: 15mins | Ready in:

Ingredients

- 11 egg whites
- 1 cup plus 2 tablespoons cake flour
- 1-1/2 cups sugar, divided
- 1-1/4 teaspoons cream of tartar
- 1 teaspoon vanilla extract
- 1/2 teaspoon salt
- 1-1/2 cups fresh or frozen blueberries
- 1 teaspoon grated lemon peel
- GLAZE:
- 1 cup confectioners' sugar
- 3 tablespoons lemon juice

Direction

- In a large bowl, add egg whites; allow to stand at room temperature for 30 minutes. Sift

together half cup of sugar and flour for three times; put aside.
- Put salt, vanilla and cream of tartar to egg whites; beat until soft peaks form on medium speed. Slowly add the rest of sugar, about 2 tablespoons at a time, beating on high until sugar dissolves and stiff glossy peaks form. Gently fold in flour mixture half cup at the time. Fold in lemon peel and blueberries.
- In paper-lined muffin cups, pour batter filling them 3/4 full. Bake at 375° until cupcakes bound back when lightly touched, about 14-17 minutes. Quickly take out from pans to wire racks to cool entirely.
- Whisk lemon juice and confectioners' sugar in a small bowl until smooth. Brush on top of cupcakes. Allow to stand to set.

Nutrition Information

- Calories: 85 calories
- Total Carbohydrate: 19g carbohydrate (15g sugars
- Cholesterol: 0 cholesterol
- Protein: 2g protein. Diabetic Exchanges: 1 starch.
- Total Fat: 0 fat (0 saturated fat)
- Sodium: 60mg sodium
- Fiber: 0 fiber)

419. Boston Cream Cupcakes

Serving: 1/2 dozen. | Prep: 25mins | Cook: 15mins | Ready in:

Ingredients

- 3 tablespoons shortening
- 1/3 cup sugar
- 1 large egg
- 1/2 teaspoon vanilla extract
- 1/2 cup all-purpose flour
- 1/2 teaspoon baking powder
- 1/4 teaspoon salt
- 3 tablespoons 2% milk
- 2/3 cup prepared vanilla pudding
- 1/2 cup semisweet chocolate chips
- 1/4 cup heavy whipping cream

Direction

- Cream sugar and shortening in a small bowl until fluffy and light. Beat in egg and vanilla. Combine the flour, salt, and baking powder; then alternately add to the creamed mixture with milk, beating properly after each addition.
- Fill half full into the paper-lined muffin cups. Bake for 15-20 minutes at 350°, or until inserting a toothpick in the center and it comes out clean. Let cool for 10 minutes before moving from pan to a wire rack to completely cool.
- In the corner of a plastic or pastry bag, cut a small hole, then insert a small tip. Next, fill the bag with pudding. To fill each cupcake, push the tip through the top.
- In a small bowl, put chocolate chips. Boil cream in a small saucepan. Pour over the chocolate and whisk until smooth. Allow to cool to room temperature or for about 10 minutes, stirring infrequently, until the ganache slightly thickens. Scoop over the cupcakes. Allow to sit until set. Keep in an airtight container in the fridge.

Nutrition Information

- Calories: 288 calories
- Protein: 4g protein.
- Total Fat: 16g fat (7g saturated fat)
- Sodium: 198mg sodium
- Fiber: 1g fiber)
- Total Carbohydrate: 35g carbohydrate (22g sugars
- Cholesterol: 53mg cholesterol

420. Bride And Groom Cupcakes

Serving: 2 dozen. | Prep: 01hours30mins | Cook: 20mins | Ready in:

Ingredients

- 1 package strawberry or yellow cake mix (regular size)
- FROSTING:
- 1 cup shortening
- 1 cup butter, softened
- 8 cups confectioners' sugar
- 7 to 8 tablespoons 2% milk, divided
- 2 teaspoons clear vanilla extract
- 1/2 cup baking cocoa
- 2 teaspoons grated lemon peel
- 1/2 teaspoon lemon extract
- DECORATIONS:
- 1 cup dark chocolate candy coating disks, melted
- 1/2 cup vanilla candy coating disks, melted
- 1 large marshmallow
- 1/2 cup green candy coating disks, melted
- White pearl dragees, flower sprinkles, white edible glitter and colored sugar
- Small piece of tulle

Direction

- Follow package instructions for cupcakes to prep and bake cake; fully cool.
- Beat butter and shortening till fluffy and light in a big bowl. Add vanilla, 6 tbsp. milk and confectioners' sugar; beat till smooth.
- In another bowl, put 1/2 frosting. To get desired consistency, add 1-2 tbsp. leftover milk and baking cocoa. To leftover frosting, add lemon extract and peel.
- Pipe 12 bow ties using melted chocolate on waxed paper. Pipe 1 1/4-in. ring using melted vanilla coating for bride's crown; put dragees onto ring immediately.
- Groom's hat: Put 1/2 tsp. round melted chocolate into 1 3/4-in. circle onto waxed paper. From top of marshmallow, cut 1/4-in. slice. Dip marshmallow into chocolate coating; put in middle of chocolate round. Pipe 12 bouquet stems on waxed paper using melted green coating; attach flower sprinkles right away. Stand decorations till set. Pipe chocolate frosting on 1/2 cupcakes then lemon frosting on leftover cupcakes. Bride: Put crown on top of lemon-frosted cupcake; for veil, attach a tulle piece. Add a bouquet; sprinkle glitter.
- Groom: Put top hat over chocolate-frosted cupcake; for buttons, attach pearl dragees then the bow tie.
- Use colored sugar, glitter, dragees, bow ties and bouquets as desired to decorate leftover cupcakes.

Nutrition Information

- Calories: 431 calories
- Total Fat: 22g fat (8g saturated fat)
- Sodium: 206mg sodium
- Fiber: 1g fiber)
- Total Carbohydrate: 59g carbohydrate (48g sugars
- Cholesterol: 47mg cholesterol
- Protein: 2g protein.

421. British Butterfly Cakes

Serving: 20 | Prep: 15mins | Cook: 15mins | Ready in:

Ingredients

- Cupcakes:
- 1/2 cup white sugar
- 7 tablespoons butter, softened
- 2 eggs
- 1 teaspoon vanilla extract
- 1 teaspoon baking powder
- 3/4 cup self-rising flour
- Frosting:
- 4 cups confectioners' sugar
- 1/2 cup butter, softened

Direction

- Start preheating the oven to 325°F (165°C). Coat with cooking spray or line paper liners on 20 muffin cups.
- In a bowl, beat together 7 tablespoons butter and white sugar with an electric mixer until they become creamy and smooth. Put in baking powder, vanilla extract, and eggs. Beat until they become smooth. Sift the flour into the creamed butter mixture until the batter becomes smooth. Spoon into each muffin cup with 2 tablespoons of batter.
- Bake in prepared oven for 15 mins or until a toothpick comes out clean when inserted in middle. Cool the cupcakes for 3 mins in tin. Then cool completely on a wire rack.
- In a bowl, mix together half a cup of butter and confectioners' sugar until the frosting becomes smooth, then spread onto the cooled cupcakes.

Nutrition Information

- Calories: 218 calories;
- Sodium: 152
- Total Carbohydrate: 33.6
- Cholesterol: 41
- Protein: 1.2
- Total Fat: 9.2

422. Brownie Graduation Caps

Serving: 4 dozen. | Prep: 55mins | Cook: 25mins | Ready in:

Ingredients

- 1 package fudge brownie mix (13-inch x 9-inch pan size)
- 48 fudge graham cookies or graham cracker halves
- 1 cup chocolate frosting
- 48 pieces red shoestring licorice
- 48 Skittles bite-size candies

Direction

- Set oven to preheat at 350°. Make brownie batter as instructed on the package for cake-y brownies. Fill it two-thirds full into miniature muffin cups lined with paper. Bake for 21-24 minutes. Allow to cool for 10 minutes before taking out of the pans to wire racks and let cool thoroughly (while cupcakes are still warm, take off the paper liners).
- Cut off 1/8-in. from each cupcake's top to level. Flip the cupcakes; use a small amount of frosting to stick a cookie to each. To make tassel, add a candy and a licorice piece atop each cookie, use frosting to stick. Let sit until set.

Nutrition Information

- Calories: 833 calories
- Protein: 4g protein.
- Total Fat: 17g fat (5g saturated fat)
- Sodium: 216mg sodium
- Fiber: 1g fiber)
- Total Carbohydrate: 166g carbohydrate (127g sugars
- Cholesterol: 28mg cholesterol

423. Butter Free Peanut Butter Cupcakes

Serving: 12 | Prep: 20mins | Cook: 20mins | Ready in:

Ingredients

- 3/4 cup soy milk
- 2 teaspoons distilled white vinegar
- 1/2 cup crunchy peanut butter
- 1/3 cup canola oil
- 2/3 cup white sugar
- 2 tablespoons honey
- 2 teaspoons vanilla extract

- 2 teaspoons flax seed meal
- 1 1/8 cups all-purpose flour
- 1 teaspoon baking powder
- 1/2 teaspoon baking soda
- 1/4 teaspoon salt

Direction

- Set the oven at 350°F (175°C) and start preheating. Grease a 12-cup muffin pan or use paper baking cups to line. In a measuring cup, mix vinegar and soy milk. Allow to sit to thicken for around 5 minutes.
- In a large bowl, mix flaxseed meal, vanilla, honey, sugar, oil and peanut butter together. Stir in soymilk. Mix together salt, baking soda, baking powder and flour; mix into the batter just till well blended. The batter may be slightly lumpy. Using a spoon, transfer the batter into the prepared cups, arranging evenly.
- Bake for 20-25 more minutes in the preheated oven, till the tops spring back when pressed lightly. Allow to cool in the pan set over a wire rack. Once cool, distribute the cupcakes onto a serving plate. Use your desired frosting to frost.

Nutrition Information

- Calories: 227 calories;
- Total Fat: 12.1
- Sodium: 202
- Total Carbohydrate: 26.5
- Cholesterol: 0
- Protein: 4.4

424. Butterfly Cakes

Serving: 16 | Prep: 20mins | Cook: 15mins | Ready in:

Ingredients

- 3/4 cup butter, softened
- 3/4 cup white sugar
- 2 tablespoons white sugar
- 3 eggs
- 1 teaspoon vanilla extract, or more to taste
- 1 1/2 cups self-rising flour
- Buttercream Filling:
- 1 cup confectioners' sugar
- 2 1/2 tablespoons confectioners' sugar
- 1/4 cup butter, softened
- 1 teaspoon vanilla extract, or to taste
- 1/2 cup raspberry jam, or as needed

Direction

- Preheat the oven to 165 degrees C/325 degrees F. Line medium-sized cupcake liners on a muffin tin.
- In a big bowl, beat 3/4 cup plus 2 tbsp. white sugar and 3/4 cup butter using an electric mixer until fluffy. Beat 1 tsp. vanilla extract and eggs in. Gradually beat flour in. Evenly divide batter in cupcake liners.
- Bake for 15-20 minutes in preheated oven until they're golden. Put on a wire rack. Cool for about 20 minutes.
- In a bowl, beat 1 tsp. vanilla extract, 1/4 cup butter and 1 cup plus 2 1/2 tbsp. confectioners' sugar to create buttercream filling.
- Scoop out some of the middle of every cupcake. Keep it in 1 piece. Fill every hole using raspberry jam. Top butter cream on cupcakes. Cut scooped-out centers to 2 pieces. Put it on the buttercream to create butterfly wings.

Nutrition Information

- Calories: 262 calories;
- Total Fat: 12.6
- Sodium: 244
- Total Carbohydrate: 35.6
- Cholesterol: 65
- Protein: 2.5

425. Buttermilk Chocolate Cupcakes

Serving: 2 dozen. | Prep: 30mins | Cook: 15mins | Ready in:

Ingredients

- 1/2 cup butter, softened
- 1-1/2 cups sugar
- 2 large eggs
- 1 teaspoon vanilla extract
- 1-1/2 cups all-purpose flour
- 1/2 cup baking cocoa
- 1 teaspoon baking soda
- 1/4 teaspoon salt
- 1/2 cup buttermilk
- 1/2 cup water
- FROSTING:
- 1/2 cup butter, softened
- 3-3/4 cups confectioners' sugar
- 2 ounces unsweetened chocolate, melted
- 2 tablespoons evaporated milk
- 1 teaspoon vanilla extract
- 1/4 teaspoon salt
- Chocolate sprinkles

Direction

- Set the oven at 375° and start preheating. Cream sugar and butter in a large bowl, till fluffy and light. Put in eggs, one per time, beating properly after each addition. Beat in vanilla. Mix together salt, baking soda, cocoa and flour. Mix water and buttermilk. Put the dry ingredients into the creamed mixture, alternately with water and buttermilk, beating properly after each addition.
- Fill into paper-lined muffin cups, 2/3 full. Bake till a toothpick comes out clean when inserted into the center, 15-20 minutes. Allow to cool for 10 minutes; take away from the pan and allow to cool completely on wire racks.
- To make the frosting, beat confectioners' sugar and butter together in a small bowl, till smooth. Beat in salt, vanilla, milk and melted chocolate. Frost the cupcakes; use chocolate sprinkles for garnish.

Nutrition Information

- Calories: 239 calories
- Sodium: 191mg sodium
- Fiber: 1g fiber)
- Total Carbohydrate: 39g carbohydrate (30g sugars
- Cholesterol: 39mg cholesterol
- Protein: 2g protein.
- Total Fat: 9g fat (5g saturated fat)

426. Cappuccino Cupcakes

Serving: | Prep: | Cook: | Ready in:

Ingredients

- 1 pkg. (2-layer size) chocolate cake mix
- brewed strong MAXWELL HOUSE Coffee, cooled
- 1/2 cup BREAKSTONE'S or KNUDSEN Sour Cream
- 2 tsp. ground cinnamon

Direction

- Turn on the oven to 350 degrees F to preheat.
- Follow the directions on package to prepare cake batter. Substitute coffer for water and blend cinnamon and sour cream in the batter, then spoon into paper-lined muffin cups.
- Bake the cupcakes following the directions on package; then let it cool completely.
- In the meantime, prepare Sour Cream Ganache Frosting or Vanilla Cream Frosting. Spread onto the cupcakes.

Nutrition Information

- Calories: 150

- Total Fat: 9 g
- Sugar: 10 g
- Cholesterol: 25 mg
- Fiber: 0.897 g
- Protein: 8 g
- Sodium: 190 mg
- Saturated Fat: 1 g
- Total Carbohydrate: 16 g

427. Carrot Blueberry Cupcakes

Serving: 16 cupcakes. | Prep: 35mins | Cook: 20mins | Ready in:

Ingredients

- 1 cup sugar
- 1/2 cup canola oil
- 2 large eggs
- 1 teaspoon vanilla extract
- 1-1/2 cups all-purpose flour
- 1 teaspoon baking powder
- 1 teaspoon ground cinnamon
- 1/2 teaspoon baking soda
- 1/2 teaspoon salt
- 1 cup finely shredded carrots
- 3/4 cup grated zucchini
- 1/2 cup unsweetened crushed pineapple, drained
- 1 cup fresh or frozen unsweetened blueberries
- FROSTING:
- 3 ounces cream cheese, softened
- 1/4 cup butter, softened
- 2-1/2 cups confectioners' sugar
- 1 teaspoon vanilla extract
- 1/2 cup chopped pecans, optional

Direction

- Beat sugar, vanilla, eggs, and oil in a small bowl. Mix salt, baking soda, cinnamon, baking powder, and flour in another large bowl; beat into the sugar mixture gradually until blended. Stir in the pineapple, zucchini, and carrots. Then fold in blueberries.
- Fill 2/3 full into the paper-lined muffin cups. Then bake for 18-22 minutes at 375°, or until inserting in the center with a toothpick and it comes out clean. Then let it cool for around 10 minutes before transferring from pans to wire racks and let it completely cool.
- To make the frosting: Whisk butter and cream cheese in a large bowl until fluffy. Then add vanilla and confectioners' sugar; continue to beat until smooth. Then frost the cupcakes. If desired, scatter with nuts. Chill the leftovers.

Nutrition Information

- Calories: 294 calories
- Sodium: 189mg sodium
- Fiber: 1g fiber)
- Total Carbohydrate: 44g carbohydrate (33g sugars
- Cholesterol: 40mg cholesterol
- Protein: 3g protein.
- Total Fat: 13g fat (4g saturated fat)

428. Carrot Cupcakes

Serving: 12 | Prep: 20mins | Cook: 15mins | Ready in:

Ingredients

- 2 cups white sugar
- 1 cup butter, softened
- 2 eggs
- 1 teaspoon vanilla extract
- 2 cups all-purpose flour
- 1/4 cup finely chopped walnuts
- 1 teaspoon ground cinnamon
- 1 teaspoon baking powder
- 1/2 teaspoon baking soda
- 1/2 teaspoon salt
- 1/2 cup milk
- 1 cup finely grated carrots

Direction

- Set the oven to 300°F (150°C) and start preheating. Grease or use paper liners to line 12 muffin cups.
- Beat butter and sugar together in a bowl with an electric mixer until creamy and smooth; beat in eggs, one at a time; beat until fully incorporated, then add the next one. Combine vanilla extract into creamed butter mixture.
- In a bowl, beat salt, cinnamon, baking soda, walnuts, baking powder and flour together. Combine 1/3 flour mixture into the creamed butter mixture until just combined; add half of the milk and mix until combined. Stir half of the rest of the flour mixture into the batter; add the rest of the milk; mix until combined. Mix the rest of the flour mixture into the batter; fold in carrots. Scoop batter into the greased/lined muffin cups.
- Bake in the prepared oven for 15-17 minutes until the inserted toothpick in the center of the cupcake comes out clean.

Nutrition Information

- Calories: 374 calories;
- Sodium: 322
- Total Carbohydrate: 51.2
- Cholesterol: 72
- Protein: 4
- Total Fat: 17.7

429. Carrot Cupcakes Or Cake With Cream Cheese Frosting

Serving: 24 | Prep: 40mins | Cook: 15mins | Ready in:

Ingredients

- 1/2 cup white sugar, or to taste
- 3/4 cup buttermilk
- 3 eggs
- 1/3 cup vegetable oil
- 2 teaspoons vanilla extract, divided
- 1 (15 ounce) can pineapple chunks, drained
- 2 cups grated carrots
- 1 cup sweetened flaked coconut
- 1 cup all-purpose flour
- 1 cup whole wheat flour
- 2 teaspoons baking soda
- 1 1/2 teaspoons salt
- 1 teaspoon ground cinnamon
- 2 cups confectioners' sugar
- 1 (8 ounce) package cream cheese, softened
- 1/2 cup butter

Direction

- Set oven temperature to 350 degrees F (175 degrees C) and preheat. Use 12 paper cupcake liners to line two 12-cup muffin tins.
- Combine buttermilk, oil, eggs, a teaspoon of vanilla extract, and sugar in a big bowl until mixed evenly. Mix in carrots, coconuts, and pineapple and stir until even.
- Mix together whole wheat flour, salt, baking soda, cinnamon, and all-purpose flour in a different bowl. Mix the contents of the flour bowl into the carrot mix bowl while stirring. Pour the batter into the muffin cups, up to 3/4 filled.
- Bake for 15 minutes in preheated oven, until an inserted toothpick can be removed without any residue. Leave aside to cool after removing from oven for 25 minutes.
- Mix together cream cheese, confectioners' sugar, the remaining 1 teaspoon of vanilla extract, and butter until creamy with an electric mixer. Put the frosting on the cooled cupcakes.

Nutrition Information

- Calories: 228 calories;
- Cholesterol: 44
- Protein: 3.3
- Total Fat: 11.9
- Sodium: 338
- Total Carbohydrate: 28.2

430. Cherry Banana Cupcakes

Serving: 5 cupcakes. | Prep: 15mins | Cook: 20mins | Ready in:

Ingredients

- 1/4 cup butter, softened
- 1/4 cup sugar
- 2 tablespoons beaten egg
- 1/4 cup mashed ripe banana
- 2 tablespoons buttermilk
- 1/2 teaspoon vanilla extract
- 1/2 cup all-purpose flour
- 1/4 cup quick-cooking oats
- 1/4 teaspoon plus 1/8 teaspoon baking soda
- 1/8 teaspoon salt
- 2 tablespoons chopped maraschino cherries, well drained
- 2 tablespoons chopped walnuts

Direction

- Cream the sugar and butter in a small bowl until smooth. Add the egg and mix the mixture well. Whisk in buttermilk, vanilla, and banana. Mix the salt, oats, flour, and baking soda, and then add the mixture into the creamed mixture until moistened. Fold the cherries into the mixture.
- Pour the mixture into the paper-lined muffin cups, filling them 3/4 full. Dust with walnuts. Bake them inside the 350° oven for 18-20 minutes or until the toothpick will come out clean. Let them cool for 5 minutes, and then transfer them from the pan onto a wire rack to completely cool.

Nutrition Information

- Calories: 229 calories
- Total Carbohydrate: 28g carbohydrate (13g sugars
- Cholesterol: 50mg cholesterol
- Protein: 4g protein.
- Total Fat: 12g fat (6g saturated fat)
- Sodium: 236mg sodium
- Fiber: 1g fiber)

431. Chocolate Cherry Cupcakes

Serving: 2 dozen. | Prep: 15mins | Cook: 20mins | Ready in:

Ingredients

- 1 package chocolate cake mix (regular size)
- 1-1/3 cups water
- 1/2 cup canola oil
- 3 large eggs
- 1 can (21 ounces) cherry pie filling
- 1 can (16 ounces) vanilla frosting
- Chocolate curls, optional

Direction

- Combine the oil, eggs, cake mix, and water in a large bowl. Whisk the mixture on low speed for 30 seconds. Whisk the mixture on medium speed for 2 more minutes.
- Pour the batter into the paper-lined muffin cups by 1/4 cupfuls. Fill the center of the cupcake with a rounded teaspoonful of pie filling. Put the remaining filling aside.
- Bake the cupcakes at 350° for 20 to 25 minutes until the inserted toothpick into the center will come out very clean. Remove them from the pans and place them on wire racks. Let them cool completely.
- Frost the cupcakes. Place a cherry from the pie filling onto each of the cupcakes. If desired, garnish the cupcake with chocolate curls. You can refrigerate any pie filling leftovers for future use.

Nutrition Information

- Calories: 252 calories
- Fiber: 1g fiber)
- Total Carbohydrate: 37g carbohydrate (28g sugars
- Cholesterol: 27mg cholesterol
- Protein: 2g protein.
- Total Fat: 11g fat (2g saturated fat)
- Sodium: 187mg sodium

432. Chocolate Orange Cupcakes

Serving: 9 cupcakes. | Prep: 15mins | Cook: 20mins | Ready in:

Ingredients

- 1-1/2 cups all-purpose flour
- 1/2 cup sugar
- 1/4 cup baking cocoa
- 1 teaspoon baking soda
- 1/4 teaspoon salt
- 1/2 cup mayonnaise
- 1 teaspoon grated orange zest
- 1 teaspoon vanilla extract
- 1/2 cup orange juice
- 1/2 cup semisweet chocolate chips
- Confectioners' sugar

Direction

- Mix the salt, baking soda, cocoa, sugar and flour in a bowl. Mix the vanilla, orange zest and mayonnaise in a separate bowl; put orange juice gradually until combined. Mix into dry mixture just until blended. Mix in chocolate chips (batter will be thick).
- Put batter in paper-lined muffin tins, about 2/3 full. Bake for 18 to 23 mins at 350°or until a toothpick comes out clean. Let cool for 10 minutes before taking out from pan to a wire rack to cool completely. Sprinkle with confectioners' sugar.

Nutrition Information

- Calories: 273 calories
- Total Fat: 13g fat (3g saturated fat)
- Sodium: 274mg sodium
- Fiber: 2g fiber)
- Total Carbohydrate: 37g carbohydrate (19g sugars
- Cholesterol: 4mg cholesterol
- Protein: 3g protein.

433. Chocolate Raspberry Tea Cakes

Serving: 1/2 dozen. | Prep: 10mins | Cook: 20mins | Ready in:

Ingredients

- 3/4 cup all-purpose flour
- 2 tablespoons sugar
- 2 tablespoons brown sugar
- 1 teaspoon baking powder
- 1/8 teaspoon salt
- 1 egg white
- 1/4 cup milk
- 1/4 cup butter, melted
- 1/2 cup milk chocolate chips
- 6 teaspoons seedless raspberry jam

Direction

- Mix salt, baking powder, sugars, and flour in a large bowl. Beat butter, milk, and egg white in a different bowl; add to dry ingredients and stir until just moistened. Then fold in the chocolate chips.
- Fill a tablespoon of batter into each of six paper-lined muffin cups. Drop a teaspoon of jam into each cup; add the rest of batter on top.
- Bake at 350 degrees until a toothpick comes out clean when inserted into the center, for 20-25 minutes. Allow to cool for 10 minutes, then

transfer from the pan onto a wire rack to cool completely.

Nutrition Information

- Calories: 255 calories
- Fiber: 1g fiber)
- Total Carbohydrate: 34g carbohydrate (21g sugars
- Cholesterol: 25mg cholesterol
- Protein: 4g protein.
- Total Fat: 12g fat (8g saturated fat)
- Sodium: 221mg sodium

434. Chocolate Zucchini Cupcakes

Serving: 21 cupcakes. | Prep: 25mins | Cook: 20mins | Ready in:

Ingredients

- 1-1/4 cups butter, softened
- 1-1/2 cups sugar
- 2 eggs
- 1 teaspoon vanilla extract
- 2-1/2 cups all-purpose flour
- 3/4 cup baking cocoa
- 1 teaspoon baking powder
- 1 teaspoon baking soda
- 1/2 teaspoon salt
- 1/2 cup plain yogurt
- 1 cup grated zucchini
- 1 cup grated carrots
- 1 can (16 ounces) chocolate frosting

Direction

- Cream sugar and butter in a large bowl, till fluffy and light. Include in eggs, one each time, beating well after each increment. Mix in vanilla. Mix salt, baking soda, baking powder, baking cocoa and flour together; put alternating with yogurt into the creamed mixture, beating well after each addition. Fold in carrots and zucchini.
- Fill paper-lined muffin cups two-thirds full. Bake at 350° till a toothpick comes out clean when inserted into the center, 18-22 minutes. Allow to cool for 10 minutes; take out of pans and place on wire racks; cool completely. Frost the cupcakes.

Nutrition Information

- Calories: 326 calories
- Fiber: 1g fiber)
- Total Carbohydrate: 40g carbohydrate (25g sugars
- Cholesterol: 50mg cholesterol
- Protein: 3g protein.
- Total Fat: 17g fat (9g saturated fat)
- Sodium: 288mg sodium

435. Chocolate Bottom Mini Cupcakes

Serving: 6 dozen. | Prep: 15mins | Cook: 20mins | Ready in:

Ingredients

- FILLING:
- 1 package (8 ounces) cream cheese, softened
- 1 large egg
- 1/3 cup sugar
- 1/8 teaspoon salt
- 1 cup (6 ounces) semisweet chocolate chips
- BATTER:
- 1 cup water
- 1/3 cup canola oil
- 1 tablespoon white vinegar
- 1 teaspoon vanilla extract
- 1-1/2 cups all-purpose flour
- 1 cup sugar
- 1/4 cup baking cocoa
- 1 teaspoon baking soda
- 1 teaspoon salt

Direction

- Whip the salt, sugar, egg and cream cheese in a big bowl until smooth. Mix in chocolate chips; put aside.
- To make the batter, mix the vanilla, vinegar, oil and water in a big bowl. Mix leftover ingredients; put into the liquid mixture and stir well (batter will be thin).
- Scoop about 2 teaspoons of the mixture into paper-lined or greased miniature muffin tins. Put about 1 teaspoon of filling on top.
- Bake for 18 to 23 mins at 350° or until a toothpick inserted in cupcake portion comes out clean. Cool for 10 minutes before taking out to wire racks to cool completely.

Nutrition Information

- Calories: 114 calories
- Total Fat: 6g fat (3g saturated fat)
- Sodium: 130mg sodium
- Fiber: 1g fiber)
- Total Carbohydrate: 15g carbohydrate (10g sugars
- Cholesterol: 13mg cholesterol
- Protein: 1g protein.

436. Chocolate Coconut Angel Cupcakes

Serving: 1-1/2 dozen. | Prep: 20mins | Cook: 30mins | Ready in:

Ingredients

- 6 large egg whites
- 2/3 cup all-purpose flour
- 1/4 cup baking cocoa
- 1/2 teaspoon baking powder
- 1-1/3 cups sugar, divided
- 1 teaspoon almond extract
- 1/2 teaspoon cream of tartar
- 1/4 teaspoon salt
- 1 cup sweetened shredded coconut
- Confectioners' sugar, optional

Direction

- Add egg whites to a large bowl; let it sit for 30 minutes at room temperature.
- Heat oven beforehand to 350°. Use cupcake liners to line 18 muffin cups. Sift together 1 cup sugar, cocoa, baking powder and flour 2 times.
- Add salt, cream of tartar and almond extract to the egg whites; on medium speed, beat until it can hold soft peaks. Gradually add in 1 tablespoon of the remaining sugar at a time, beating on high after each time you add until sugar dissolves. Keep on beating until it holds stiff glossy peaks. Gradually fold in about 1/2 cup of the flour mixture at a time. Fold in the coconut gently.
- Fill two-thirds full into the prepared cups. Bake till top looks dry for 30-35 minutes.
- Cool for 10 minutes in pan. Take out to wire racks; cool thoroughly. If you wish, dust with confectioners' sugar.

Nutrition Information

- Calories: 110 calories
- Cholesterol: 0 cholesterol
- Protein: 2g protein. Diabetic Exchanges: 1-1/2 starch.
- Total Fat: 2g fat (2g saturated fat)
- Sodium: 78mg sodium
- Fiber: 1g fiber)
- Total Carbohydrate: 22g carbohydrate (17g sugars

437. Cinnamon Mocha Cupcakes

Serving: 8 cupcakes. | Prep: 15mins | Cook: 20mins | Ready in:

Ingredients

- 1/4 cup butter, softened
- 2/3 cup sugar
- 1 egg
- 1/2 teaspoon vanilla extract
- 3/4 cup plus 2 tablespoons all-purpose flour
- 1/4 cup baking cocoa
- 1/2 teaspoon baking soda
- 1/2 teaspoon salt
- 1/4 teaspoon baking powder
- 1/4 teaspoon ground cinnamon
- 1/4 cup strong brewed coffee, room temperature
- 3 tablespoons buttermilk
- 1 cup chocolate frosting
- 3/4 teaspoon instant coffee granules
- 1 teaspoon hot water

Direction

- In a small bowl, cream the sugar and butter until fluffy and light. Beat in egg and vanilla. Combine the baking soda, baking powder, flour, cinnamon, salt, and cocoa; add buttermilk and coffee to the creamed mixture alternately; after each addition, beating well.
- Fill with batter to half full of paper-lined muffin cups. Bake at 350° until a toothpick comes out clean or for 18 to 20 minutes. Allow 5 minutes to cool before taking away from pan to a wire rack for completely cooling.
- In a bowl, place the frosting. Place coffee granules in hot water to dissolve; stir into frosting until smooth. Frost cupcakes.

Nutrition Information

- Calories: 325 calories
- Protein: 3g protein.
- Total Fat: 13g fat (5g saturated fat)
- Sodium: 391mg sodium
- Fiber: 1g fiber)
- Total Carbohydrate: 50g carbohydrate (35g sugars
- Cholesterol: 42mg cholesterol

438. Citrus Chocolate Cupcakes

Serving: 1 dozen. | Prep: 20mins | Cook: 15mins | Ready in:

Ingredients

- 1/2 cup orange juice
- 1/3 cup water
- 3 tablespoons canola oil
- 1 tablespoon white vinegar
- 1 teaspoon vanilla extract
- 1-1/2 cups all-purpose flour
- 1/2 cup sugar
- 1/4 cup baking cocoa
- 1 teaspoon baking soda
- 1/2 teaspoon salt
- 1/3 cup miniature semisweet chocolate chips
- 1-1/2 teaspoons confectioners' sugar

Direction

- In a small bowl, beat together the vanilla, vinegar, oil, water and orange juice. Combine the salt, baking soda, cocoa, sugar, and flour in a large bowl; beat them into the orange juice mixture slowly until combined. Mix in the chocolate chips.
- Use cooking spray or paper liners to coat muffin cups; fill batter half full into them. Bake at 375° for 13-16 minutes or until a toothpick comes out clean. Allow to cool for 5 minutes then take out of pan to a wire rack to cool down thoroughly. Sprinkle confectioners' sugar on top before serving.

Nutrition Information

- Calories: 155 calories
- Total Fat: 5g fat (1g saturated fat)
- Sodium: 204mg sodium
- Fiber: 1g fiber)
- Total Carbohydrate: 26g carbohydrate (0 sugars

- Cholesterol: 0 cholesterol
- Protein: 2g protein. Diabetic Exchanges: 1-1/2 starch

439. Cone Cupcakes

Serving: 24 | Prep: | Cook: | Ready in:

Ingredients

- 1/2 cup butter, softened
- 1 cup white sugar
- 2 eggs
- 1 teaspoon vanilla extract
- 1 3/4 cups all-purpose flour
- 2 1/2 teaspoons baking powder
- 1/4 teaspoon salt
- 2/3 cup milk
- 24 flat bottomed ice cream cones

Direction

- Set the oven to 190°C or 375°F to preheat.
- In a mixing bowl, cream sugar and butter together well, then beat in one egg at a time. Add in vanilla and mix well. In a small bowl, measure salt, baking powder and flour, then stir. Put into the butter mixture with milk in 2 parts together with 3 parts of the flour mixture, alternately. Starting and finishing with flour.
- Fill batter into cones until 3/4 full while leaving the batter 1/2 inch from top. Put on a baking tray with filled cones and bake in the oven until an inserted toothpick exits clean, about 15-20 minutes.

Nutrition Information

- Calories: 126 calories;
- Total Carbohydrate: 19
- Cholesterol: 26
- Protein: 2.1
- Total Fat: 4.7

- Sodium: 117

440. Cookout Brownies

Serving: varies. | Prep: 02hours00mins | Cook: 0mins | Ready in:

Ingredients

- Brownie cupcakes or chocolate cupcakes
- Orange colored sugar
- 1 tube (4-1/4 ounces) black decorating icing
- Caramel cream candies, gumdrops and Hot Tamales
- Colored toothpicks

Direction

- Scatter colored sugar on top of brownies to look like hot coals. Pipe grill grates onto brownies with icing.
- Slice caramel candies into slices, indent lightly to make steaks. Slice gum drops into 2 parts and slice a caramel candy into tiny pieces, then thread alternately onto toothpicks to make kabobs. Place kabobs, steaks and hot dogs (Hot Tamales) on brownies. Use icing to pipe grill marks on the surface.

Nutrition Information

- Calories:
- Sodium:
- Fiber:
- Total Carbohydrate:
- Cholesterol:
- Protein:
- Total Fat:

441. Cream Cheese Chocolate Cupcakes

Serving: 1-1/2 dozen. | Prep: 20mins | Cook: 25mins | Ready in:

Ingredients

- 1 package (8 ounces) cream cheese, softened
- 1/3 cup sugar
- 1 large egg
- 1/8 teaspoon salt
- 1 cup semisweet chocolate chips
- 1 cup peanut butter chips
- CUPCAKES:
- 1 cup sugar
- 1 cup water
- 1/3 cup canola oil
- 1 tablespoon white vinegar
- 1 teaspoon vanilla extract
- 1-1/2 cups all-purpose flour
- 1/4 cup baking cocoa
- 1 teaspoon baking soda
- 1/2 teaspoon salt

Direction

- Beat cream cheese in a large bowl till fluffy. Beat in salt, egg and sugar till smooth. Mix in peanut butter chips and chocolate chips; set aside.
- For the cupcakes: Beat together vanilla, vinegar, oil, water and sugar in a large bowl till well-blended. Mix together salt, baking soda, cocoa and flour in a large bowl; slowly beat into the sugar mixture; stir properly.
- Fill the batter into paper-lined muffin cups, 1/2 full. Place around 2 tablespoons of the cream cheese mixture on top of each. Bake at 350° till a toothpick comes out clean when inserted into the cupcake, 25-30 minutes. Allow to cool for 10 minutes; take away from the pans and allow to cool completely on wire racks.

Nutrition Information

- Calories: 274 calories
- Fiber: 2g fiber
- Total Carbohydrate: 34g carbohydrate (23g sugars
- Cholesterol: 26mg cholesterol
- Protein: 5g protein.
- Total Fat: 14g fat (6g saturated fat)
- Sodium: 217mg sodium

442. Cream Cheese Cupcakes

Serving: 24 | Prep: | Cook: |Ready in:

Ingredients

- 3 (8 ounce) packages cream cheese
- 1 cup white sugar
- 1 1/2 teaspoons vanilla extract
- 5 eggs
- 3 1/2 cups apple pie filling

Direction

- Set the oven at 165°C (325°F) to preheat. Use paper liners to line 12 muffin cups (2 muffin tins).
- Mix sugar and cream cheese in a large bowl. Blend until soft. Put in the eggs and blend. Add vanilla.
- Evenly distribute into 12 lined muffin cups (2 muffin tins) and bake for 35 minutes in the preheated oven.
- When finished, the centers will fall in a little while cooling. Once cool, fill with 2-3 tbsp. of your favorite fruit pie filling into depressions. Keep in the fridge.

Nutrition Information

- Calories: 183 calories;
- Total Fat: 10.8
- Sodium: 114
- Total Carbohydrate: 18.9
- Cholesterol: 70

- Protein: 3.5

443. Cream Cheese Cupcakes With Sour Cream Topping

Serving: 18 | Prep: 15mins | Cook: 40mins | Ready in:

Ingredients

- Cupcakes:
- 3 (8 ounce) packages cream cheese, at room temperature
- 5 eggs, at room temperature
- 1 cup white sugar
- 1 1/2 teaspoons vanilla extract
- Topping:
- 1/2 pint sour cream
- 2 tablespoons white sugar
- 1/4 teaspoon vanilla extract

Direction

- Set the oven to 350°F (175°C), and start preheating. Line paper liners on 18 muffin cups.
- In a bowl, beat cream cheese with an electric mixer until smooth; put it eggs, 1 at a time, making sure that each is fully blended before each adding. Beat in 1 1/2 teaspoons vanilla extract and 1 cup sugar until smooth; add the mixture in muffin cups until reaching 1/8 inch of the top.
- Bake in the prepped oven until set in the center, about 35 minutes.
- In a bowl, combine 1/4 teaspoon vanilla extract, 2 tablespoons sugar and sour cream together. In the cupcakes, drop a teaspoonful of sour cream mixture.
- Bake the cupcakes in the oven for an additional 5 minutes. Allow to cool to room temperature and chill in the fridge.

Nutrition Information

- Calories: 227 calories;
- Total Fat: 17.1
- Sodium: 137
- Total Carbohydrate: 14.2
- Cholesterol: 98
- Protein: 5

444. Cream Filled Pumpkin Cupcakes

Serving: about 1-1/2 dozen. | Prep: 35mins | Cook: 20mins | Ready in:

Ingredients

- 2 cups sugar
- 3/4 cup canola oil
- 1 can (15 ounces) solid-pack pumpkin
- 4 eggs
- 2 cups all-purpose flour
- 2 teaspoons baking soda
- 1 teaspoon salt
- 1 teaspoon baking powder
- 1 teaspoon ground cinnamon
- FILLING:
- 1 tablespoon cornstarch
- 1 cup milk
- 1/2 cup shortening
- 1/4 cup butter, softened
- 2 cups confectioners' sugar
- 1/2 teaspoon vanilla extract, optional
- Whole cloves, optional

Direction

- Set the oven to 350° and start preheating. Beat eggs, pumpkin, oil and sugar until well blended in a large bowl. Mix cinnamon, baking powder, salt, baking soda and flour; beat into pumpkin mixture gradually until well blended.
- Fill 2/3 full of paper-lined muffin cups. Bake until the inserted toothpick in the center is clean when coming out or for 18-22 minutes.

Cool 10 minutes; transfer from pans to wire racks to completely cool.
- To prepare filling: In a small saucepan, mix milk and cornstarch until smooth. Bring to boiling; stir constantly. Take out of the heat; cool to room temperature.
- Cream confectioners' sugar, butter and shortening until fluffy and light in a large bowl. Beat in vanilla if preferred. Add cornstarch mixture gradually; beat until smooth.
- Cut a 1-in. circle 1 in. deep with a sharp knife in the top of each cupcake. Remove tops carefully; put aside. Pipe or scoop filling into cupcakes. Place tops on top. If preferred, add a clove "pumpkin stem" to the tops.

Nutrition Information

- Calories:
- Total Fat:
- Sodium:
- Fiber:
- Total Carbohydrate:
- Cholesterol:
- Protein:

445. Creme De Menthe Cupcakes

Serving: about 1 dozen. | Prep: 30mins | Cook: 15mins | Ready in:

Ingredients

- 3/4 cup butter, softened
- 1 cup granulated sugar
- 2 large eggs, room temperature
- 1/2 teaspoon mint extract
- 1-1/2 cups cake flour
- 1-1/2 teaspoons baking powder
- 1/4 teaspoon salt
- 2/3 cup 2% milk
- 2 tablespoons white (clear) creme de menthe
- Green paste food coloring
- FROSTING:
- 1 carton (8 ounces) mascarpone cheese
- 1/3 cup heavy whipping cream
- 1/4 cup confectioners' sugar
- 4 teaspoons white (clear) creme de menthe
- Green paste food coloring

Direction

- Set the oven to 350 degrees to preheat. Cream granulated sugar and butter together until fluffy and light. Put in 1 egg at a time while beating well between additions. Put in mint extract. Whisk together salt, baking powder and flour in a separate bowl, then put into creamed mixture together with crème de menthe and milk, alternately, while beating well between additions. Remove 2 cups of batter to a separate bowl, then mix into leftover batter with food coloring paste.
- Cut in the tip of a pastry bag or in a corner of a food-safe plastic bag with a small hole, then insert a #12 round tip. Scoop batters into bag, alternately. Pipe into 12 muffin cups lined with paper with batter, 3/4 full. Bake for 15 to 20 minutes, until a toothpick exits clean. Allow to cool about 10 minutes, then transfer from pan to a wire rack to cool thoroughly.
- To make frosting, stir whipping cream and mascarpone together until smooth, then put in crème de menthe and confectioners' sugar, stirring until combined. Remove 1/2 of the frosting to a separate bowl and mix into leftover frosting with food coloring paste. Stir each portion forcefully until forming stiff peaks but avoid over-mixing.
- In the tip of a pastry bag or in a corner of a food-safe plastic bag, cut a small hole, then insert a #12 round tip. Scoop into bag alternately with frostings, then pipe frosting over cupcakes. Chill leftovers.

Nutrition Information

- Calories: 372 calories
- Protein: 5g protein.

- Total Fat: 24g fat (14g saturated fat)
- Sodium: 222mg sodium
- Fiber: 0 fiber
- Total Carbohydrate: 35g carbohydrate (21g sugars)
- Cholesterol: 95mg cholesterol

446. Double Chocolate Cupcakes

Serving: 12 | Prep: 40mins | Cook: | Ready in:

Ingredients

- Cupcakes
- ¾ cup cake flour
- ¾ cup whole-wheat pastry flour
- ½ cup unsweetened cocoa powder
- ½ teaspoon baking soda
- ½ teaspoon salt
- ¼ teaspoon baking powder
- 1 cup granulated sugar
- ½ cup butter or coconut oil, softened
- 2 large eggs
- 1 teaspoon vanilla extract
- ¾ cup buttermilk
- Frosting
- 6 ounces bittersweet or semisweet chocolate, finely chopped
- ⅓ cup heavy cream
- ½ teaspoon vanilla extract
- 2 tablespoons mini chocolate chips (optional)

Direction

- For cupcakes: Set oven to 350°F to preheat. Line 12 (1/2-cup) muffin tins with paper liners.
- Whip baking powder, salt, baking soda, cocoa, whole-wheat flour and cake flour in a medium bowl.
- Whip butter (or coconut oil) and sugar in a big mixing bowl with an electric mixer on medium speed until blended. Whip in eggs, 1 at a time, until thoroughly mixed. Put in vanilla. Blend in the dry ingredients and buttermilk alternately with the mixer on low, starting and ending with dry ingredients and scraping the sides of the bowl as necessary, until just mixed. Split the batter among the lined cups. (They should be about 3/4 full.)
- Bake the cupcakes for 18 to 22 minutes until a cake tester inserted into the center exits clean. Cool for 5 minutes in the pan. Put to a wire rack and cool completely.
- In the meantime, for frosting: In a heatproof medium bowl, put chocolate. Heat vanilla and cream in a small saucepan over medium heat until simmering (don't let it boil). Add the cream on top of the chocolate and let sit for 3 minutes. Mix until smooth, then blend using an electric mixer for 1 to 2 minutes until fluffy and very slightly lightened in color.
- Smear the frosting on the cooled cupcakes and top with mini chips, if preferred.

Nutrition Information

- Calories: 295 calories;
- Fiber: 3
- Protein: 5
- Total Fat: 15
- Saturated Fat: 9
- Sodium: 204
- Cholesterol: 59
- Total Carbohydrate: 40
- Sugar: 23

447. Easy Chocolate Zucchini Cupcakes

Serving: 24 | Prep: 15mins | Cook: 22mins | Ready in:

Ingredients

- 1 (18.25 ounce) package devil's food cake mix
- 1 (3.9 ounce) package instant chocolate pudding mix

- 1 cup pureed zucchini
- 3 large eggs (such as omega-3 eggs)
- 1/2 cup reduced-fat sour cream
- 1/2 cup applesauce
- 1 cup miniature semisweet chocolate chips (optional)

Direction

- Preheat an oven to 175 °C or 350 °F. Line paper liners on 2-dozen muffin cups.
- In a bowl, combine applesauce, sour cream, eggs, zucchini, pudding mix and cake mix together till batter is thick and velvety; fold in the chocolate chips. Into the prepped muffin cups, scoop the batter.
- In the prepped oven, bake for 22 to 25 minutes till a toothpick pricked in the middle of a cupcake comes out clean.

Nutrition Information

- Calories: 164 calories;
- Sodium: 236
- Total Carbohydrate: 24.7
- Cholesterol: 29
- Protein: 3.1
- Total Fat: 6.5

---

448. Easy Strawberry Cupcakes

Serving: 24 | Prep: 10mins | Cook: 15mins | Ready in:

Ingredients

- 2 cups white sugar
- 1 3/4 cups pureed strawberries
- 3/4 cup vegetable oil
- 4 large eggs
- 2 teaspoons vanilla extract
- 3 cups self-rising flour
- 3 drops red food coloring, or as needed (optional)

Direction

- Heat oven to 325°F (165°C). Line 24 muffin tins with paper muffin liners or grease the tins.
- In a bowl, whip vanilla extract, eggs, oil, pureed strawberries and sugar with an electric mixer until smooth. Put in flour, stirring just to combine. Mix food coloring into batter until evenly colored. Split between lined muffin tins.
- Bake in the heated oven 15 to 20 minutes until it tests done (a tester comes out clean when inserted in the middle). Cool in the pans for about 10 minutes before taking out to cool entirely on a wire rack.

Nutrition Information

- Calories: 198 calories;
- Sodium: 210
- Total Carbohydrate: 29.7
- Cholesterol: 31
- Protein: 2.7
- Total Fat: 7.8

---

449. Fluffernutter Cupcakes

Serving: 12 | Prep: 30mins | Cook: 20mins | Ready in:

Ingredients

- Cupcake:
- 1 2/3 cups all-purpose flour
- 1 teaspoon baking powder
- 1/2 teaspoon baking soda
- 1/2 teaspoon salt
- 3/4 cup firmly packed light brown sugar
- 5 tablespoons creamy natural peanut butter
- 2 tablespoons unsalted butter, softened
- 3/4 cup mashed ripe bananas
- 2 large eggs
- 1 1/2 teaspoons vanilla extract
- 1/2 cup milk
- Frosting:

- 3/4 cup marshmallow fluff
- 2 tablespoons unsalted butter, softened
- 2 tablespoons vegetable shortening
- 1 teaspoon vanilla extract
- 1 1/2 cups confectioners' sugar, or as needed
- 2 tablespoons milk

Direction

- Preheat an oven to 175°C/350°F; use paper liners to line 12 muffin cups.
- Sift together salt, baking soda, baking powder and flour into bowl.
- Beat 2 tbsp. butter, peanut butter and brown sugar, using an electric mixer at medium speed, for about 1 minute till creamy in a bowl; beat 1 1/2 tsp. vanilla extract, eggs and banana into the creamed peanut butter mixture for about 1 minute till incorporated.
- Alternating with 1/2 cup of milk, beat flour mixture into the creamed peanut butter mixture till batter is combined well; put into muffin cups.
- In preheated oven, bake for 20-23 minutes till an inserted toothpick in middle of cake exits with moist crumbs; cool cupcakes for 15 minutes in tin. Transfer onto wire rack; fully cool.
- Beat 1 tsp. vanilla extract, shortening, 2 tbsp. butter and marshmallow fluff using an electric mixer till smooth in a bowl; alternating with 2 tbsp. milk, beat confectioners' sugar slowly into marshmallow mixture till you get desired thickness. Chill for about 15 minutes in the fridge till thick.
- Spread frosting on cupcakes/pipe through pastry bag.

Nutrition Information

- Calories: 322 calories;
- Total Fat: 10.6
- Sodium: 234
- Total Carbohydrate: 52.9
- Cholesterol: 42
- Protein: 5.1

450. French Toast Cupcakes

Serving: 24 | Prep: 15mins | Cook: 20mins | Ready in:

Ingredients

- 1 1/4 cups all-purpose flour
- 2/3 cup milk
- 1/2 cup yogurt
- 1/2 cup white sugar
- 1/2 cup butter, melted
- 1/2 cup raisins
- 1/3 cup dark brown sugar
- 2 tablespoons maple syrup, or more to taste
- 1 1/2 teaspoons vanilla extract
- 1 teaspoon baking powder
- 1 teaspoon ground cinnamon
- 1/2 teaspoon baking soda
- 1/2 teaspoon salt

Direction

- Set the oven to 350°F or 175°C for preheating. Grease the 24 muffin cups or use the paper muffin liners to line the cups.
- In a bowl, mix the yogurt, raisins, maple syrup, baking powder, salt, baking soda, flour, white sugar, vanilla extract, brown sugar, cinnamon, butter, and milk until it forms a batter. Pour the batter into the prepared muffin cups.
- Bake them inside the preheated oven for 20-25 minutes until they turn golden and their tops spring back once they are pressed lightly.

Nutrition Information

- Calories: 106 calories;
- Sodium: 125
- Total Carbohydrate: 16.5
- Cholesterol: 11
- Protein: 1.3
- Total Fat: 4.1

451. Fresh Strawberry Shortcake Cupcakes

Serving: 24 | Prep: 45mins | Cook: 20mins | Ready in:

Ingredients

- Cupcakes:
- 1 1/2 cups all-purpose flour
- 2 teaspoons baking powder
- 1/2 teaspoon salt
- 1 cup butter, softened
- 1 cup white sugar
- 2 eggs
- 1/2 teaspoon vanilla extract
- 1/2 cup milk
- Filling:
- 1 (8 ounce) container strawberry-flavored cream cheese
- 1/3 cup white sugar
- 2 tablespoons heavy whipping cream
- 1 teaspoon strawberry jam
- 8 strawberries
- Topping:
- 1 (7 ounce) can whipped cream
- 10 strawberries, sliced crosswise

Direction

- Set oven to preheat at 165 o C (325 o F). Use paper liners to line two 12-cup muffin tins.
- In a bowl, whisk together salt, baking powder, and flour.
- Combine 1 cup sugar and butter in a bowl; use an electric mixer to beat until creamy. Beat in eggs one by one. Mix in the vanilla extract. Add the milk and flour mixture alternately, briefly beating the batter after each time you add them.
- Evenly pour batter into the lined cups.
- In the preheated oven, bake until a toothpick comes out clean when inserted into the middle, about 20 minutes. Allow to cool for 5 minutes in the tins. Move to a wire rack to cool down entirely.
- In a bowl, combine strawberry jam, 1/3 cup sugar, heavy cream, and cream cheese; use an electric mixer to beat until creamy.
- Remove seeds of 8 strawberries by slicing off their sides. In a small bowl, use a fork to mash strawberries. Beat into the cream cheese mixture until completely combined.
- For each cooled cupcake, cut a small hole in its center; take out about 1/2 inch of cake. Use a spoonful of cream cheese frosting to fill each hole.
- Swirl whipped cream on top of each cupcake. Put 1 strawberry slice in each cupcake's center.

Nutrition Information

- Calories: 204 calories;
- Total Fat: 12.9
- Sodium: 198
- Total Carbohydrate: 21.2
- Cholesterol: 51
- Protein: 2.2

452. Frost Me Nots

Serving: 15 | Prep: | Cook: | Ready in:

Ingredients

- 1 cup butter
- 1/2 cup semisweet chocolate chips
- 4 eggs
- 1 teaspoon vanilla extract
- 1 1/2 cups white sugar
- 1 cup all-purpose flour

Direction

- Set the oven to 325°F (165°C) for preheating. Use paper liners to line the muffin cups.
- Melt the chocolate chips and butter. Whisk the mixture and put it aside to cool.
- Mix the flour, eggs, sugar, and vanilla in a separate bowl.

- Pour in the butter-chocolate mixture; mix well.
- Fill the paper-lined muffin pans with the mixture, about 2/3 full. Bake them inside the preheated oven for 25 minutes.

Nutrition Information

- Calories: 263 calories;
- Cholesterol: 82
- Protein: 2.9
- Total Fat: 15.4
- Sodium: 107
- Total Carbohydrate: 30

453. Gluten Free Banana Cupcakes

Serving: 18 | Prep: 20mins | Cook: 20mins | Ready in:

Ingredients

- 1 1/2 cups white sugar
- 1/2 cup palm oil shortening
- 2 eggs
- 2 1/4 cups gluten-free flour blend (such as Namaste Perfect Flour Blend)
- 4 ripe bananas
- 1/4 cup buttermilk
- 1 teaspoon sea salt
- 3/4 teaspoon baking soda
- 1/4 teaspoon baking powder

Direction

- Set the oven to 350°F or 175°C for preheating. Use paper liners to line the muffin tin.
- In a large bowl, whisk the shortening and sugar using the electric mixer until fluffy and light. Whisk in eggs, one at a time.
- Sift the flour into the shortening mixture, and then add the buttermilk, baking powder, bananas, baking soda, and salt. Whisk the mixture until well-blended. Pour the batter into the prepared muffin tin, filling each to 2/3 full.
- Bake them inside the preheated oven for 20-22 minutes until the inserted toothpick into the center will come out clean.

Nutrition Information

- Calories: 203 calories;
- Sodium: 168
- Total Carbohydrate: 35.3
- Cholesterol: 18
- Protein: 2.7
- Total Fat: 6.9

454. Gluten Free, Vegan, Banana Chocolate Cupcakes

Serving: 18 | Prep: 20mins | Cook: 18mins | Ready in:

Ingredients

- 3 3/4 cups gluten-free flour blend
- 1 cup white sugar
- 1/4 cup unsweetened cocoa powder
- 1 teaspoon baking soda
- 1/2 teaspoon baking powder
- 1/4 teaspoon salt
- 1 very ripe banana
- 1 cup freshly brewed coffee, cooled to room-temperature
- 1/3 cup canola oil
- 1 1/2 tablespoons almond milk
- 1 tablespoon apple cider vinegar
- 2 teaspoons vanilla extract

Direction

- Set the oven to 350°F or 175°C for preheating. Use paper liners to line the 12-cup muffin tin.
- In a large bowl, beat the cocoa powder, baking powder, baking soda, gluten-free flour blend, salt, and sugar.

- In a bowl, mash the banana, and then add the almond milk, vanilla extract, apple cider vinegar, oil, and cooled coffee. Whisk the mixture until blended. Pour the mixture into the flour mixture and mix it slowly until just blended and the batter is gummy and thick.
- Fill the cups of the lined muffin tin with batter, about 2/3 full.
- Bake it inside the preheated oven for 18-20 minutes until the inserted toothpick into the center comes out clean.

Nutrition Information

- Calories: 185 calories;
- Total Fat: 5.3
- Sodium: 117
- Total Carbohydrate: 34.2
- Cholesterol: 0
- Protein: 3.2

455. Green Tea Cupcakes

Serving: 12 | Prep: 25mins | Cook: 20mins | Ready in:

Ingredients

- 1/4 cup butter
- 1/4 cup vegetable oil butter spread (such as Smart Balance®)
- 1/2 cup granular no-calorie sucralose sweetener (such as Splenda®)
- 1/2 cup white sugar
- 3 egg whites
- 1 teaspoon vanilla extract
- 1 teaspoon almond extract
- 1 1/2 cups cake flour
- 2 teaspoons baking powder
- 2 tablespoons green tea powder (matcha)
- 1/2 cup nonfat milk

Direction

- Preheat the oven to 350°F (175°C). Coat 12 muffin cups with oil, or line using paper muffin liners.
- In a large bowl, beat sugar, sweetener, vegetable oil butter spread and butter with an electric mixer until fluffy and light. The mixture should be clearly lighter in color. Put in the room-temperature egg whites, one at a time, make sure to blend each egg into the butter mixture prior to putting the next. Beat in almond extracts and vanilla along with the last egg. In a small bowl, mix green tea powder, baking powder and cake flour together. Add in the flour mixture, alternately with the milk, stirring until just combined. Add the batter into prepared pan.
- Bake in the preheated oven for about 20 minutes, until a toothpick put into the middle goes out clean. Allow to cool down in pans for 10 minutes, then transfer to completely cool on a wire rack.

Nutrition Information

- Calories: 168 calories;
- Total Fat: 6.9
- Sodium: 174
- Total Carbohydrate: 23.3
- Cholesterol: 11
- Protein: 2.9

456. Halfway Healthy Hanukkah Cupcakes

Serving: 6 | Prep: 20mins | Cook: 20mins | Ready in:

Ingredients

- 1/2 cup butter, softened
- 1/2 cup white sugar
- 1 egg
- 1 teaspoon vanilla extract
- 3/4 cup whole wheat flour
- 1/2 teaspoon baking powder

- 1/3 cup almond milk
- 3/4 cup vanilla frosting, divided
- 4 drops blue food coloring, or as needed

Direction

- Preheat an oven to 175 degrees C (350 degrees F). Line paper liners onto 6 muffin cups.
- Use an electric mixer to beat sugar and butter together in bowl until creamy. Beat in vanilla extract and egg. Mix baking powder and flour into the creamed butter mixture until blended. Mix in almond milk until the batter is smooth. Pour the batter into the lined muffin cups.
- Bake for 20 to 25 minutes in oven until the cupcakes are browned lightly. Let the cupcakes cool completely for about 30 minutes.
- In a bowl, combine food coloring and 1/2 cup frosting together until the color is even. Pour remaining 1/4 cup of frosting into small plastic bag and then make a small hole at bottom corner.
- Use the blue frosting to frost cooled cupcakes and then use the white frosting piping bag to draw a star at the top.

Nutrition Information

- Calories: 386 calories;
- Protein: 3.3
- Total Fat: 21.2
- Sodium: 223
- Total Carbohydrate: 47.4
- Cholesterol: 72

457. Hazelnut Truffle Cupcakes

Serving: 24 | Prep: 20mins | Cook: 25mins | Ready in:

Ingredients

- 2 1/4 cups all-purpose flour
- 1/2 cup unsweetened cocoa powder
- 1 tablespoon baking powder
- 3/4 cup milk
- 1/4 cup hazelnut liqueur
- 1 teaspoon vanilla extract
- 1 cup butter
- 1 1/2 cups white sugar
- 3 eggs
- 24 chocolate-hazelnut truffles (such as Ferrero Rocher®)
- 1 (13 ounce) jar chocolate-hazelnut spread (such as Nutella®)
- 1/4 cup chopped hazelnuts

Direction

- Preheat an oven to 175°C or 350°F. Line foil liners or paper on a muffin pan. Sift baking powder, cocoa and flour together then put aside. In a small bowl, combine vanilla, liqueur and milk.
- In a large bowl, use an electric mixer to beat sugar and butter till fluffy and light. The color of the mixture should be noticeably lighter. Add one room-temperature egg at a time, let each egg blend into the mixture before the next addition. Place in flour mixture alternating with milk, mix to incorporate and end with the flour. Pour about 1/2 cup of batter into each of the prepped cups.
- In the bottom of each cupcake, press an unwrapped truffle and spread over each truffle with the batter. Bake for 20-25 minutes in the preheated oven till the top springs back when touched. Let the cupcakes cool for 5-10 minutes in the pan then place on a wire rack till completely cool.
- Frost chocolate-hazelnut spread over the cooled cupcakes and add chopped hazelnuts for garnish.

Nutrition Information

- Calories: 345 calories;
- Total Carbohydrate: 39.3
- Cholesterol: 44
- Protein: 5.2

- Total Fat: 18.9
- Sodium: 135

458. Honey Cupcakes With Strawberries

Serving: 12 | Prep: 20mins | Cook: 25mins | Ready in:

Ingredients

- 1/4 cup butter, softened
- 1/4 cup white sugar
- 3/4 cup honey
- 2 eggs
- 1/2 cup buttermilk
- 1/2 teaspoon vanilla extract
- 2 cups all-purpose flour
- 1 tablespoon baking powder
- 1/4 teaspoon salt
- 3/4 cup heavy cream
- 2 tablespoons confectioners' sugar (optional)
- 1 pint strawberries, sliced

Direction

- Turn the oven to 350°F (175°C) to preheat. Coat a 12-cup muffin pan with oil or use paper baking cups to line.
- Use an electric mixer to whisk sugar and butter together in a medium-sized bowl until fluffy and light. Stir in vanilla, buttermilk, eggs, and honey. Mix together salt, baking powder, and flour; mix into the batter until barely combined. Evenly distribute the batter to the prepared cups.
- Put in the preheated oven and bake for 20-25 mins until the tops are springy to the touch. Put pan with the cupcakes on a wire rack to cool. Once cool, put the cupcakes on a serving dish.
- In a cold bowl, use an electric mixer to whip heavy cream until forming a stiff peak. Add confectioners' sugar to sweeten if you like. Put onto the cupcakes and put sliced strawberries on top right before eating.

Nutrition Information

- Calories: 273 calories;
- Total Fat: 10.6
- Sodium: 227
- Total Carbohydrate: 42.3
- Cholesterol: 62
- Protein: 4.1

459. How To Decorate Soccer Cupcakes

Serving: 12 | Prep: 30mins | Cook: | Ready in:

Ingredients

- 12 unfrosted cupcakes, cooled
- 1 1/2 cups prepared vanilla frosting
- 1 1/2 cups prepared chocolate frosting
- 2 drops blue food coloring, or as needed

Direction

- Use a thin layer of vanilla frosting to frost each of the cupcakes. Place them inside the fridge for 1 hour so that you can decorate them easily.
- For a darker chocolate frosting, add some 1-2 drops of blue food coloring. Pour the frosting into the piping bag with a small round tip attached to it. Create an outline of a small pentagon shape on top of the cupcakes. Pipe the chocolate frosting into the pentagons, making sure to start at the pentagon shapes' points. Draw lines toward the edges of each cupcake halfway. At the bottom of each line, draw a triangle that connects one of the corners to the line, indicating a partial pentagon shape that surrounds the edges of each cupcake. Fill the triangles with the chocolate frosting.

Nutrition Information

- Calories: 399 calories;
- Total Carbohydrate: 62.3
- Cholesterol: 18
- Protein: 2.2
- Total Fat: 16.5
- Sodium: 241

460. Irish Cream Cupcakes

Serving: 2 dozen. | Prep: 25mins | Cook: 20mins | Ready in:

Ingredients

- 1/2 cup butter, softened
- 1-1/2 cups sugar
- 2 large eggs
- 3/4 cup unsweetened applesauce
- 2 teaspoons vanilla extract
- 2-1/2 cups all-purpose flour
- 3 teaspoons baking powder
- 1/2 teaspoon salt
- 1/2 cup Irish cream liqueur
- FROSTING:
- 1/3 cup butter, softened
- 4 ounces reduced-fat cream cheese
- 6 tablespoons Irish cream liqueur
- 4 cups confectioners' sugar

Direction

- Beat the sugar and butter in a large bowl for 2 minutes until crumbly. Add the eggs, one at a time and whisking well after every addition.
- Mix in the vanilla and applesauce until the mixture looks curdled. Combine the baking powder, flour, and salt and add the mixture to the creamed mixture alternately with the liqueur. Make sure to whisk the mixture well after every addition.
- Pour the mixture into the paper-lined muffin cups, filling them to 2/3 full. Bake them at 350° for 18 to 22 minutes until the inserted toothpick into the center comes out very clean. Let them cool for 10 minutes. Remove them from the pans and place them on wire racks. Let them cool completely.
- Beat the cream cheese and butter in a large bowl for the frosting until fluffy. Mix in the liqueur. Add the confectioners' sugar and whisk the mixture until smooth. Pipe the mixture all over the cupcakes' tops. Refrigerate any leftovers.

Nutrition Information

- Calories: 273 calories
- Total Fat: 9g fat (5g saturated fat)
- Sodium: 170mg sodium
- Fiber: 0 fiber)
- Total Carbohydrate: 45g carbohydrate (33g sugars
- Cholesterol: 38mg cholesterol
- Protein: 2g protein.

461. Key Lime Coconut Cupcakes

Serving: 12 | Prep: 10mins | Cook: 25mins | Ready in:

Ingredients

- Cake:
- 1 1/2 cups sifted all-purpose flour
- 1 1/2 teaspoons baking powder
- 1/4 teaspoon salt
- 1 cup white sugar
- 1/2 cup virgin coconut oil
- 3 tablespoons Key lime juice
- 1 1/2 teaspoons Key lime zest
- 1 teaspoon vanilla extract
- 2 eggs
- 1/2 cup milk
- Frosting:
- 1 (4 ounce) package cream cheese, softened
- 1/4 cup virgin coconut oil
- 1 1/2 teaspoons Key lime juice

- 1/2 teaspoon Key lime zest
- 1 1/2 cups confectioners' sugar
- Topping:
- 1 cup sweetened flaked coconut

Direction

- Set an oven to 175°C (350°F) and start preheating. Coat a 12-cup muffin tin with cooking spray.
- In a bowl, mix salt, baking powder and flour.
- In a large bowl, whisk 1/2 cup of coconut oil and white sugar with an electric mixer for 3-4 minutes until airy and light. Put in the vanilla extract, 1 1/2 teaspoons of Key lime zest and 3 tablespoons of Key lime juice. Put in one egg at a time and whisk thoroughly between additions.
- Turn down the speed of the mixer to low. Whisk in flour, 1/3 at a time, alternate with half of the milk and finish with the last 1/3 of the flour mixture. Combine just until they are blended but don't overmix. Fill in 2/3-full of the muffin cups with batter.
- In the prepared oven, bake for 20-25 minutes until the tops spring back once you press them lightly. Leave in the tin to cool for 5 minutes. Place onto a wire tack to cool entirely for 20 minutes.
- In a bowl, use an electric mixer to whisk together 1/4 cup of coconut oil and cream cheese until they are mixed thoroughly and creamy. Combine in 1/2 teaspoon of Key lime zest and 1 1/2 teaspoons of Key lime juice. Gradually mix in the confectioners' sugar. Then frost the cooled cupcakes.
- Set a non-stick skillet on medium heat and start heating. Stir and cook the flaked coconut for 4 minutes until toasted slightly. Take out of the pan to cool for 5 minutes. Put the coconut atop the frosted cupcakes and lightly press in.

Nutrition Information

- Calories: 380 calories;
- Protein: 3.9
- Total Fat: 19.8
- Sodium: 171
- Total Carbohydrate: 48.8
- Cholesterol: 42

462. Lemon Sparkle Cupcakes

Serving: about 1-1/4 dozen. | Prep: 15mins | Cook: 20mins | Ready in:

Ingredients

- 2/3 cup shortening
- 1 cup sugar
- 3 eggs
- 1-2/3 cups all-purpose flour
- 2-1/2 teaspoons baking powder
- 1/2 teaspoon salt
- 2/3 cup 2% milk
- 1 tablespoon grated lemon peel
- TOPPING:
- 1/4 cup sugar
- 1 tablespoon grated lemon peel
- 1/8 teaspoon ground nutmeg

Direction

- Set oven to 350 degrees and start preheating. Beat sugar and shortening in a big bowl until fluffy and light. Put in eggs, 1 at a time, mixing thoroughly between additions. Mix together salt, baking powder and flour; alternately pour into the beaten mixture with milk, mixing thoroughly between additions. Mix in lemon peel.
- Pour batter into muffin cups lined with paper until 2/3 full. Mix together ingredients for the topping and on top of each cupcake, sprinkle a rounded half teaspoon of the topping.
- Bake until a toothpick comes out clean when pierced into the middle, or about 20 to 24 minutes. Allow to cool for 10 minutes, then transfer to wire racks and let cool fully.

Nutrition Information

- Calories: 215 calories
- Protein: 3g protein.
- Total Fat: 10g fat (3g saturated fat)
- Sodium: 164mg sodium
- Fiber: 0 fiber)
- Total Carbohydrate: 28g carbohydrate (17g sugars
- Cholesterol: 44mg cholesterol

- Calories: 301 calories
- Total Fat: 15g fat (4g saturated fat)
- Sodium: 218mg sodium
- Fiber: 0 fiber)
- Total Carbohydrate: 38g carbohydrate (30g sugars
- Cholesterol: 42mg cholesterol
- Protein: 3g protein.

463. Mardi Gras Cupcakes

Serving: 2 dozen. | Prep: 25mins | Cook: 20mins |Ready in:

Ingredients

- 1 package white cake mix (regular size)
- 1 cup (8 ounces) sour cream
- 2/3 cup canola oil
- 1/3 cup sugar
- 4 large eggs
- 3 tablespoons each lemon, lime and grape gelatin powder
- 1 can (16 ounces) cream cheese frosting
- Purple, green and yellow sprinkles

Direction

- Combine eggs, sugar, oil, sour cream and cake mix together in a large bowl; beat for 30 seconds on low speed. Beat for 2 minutes on medium. Evenly distribute among 3 bowls.
- Mix one flavor of gelatin powder into each bowl till well-blended. Fill a scant 2 tablespoons of each flavored batter into muffin cups lined with paper.
- Bake at 350° till a toothpick comes out clean when inserted into the center, 18-22 minutes. Allow to cool for 10 minutes; take away from pans and let cool completely on wire racks. Use cream cheese frosting to frost. Decorate with sprinkles.

Nutrition Information

464. Marissa's Gluten Free Strawberry Banana Coconut Cupcakes

Serving: 12 | Prep: 15mins | Cook: 15mins |Ready in:

Ingredients

- 1/2 cup unsalted butter, at room temperature
- 1 cup white sugar
- 2 large eggs, at room temperature
- 1 teaspoon coconut extract
- 1 1/2 cups gluten-free all purpose baking flour
- 1 1/2 teaspoons baking powder
- 1/4 teaspoon salt
- 1/2 cup coconut milk
- 1 pint strawberries, hulled and sliced
- 1 banana, sliced into 12 rounds

Direction

- Set the oven to 350°F (175°C), and start preheating. Line paper liners on twelve muffin cups.
- In a bowl, beat butter with an electric mixer until creamy and smooth; put in sugar and beat until fluffy and light. Put in eggs, 1 at a time, beating well after each addition. Pour in coconut extract and mix well.
- In another bowl, combine salt, baking powder and flour together. Beat one-third the flour mixture on low speed into the creamed butter mixture just until incorporated. Then pour in half of coconut milk and beat on low speed until the mixture is just incorporated. Beat in

one third the flour mixture, then the remaining of coconut milk and 1/3 flour mixture just until mixed.
- In each muffin cup, add 2 tablespoons of batter using a spoon; add 1 strawberry slice on top. Scoop 1 tablespoon of batter over the strawberry layer; then top with banana slice. Scoop batter over the banana layer to completely fill the muffin cup.
- Bake in the prepared oven for 15-20 minutes, until a toothpick put in the middle goes out clean.

Nutrition Information

- Calories: 239 calories;
- Sodium: 124
- Total Carbohydrate: 34.2
- Cholesterol: 51
- Protein: 3.3
- Total Fat: 11.2

465. Mini Coconut Cupcakes With Passion Fruit Icing

Serving: 12 | Prep: 20mins | Cook: 15mins | Ready in:

Ingredients

- Cupcakes:
- 1 1/4 cups cake flour
- 1 1/4 teaspoons baking powder
- 1/4 teaspoon salt
- 1/3 cup unsalted butter, softened
- 1/3 cup white sugar
- 1 large egg
- 1/2 teaspoon vanilla extract
- 1/2 cup unsweetened coconut milk
- 1/2 cup sweetened shredded coconut
- Icing:
- 1 cup confectioners' sugar
- 2 tablespoons passion fruit nectar
- 1 teaspoon heavy whipping cream
- 24 edible flowers (such as violets or pansies)

Direction

- Set the oven to 350°F or 175°C for preheating. Use the mini paper liners to line the two mini muffin tins.
- In a bowl, sift the baking powder, salt, and flour. In a separate bowl, beat the white sugar, vanilla extract, butter, and egg using the electric mixer at medium speed for 3 minutes until creamy. Whisk the flour mixture into the creamed butter mixture using the mixer at low speed until smooth. Pour in the coconut milk. Beat the mixture until the batter is smooth. Fold in the shredded coconut.
- Fill the prepared muffin cups with rounded tablespoons of batter.
- Position the tins on the center rack of the preheated oven. Bake the cupcakes for 15-18 minutes until the inserted toothpick into their centers comes out clean. Place the cupcakes onto a rack. Let them cool entirely for 20-30 minutes.
- In a small bowl, mix the cream, confectioners' sugar, and passion fruit nectar until smooth. Dip each cupcake's top into the icing, allowing the excess to drip off. Allow the icing to set for 2 minutes. Garnish each with flowers.

Nutrition Information

- Calories: 204 calories;
- Cholesterol: 30
- Protein: 2.1
- Total Fat: 8.7
- Sodium: 103
- Total Carbohydrate: 30

466. Moist Banana Cupcakes

Serving: 1 dozen. | Prep: 15mins | Cook: 20mins | Ready in:

Ingredients

- 1/3 cup shortening
- 2/3 cup sugar
- 1 egg
- 1 teaspoon vanilla extract
- 3/4 cup mashed ripe bananas (about 2 small bananas)
- 1-1/3 cups cake flour
- 1 teaspoon baking powder
- 1/2 teaspoon salt
- 1/2 teaspoon baking soda
- 1/2 teaspoon ground cinnamon
- 1/2 teaspoon ground cloves
- 1/4 teaspoon ground nutmeg
- 1 tablespoon confectioners' sugar

Direction

- Cream sugar and shortening in a big bowl until the mixture is fluffy and light. Beat in bananas, vanilla and egg. Mix nutmeg, cloves, cinnamon, baking soda, salt, baking powder and flour; put into creamed mixture just until combined.
- Pour into muffin cups lined with papers, filling each two-thirds full. Bake for 18 to 20 minutes at 375 degrees or until a toothpick comes out clean. Let it cool for 10 minutes before transferring from the pan to a wire rack to cool completely. Sprinkle with confectioners' sugar.

Nutrition Information

- Calories: 154 calories
- Total Carbohydrate: 24g carbohydrate (0 sugars
- Cholesterol: 18mg cholesterol
- Protein: 2g protein. Diabetic Exchanges: 1-1/2 starch
- Total Fat: 6g fat (2g saturated fat)
- Sodium: 175mg sodium
- Fiber: 1g fiber)

467. Mountain Dew® Strawberry Cupcakes

Serving: 24 | Prep: 10mins | Cook: 15mins | Ready in:

Ingredients

- 1 (18.25 ounce) package strawberry cake mix
- 12 ounces citrus-flavored soda (such as Mountain Dew®)
- 2 tablespoons chocolate chips (optional)

Direction

- Set the oven to 350°F or 175°C for preheating. Grease 48-miniature cups.
- In a bowl, mix the citrus-flavored soda and strawberry cake mix until the batter is smooth. Pour the mixture into the prepared muffin cups. Top each cupcake with a chocolate chip.
- Bake the cupcakes inside the preheated oven for 15-20 minutes until the inserted toothpick into the center will come out clean.

Nutrition Information

- Calories: 88 calories;
- Total Carbohydrate: 17.9
- Cholesterol: 0
- Protein: 0.5
- Total Fat: 1.7
- Sodium: 136

468. One Bowl Vanilla Cupcakes For Two

Serving: 2 | Prep: 15mins | Cook: 10mins | Ready in:

Ingredients

- 1 egg white
- 2 tablespoons white sugar
- 2 tablespoons butter, melted
- 1 teaspoon vanilla extract

- 1/4 cup all-purpose flour
- 1/4 teaspoon baking powder
- 1 pinch salt
- 1 1/2 tablespoons milk

Direction

- Set the oven to 350°F or 175°C for preheating. Use paper liners to line the 2 cups in the muffin pan.
- In a bowl, beat the sugar and egg white. Mix in the vanilla extract and melted butter until smooth. Add the salt, flour, and baking powder; stir well. Pour in the milk and stir the mixture until smooth. Distribute the batter evenly among the two prepared cups in the muffin pan.
- Bake them inside the preheated oven for 10-12 minutes until the cake is set.

Nutrition Information

- Calories: 227 calories;
- Total Fat: 11.9
- Sodium: 253
- Total Carbohydrate: 25.5
- Cholesterol: 31
- Protein: 3.9

469. Orange Pudding Cakes With Marmalade Drizzle

Serving: 8 | Prep: | Cook: | Ready in:

Ingredients

- 2 tablespoons very soft butter
- 3/4 cup sugar, divided
- 1 1/2 teaspoons finely grated orange zest
- 1/4 cup juice from a large orange
- 4 eggs, separated
- 1/4 cup instant flour (Wondra)
- 4 tablespoons fresh lemon juice, divided
- 1 cup milk
- 6 tablespoons orange marmalade
- 2 tablespoons orange-flavored liqueur

Direction

- Grease eight 6-ounce ovenproof custard cups (such as Pyrex) with vegetable cooking spray. Put them in two 9-inch square or round baking pans. In a tea kettle, boil 1 1/2 quarts of water. Set oven to 325 ° to heat.
- Whisk zest, 1/2 cup sugar and butter until smooth. Mix in egg yolks, then flour, until smooth. Then whisk in 2 tablespoons lemon juice and 1/4 cup orange juice, then milk, to make a thin batter.
- In a different bowl, use a hand mixer to beat egg whites until foamy. Slowly add 1/4 cup of leftover sugar, until the whites are firm enough hold peak. Softly fold the whites into the batter just until smooth.
- Put the batter into each custard cup. Put pans on oven rack, then carefully add hot water to each pan, make sure water is not leaking into the cakes. Bake for 25-35 minutes, until tops turn golden brown and bounce back to the touch. Take pans out of oven; allow custard cups to sit in the water just until warm. Put a dessert plate over each custard cup; turn cake over to plate. Combine 2 tablespoons of leftover lemon juice, liqueur and marmalade. Drizzle sauce over cakes.

Nutrition Information

- Calories: 220 calories;
- Protein: 4.7
- Total Fat: 6
- Sodium: 77
- Total Carbohydrate: 36.9
- Cholesterol: 103

470. Paleo Jelly Donut Cupcakes

Serving: 12 | Prep: 15mins | Cook: 25mins | Ready in:

Ingredients

- 1/2 cup applesauce
- 1/2 cup coconut oil, melted
- 3 eggs
- 3 tablespoons honey
- 1 tablespoon vanilla extract
- 1/2 cup coconut flour
- 1/2 teaspoon salt
- 1/4 teaspoon baking soda
- 1 tablespoon almond milk, or as needed (optional)
- 1/2 cup raspberry jam, or as needed

Direction

- Preheat an oven to 175°C/350°F. Line paper liners on 12 muffin cups.
- Blend vanilla extract, honey, eggs, coconut oil and applesauce with immersion blender/in food processor. Put mixture in big bowl; mix baking soda, salt and coconut flour in till batter is solid but easily spooned. If needed, use almond milk to thin mixture. Use batter to fill prepped muffin cups to 2/3 full. Spoon then swirl raspberry jam in each cup.
- In preheated oven, bake for 25 minutes till an inserted toothpick in cupcake exits clean.

Nutrition Information

- Calories: 157 calories;
- Sodium: 142
- Total Carbohydrate: 14.9
- Cholesterol: 46
- Protein: 1.6
- Total Fat: 10.6

471. Perfect Cake Mix Cupcakes

Serving: 2 dozen. | Prep: 10mins | Cook: 15mins | Ready in:

Ingredients

- 1 package white cake mix (regular size)
- 1 cup buttermilk
- 4 eggs
- 1/3 cup canola oil

Direction

- Mix all ingredients in a big bowl. Combine by beating on low speed settings until texture is moist, then increase to high and continue beating for an additional 2 minutes.
- Fill a large re-sealable bag with half of the batter and make a cut at one corner of the bag, measuring 1/4 inches. Fill muffin cups that are lined with paper up to two-thirds full. Continue filling with the rest of the batter. Bake for 15-20 minutes at 350 degrees or until an inserted toothpick can be removed cleanly without any residue sticking.
- Allow to cool for 10 minutes before taking them out of the trays to cool completely on wire racks. Use frosting and decoration as preferred.

Nutrition Information

- Calories: 134 calories
- Sodium: 168mg sodium
- Fiber: 0 fiber)
- Total Carbohydrate: 18g carbohydrate (10g sugars
- Cholesterol: 36mg cholesterol
- Protein: 2g protein. Diabetic Exchanges: 1 starch
- Total Fat: 6g fat (1g saturated fat)

472. Pineapple Marzipan Cupcakes

Serving: 16 cupcakes. | Prep: 30mins | Cook: 20mins | Ready in:

Ingredients

- 3/4 cup butter, softened
- 1 package (7 ounces) marzipan, crumbled
- 1/2 cup sugar
- 1/4 cup packed brown sugar
- 3 large eggs
- 1 teaspoon vanilla extract
- 2 cups all-purpose flour
- 2 teaspoons baking powder
- 1 can (8 ounces) crushed pineapple, drained
- TOPPING:
- 8 ounces semisweet chocolate, chopped
- 2 tablespoons butter
- Pineapple tidbits, patted dry

Direction

- Set the oven to 350° for preheating. Use paper or foil liners to line the 16 muffin cups.
- Beat the marzipan, sugars, and butter in a large bowl until well-blended. Add the eggs, one at a time and whisk the mixture well every after addition. Whisk in the vanilla. In a separate bowl, beat the baking powder and flour, and then whisk this mixture gradually into the butter mixture. Fold in the crushed pineapple.
- Distribute the mixture among the prepared cups, filling the cup 2/3 full. Bake them for 20-25 minutes or until the inserted toothpick in the center comes out clean. Let them cool in pans for 10 minutes, and then transfer them onto the wire racks to let them cool completely.
- Melt the butter and chocolate in a small heavy saucepan over very low heat. Stir the mixture until smooth. Allow the mixture to cool slightly until it has a thick spreading consistency. Lather mixture over the cupcakes and place the pineapple on each top.

Nutrition Information

- Calories: 326 calories
- Sodium: 136mg sodium
- Fiber: 2g fiber)
- Total Carbohydrate: 40g carbohydrate (26g sugars
- Cholesterol: 66mg cholesterol
- Protein: 5g protein.
- Total Fat: 17g fat (9g saturated fat)

473. Posy Cupcakes

Serving: 2 dozen. | Prep: 15mins | Cook: 20mins | Ready in:

Ingredients

- 1 package white or yellow cake mix (regular size)
- 1 can (16 ounces) white or vanilla frosting
- 40 to 50 Candied Flowers

Direction

- Follow the package directions to prepare the cake batter.
- Fill the greased, paper or foil-lined muffin cups with 2/3 full of batter. Bake them at 350°F for 18 to 24 minutes until the toothpick will come out clean. Let them cool for 5 minutes. Transfer them from the pans to wire racks. Let them cool completely before frosting them. Garnish them with candied flowers.

Nutrition Information

- Calories:
- Total Fat:
- Sodium:
- Fiber:
- Total Carbohydrate:
- Cholesterol:

- Protein:

474. Pudding Filled Butterfly Cupcakes

Serving: 2 dozen. | Prep: 30mins | Cook: 20mins | Ready in:

Ingredients

- 1 package chocolate cake mix (regular size)
- 1 cup cold milk
- 1 package (3.9 ounces) instant chocolate pudding mix
- 1 carton (8 ounces) frozen whipped topping, thawed
- Pastel sprinkles
- Black shoestring licorice, cut into 2-inch pieces

Direction

- Follow the package instructions to prepare and bake the cake mix for the cupcakes. Let them cool completely before slicing the top fourth of each cupcake off. Divide the slices in half; put aside.
- Whisk the pudding mix with milk in a large bowl for 2 minutes until thick. Fold in the whipped topping. Drizzle 2 tbsp. of the pudding mixture over each of the cupcakes.
- Put 2 reserved cupcake halves into the pudding mixture, arranging the rounded edges together for the wings. Press the sprinkles gently into the wings. The cupcakes must be moist enough so that the candy will stick. Insert 2 pieces of licorice into each cupcake for the antennae.

Nutrition Information

- Calories:
- Sodium:
- Fiber:
- Total Carbohydrate:
- Cholesterol:
- Protein:
- Total Fat:

475. Pumpkin Chip Cupcakes

Serving: 15 cupcakes. | Prep: 20mins | Cook: 20mins | Ready in:

Ingredients

- 1 cup all-purpose flour
- 3/4 cup whole wheat flour
- 1 teaspoon baking powder
- 1 teaspoon baking soda
- 1/2 teaspoon salt
- 1/2 teaspoon ground cinnamon
- 1/4 teaspoon ground nutmeg
- 2 large eggs, lightly beaten
- 1 cup canned pumpkin
- 1/2 cup canola oil
- 1/2 cup honey
- 1/3 cup water
- 1/2 cup chopped walnuts or pecans
- 1 cup miniature chocolate chips
- FROSTING:
- 1 package (8 ounces) cream cheese, softened
- 1/4 cup butter, softened
- 1 teaspoon vanilla extract
- 2 cups confectioners' sugar

Direction

- Mix the first 7 ingredients together in a big bowl. Mix together water, honey, oil, pumpkin, and eggs. Mix into the dry ingredients until just blended, fold in chocolate chips and walnuts.
- Fill muffin cups lined with foil or coated with oil until 3/4 full. Bake at 350° a toothpick will come out clean when you insert it into the middle, about 20-25 minutes. Let cool for 10 minutes, and then transfer from the pans to wire racks to fully cool.

- To prepare the frosting, whisk vanilla, butter, and cream cheese together in a small bowl until fluffy. Slowly whisk in confectioners' sugar until smooth. Frost the cupcakes.

Nutrition Information

- Calories: 388 calories
- Sodium: 276mg sodium
- Fiber: 3g fiber)
- Total Carbohydrate: 46g carbohydrate (31g sugars
- Cholesterol: 53mg cholesterol
- Protein: 5g protein.
- Total Fat: 22g fat (9g saturated fat)

476.   Raspberry Cup Cakes

Serving: 12 | Prep: 15mins | Cook: |Ready in:

Ingredients

- 3/4 cup graham cracker crumbs
- 1/4 cup chopped pecans
- 3 tablespoons butter, melted
- 3/4 cup fresh raspberries, crushed
- 1/2 (8 ounce) package cream cheese
- 10 1/2 fluid ounces sweetened condensed milk
- 1 cup frozen whipped topping, thawed

Direction

- Use paper cup liners to line 12-cup muffin pan. Mix melted margarine, crushed pecans and graham cracker crumbs well to blend in a medium bowl; evenly put into paper cup liners-lined 12-cup muffin pan. To firm bottom, use a spoon to press mixture. Puree raspberries; put aside.
- Beat cream cheese till fluffy. Add 1/2 cup raspberry puree and condensed milk; mix till blended well. Fold in whipped topping.
- Evenly put in baking cups; freeze for 5 hours minimum. Remove paper liners for serving

time. Invert cake onto the individual serving plates. Drizzle leftover raspberry puree on cakes. Use few whole raspberries to garnish; serve frozen.

Nutrition Information

- Calories: 227 calories;
- Total Fat: 12.8
- Sodium: 124
- Total Carbohydrate: 25.1
- Cholesterol: 29
- Protein: 4.1

477.   Real Pistachio Cupcakes

Serving: 24 | Prep: 15mins | Cook: 15mins |Ready in:

Ingredients

- 1 cup roasted pistachio nut meats
- 1 1/2 cups white sugar, divided
- 3/4 cup all-purpose flour
- 3/4 cup cake flour
- 2 teaspoons baking powder
- 3/4 teaspoon salt
- 3/4 cup unsalted butter, at room temperature
- 4 large eggs
- 2/3 cup milk, at room temperature
- 2 teaspoons vanilla

Direction

- Set an oven to preheat to 175°C (350°F). Use paper liners to line the 24 muffin cups.
- In a blender, blend 1/2 cup sugar and pistachios until ground finely.
- In a bowl, sift together the salt, baking powder, cake flour and all-purpose flour.
- In a big bowl, beat the butter and 1 cup sugar together using an electric mixer, until it becomes fluffy and light. Beat the egg into the creamy butter mixture, one at a time,

incorporating each egg thoroughly prior to adding the next one.
- In another bowl, mix together the vanilla extract and milk.
- Stir the flour mixture alternately with the milk mixture into the butter mixture in small amounts, starting and ending with the flour mixture, then mix just until it gathers together into a batter. Fold in the ground pistachios on the batter, then scoop the batter on the prepped muffin cups to approximately two-thirds full.
- Let it bake in the preheated oven for 15-18 minutes, until an inserted toothpick in the middle exits clean. Let it cool for 5 minutes in the muffin cups prior to taking it out to fully cool on a wire rack.

Nutrition Information

- Calories: 175 calories;
- Total Carbohydrate: 20.9
- Cholesterol: 47
- Protein: 3.2
- Total Fat: 9.1
- Sodium: 151

478. Rosy Rhubarb Cupcakes

Serving: 1-1/2 dozen. | Prep: 15mins | Cook: 30mins | Ready in:

Ingredients

- 1/2 cup shortening
- 1 cup packed brown sugar
- 1/4 cup sugar
- 1 large egg
- 2 cups all-purpose flour
- 1/2 teaspoon baking soda
- 1/4 teaspoon baking powder
- 1/4 teaspoon ground nutmeg
- 1 cup buttermilk
- 1-1/2 cups finely chopped fresh or frozen rhubarb, thawed
- Cream cheese frosting, optional

Direction

- Cream sugars and shortening together in a big bowl until fluffy and light. Beat in egg. Mix together nutmeg, baking powder, baking soda, and flour; add to the creamed mixture, switching with buttermilk, beating thoroughly between additions. Fold in rhubarb.
- Fill muffin cups lined with paper until 2/3 full. Bake at 350° until a toothpick will come out clean when you insert it into the middle, about 30-35 minutes. Frost if you want.

Nutrition Information

- Calories: 168 calories
- Sodium: 64mg sodium
- Fiber: 1g fiber)
- Total Carbohydrate: 26g carbohydrate (16g sugars
- Cholesterol: 12mg cholesterol
- Protein: 2g protein.
- Total Fat: 6g fat (2g saturated fat)

479. Salted Caramel Cupcakes

Serving: 10 cupcakes. | Prep: 25mins | Cook: 20mins | Ready in:

Ingredients

- 1/2 cup butter, softened
- 1/2 cup packed brown sugar
- 1/4 cup sugar
- 2 large eggs
- 1 teaspoon vanilla extract
- 1-1/4 cups all-purpose flour
- 3/4 teaspoon baking powder
- 1/4 teaspoon salt
- 1/2 cup 2% milk

- FROSTING:
- 1/3 cup sugar
- 4 teaspoons water
- 1/8 teaspoon salt
- 1-1/3 cups heavy whipping cream

Direction

- Set oven temperature to 350 degrees and leave aside to preheat. Add sugar and butter into a big bowl and cream until appearance is fluffy and light. Beat in eggs one by one, ensuring they are mixed well after each egg. Add vanilla and beat together. Mix baking powder, salt, and flour, and combine alternately with milk into the creamed mixture, ensuring the mixture is beaten well after each addition.
- Pour batter into 10 muffin cups which are lined with paper, up to 3/4 full. Bake until an inserted toothpick can be removed cleanly from the center without any residue sticking on it, or for 18-22 minutes. Leave to cool for 10 minutes before transferring to a wire rack to fully cool.
- Mix water, salt, and sugar in a big heavy saucepan. Cook at medium-low heat until the sugar starts to melt. Pull the melted sugar to the pan's center until the sugar has melted evenly. Continue cooking without stirring until the appearance is amber in color.
- Turn off heat source and add cream in small amounts while stirring until consistency is smooth. Move mixture into a small bowl, keep covered and refrigerated for 4 hours. Beat until there is a formation of stiff peaks. Apply as frosting on cupcakes.

Nutrition Information

- Calories: 416 calories
- Fiber: 0 fiber)
- Total Carbohydrate: 52g carbohydrate (39g sugars
- Cholesterol: 111mg cholesterol
- Protein: 4g protein.
- Total Fat: 22g fat (14g saturated fat)
- Sodium: 224mg sodium

480. Shoofly Cupcakes

Serving: 2 dozen. | Prep: 15mins | Cook: 20mins | Ready in:

Ingredients

- 4 cups all-purpose flour
- 2 cups packed brown sugar
- 1/4 teaspoon salt
- 1 cup cold butter, cubed
- 2 teaspoons baking soda
- 2 cups boiling water
- 1 cup molasses

Direction

- Set the oven to 350° for preheating. Mix the flour, salt, and brown sugar in a large bowl. Cut in the butter until the mixture is crumbly. Reserve 1 cup of the mixture for the topping. Add baking soda to the remaining crumb mixture, and then mix in the molasses and water.
- Fill the paper-lined muffin cups with the mixture, about 2/3 full. Sprinkle each cup with the reserved crumb mixture. Let them bake for 20 to 25 minutes or until the inserted toothpick into the center comes out clean. Let them cool for 10 minutes, and then transfer them from pans onto the wire racks; cool.

Nutrition Information

- Calories: 248 calories
- Protein: 2g protein.
- Total Fat: 8g fat (5g saturated fat)
- Sodium: 219mg sodium
- Fiber: 1g fiber)
- Total Carbohydrate: 43g carbohydrate (26g sugars
- Cholesterol: 20mg cholesterol

481. Shortcake Cupcakes With Berries

Serving: 6 | Prep: 20mins | Cook: 30mins | Ready in:

Ingredients

- 2 cups evaporated milk
- 2 cups all-purpose flour
- 2 cups white sugar, divided
- 2 eggs
- 2 tablespoons vanilla extract
- 4 cups whipped cream, divided
- 1 cup strawberries, halved
- 1 cup blueberries
- 1 cup blackberries

Direction

- Set the oven to 400 0 F (200 0 C) and preheat. Coat a 6-cup muffin tin with grease or use paper liners to line cups.
- Pour vanilla extract, eggs, 1 cup of sugar, flour, and evaporated milk into a bowl. Mix until no more chunks. Pour the batter into the greased muffin tin. Create a divot in the center of each cupcake with a spoon.
- Put in the prepared oven and bake for about 30 minutes until an inserted toothpick in the center of a cupcake comes out clean. Let cool fully, about 30 minutes longer. Halve cupcakes horizontally.
- On the cut surface of the bottom half of each cupcake, layer a half cup of whipped cream. Replace the top of each cupcake. Put filled cupcakes in the refrigerator for 10 minutes.
- In a bowl, mix together blackberries, blueberries and strawberries. Stir in remaining cup of whipped cream and remaining cup of sugar. Spread mixture evenly on top of the cupcakes. Put in the refrigerator for 10 minutes. Serve chilled.

Nutrition Information

- Calories: 694 calories;
- Total Fat: 17.6
- Sodium: 166
- Total Carbohydrate: 120.3
- Cholesterol: 117
- Protein: 14.1

482. Simple White Cake

Serving: 12 | Prep: 20mins | Cook: 30mins | Ready in:

Ingredients

- 1 cup white sugar
- 1/2 cup butter
- 2 eggs
- 2 teaspoons vanilla extract
- 1 1/2 cups all-purpose flour
- 1 3/4 teaspoons baking powder
- 1/2 cup milk

Direction

- Preheat the oven to 350°F (175°C). Place paper liners on a muffin pan or grease and flour the surface of a 9x9 inch pan.
- Mix the butter and sugar together in a mid-sized bowl until fluffy and add the eggs in one by one, beating until combined then whisk the vanilla in. blend the baking powder and flour together then add to the mixture finally pour milk into the batter and stir until it is smooth. Place batter into the prepped pan.
- Insert the pan into the preheated oven and bake for 30 to 40 minutes or 20 to 25 minutes for cupcakes. If the cake springs back upon touch it is done.

Nutrition Information

- Calories: 209 calories;
- Sodium: 142
- Total Carbohydrate: 29.4
- Cholesterol: 52

- Protein: 3.1
- Total Fat: 8.9

483. Sour Cream Cupcakes

Serving: 16 | Prep: 10mins | Cook: 20mins | Ready in:

Ingredients

- 1 1/2 cups all-purpose flour
- 2 teaspoons baking powder
- 1/4 teaspoon baking soda
- 1/3 cup vegetable shortening (such as Crisco®)
- 3/4 cup white sugar
- 2 eggs
- 1/3 cup sour cream
- 1 teaspoon vanilla extract

Direction

- Start preheating oven to 375°F (190°C). Lightly coat or line paper liners on the muffin pans.
- In a bowl, whisk together baking soda, flour and baking powder. Put aside.
- In a bowl, beat together sugar and the shortening until creamy. Beat in 1 egg at a time, then the vanilla extract and sour cream. Mix in flour mixture until no dry lumps remain. Transfer to prepared muffin pans.
- Bake in the preheated oven for 15-20 minutes until toothpick comes out clean when inserted into middle and golden. Place on the wire rack to cool completely. Then serve.

Nutrition Information

- Calories: 137 calories;
- Total Carbohydrate: 18.8
- Cholesterol: 25
- Protein: 2.1
- Total Fat: 6
- Sodium: 92

484. Spice Cupcakes With Dates

Serving: 16 cupcakes. | Prep: 25mins | Cook: 15mins | Ready in:

Ingredients

- 1 cup quick-cooking oats
- 1 cup finely chopped dates
- 1 cup hot water
- 1/2 cup shortening
- 1 cup packed brown sugar
- 1/2 cup sugar
- 2 eggs
- 1 teaspoon vanilla extract
- 1-1/4 cups all-purpose flour
- 1 teaspoon baking soda
- 1/2 teaspoon salt
- 1/2 teaspoon ground cinnamon
- 1/2 teaspoon ground cloves
- 1/4 teaspoon ground nutmeg
- 1/2 cup finely chopped nuts
- Caramel Frosting or frosting of your choice

Direction

- Combine the dates and oats in a small bowl. Pour in water. Allow the mixture to stand for 10 minutes. In the meantime, whisk the sugars and shortening in a small bowl for 2 minutes until crumbly. Add the eggs, one at a time and whisking well after every addition.
- Add the vanilla and oat mixture. Whisk it at low speed until well-blended. Combine the salt, nutmeg, baking soda, flour, cloves, and cinnamon and whisk the mixture into the sugar mixture until combined. Mix in the nuts.
- Pour the mixture into the paper-lined muffin cups, filling them to 2/3 full. Bake them at 375° for 15 to 20 minutes until a toothpick will come out from the cups clean. Let them cool for 10 minutes. Remove them from the pans and let them cool on wire racks completely. Frost the cupcakes.

Nutrition Information

- Calories: 251 calories
- Sodium: 167mg sodium
- Fiber: 2g fiber)
- Total Carbohydrate: 39g carbohydrate (27g sugars
- Cholesterol: 27mg cholesterol
- Protein: 4g protein.
- Total Fat: 9g fat (2g saturated fat)

485. Spiced Cocoa Cupcakes

Serving: 1 dozen. | Prep: 15mins | Cook: 20mins | Ready in:

Ingredients

- 1-1/2 cups all-purpose flour
- 3/4 cup sugar
- 1/4 cup baking cocoa
- 3/4 teaspoon baking soda
- 1/4 teaspoon salt
- 1/4 teaspoon ground cinnamon
- 1/4 teaspoon ground nutmeg
- 1 large egg
- 3/4 cup applesauce
- 1/4 cup butter, melted
- 1/2 cup dried cranberries
- 1 cup confectioners' sugar
- 4-1/2 teaspoons whole milk

Direction

- Mix the first 7 ingredients together in a big bowl. Whisk butter, applesauce and egg in a separate bowl, then stir into dry ingredients just until blended. Fold in the cranberries.
- Pour batter into paper-lined or greased muffin cups until 2/3 full. Bake at 350 degrees until a toothpick pricked in the center exits clean, about 18 to 20 minutes. Allow to cool about 5 minutes, then take out of pan and place onto a wire rack to cool fully.
- Mix milk and confectioners' sugar in a small bowl until smooth, then sprinkle over cupcakes.

Nutrition Information

- Calories: 212 calories
- Sodium: 173mg sodium
- Fiber: 1g fiber)
- Total Carbohydrate: 41g carbohydrate (27g sugars
- Cholesterol: 28mg cholesterol
- Protein: 3g protein.
- Total Fat: 5g fat (3g saturated fat)

486. Spiced Cupcakes With Cinnamon Cream Cheese Frosting

Serving: 18 | Prep: 30mins | Cook: 25mins | Ready in:

Ingredients

- Cupcakes:
- 1/2 cup unsalted butter, softened
- 1 cup sugar
- 1 egg
- 1 cup MUSSELMAN'S® Apple Butter
- 1/2 cup plain Greek yogurt (or sour cream)
- 1 teaspoon vanilla extract
- 1/2 teaspoon ground nutmeg
- 1 teaspoon ground cinnamon
- 2 cups flour
- 1 teaspoon baking powder
- 1 teaspoon salt
- Frosting:
- 3 tablespoons unsalted butter, softened
- 6 ounces cream cheese, softened
- 1/2 teaspoon ground cinnamon
- 1/8 teaspoon salt
- 2 1/4 cups powdered sugar
- 1 teaspoon vanilla extract

Direction

- Set oven to 350 degrees F and start preheating.
- Cream sugar and butter together in a big bowl. Whisk in vanilla, yogurt, apple butter, and egg.
- Combine salt, baking powder, nutmeg, cinnamon and flour in a medium bowl.
- Slowly blend dry ingredients into wet ingredients.
- Distribute batter into 18 standard muffin tins lined with paper liners. Bake until cooked through, about 25-27 minutes.
- Remove to rack, let cool completely before frosting.
- Whip cream cheese and butter with a mixer, about 2 minutes.
- Put in powdered sugar, one cup per time, whisking 1 minute between each addition.
- Blend in salt, vanilla and cinnamon. Whisk until fluffy and light, about 1-2 minutes longer.
- Chill frosting in the fridge 15-30 minutes; then pipe onto cupcakes.
- Chill cupcakes in the fridge until about to serve.

Nutrition Information

- Calories: 288 calories;
- Total Fat: 11.3
- Sodium: 209
- Total Carbohydrate: 44.6
- Cholesterol: 41
- Protein: 2.9

487. Steamed Rainbow Cupcakes

Serving: 20 | Prep: 15mins | Cook: 25mins | Ready in:

Ingredients

- 2 1/3 cups all-purpose flour
- 1/2 teaspoon baking soda
- 1 1/4 cups white sugar
- 5 egg yolks
- 4 egg whites
- 3/4 cup soda water
- 1/2 teaspoon vanilla extract
- 5 drops yellow food coloring, or as needed
- 5 drops green food coloring, or as needed
- 5 drops red food coloring, or as needed

Direction

- In a saucepan, set a steamer insert and pour in water filling to barely under the base of steamer. Boil the water. Line paper liners on 20 small ramekins or muffin cups.
- Sift together the baking soda and flour in bowl.
- Use an electric mixer to whip vanilla extract, egg whites, egg yolks and sugar in another bowl till extremely fluffy. Mix in soda and flour mixture slowly; stir thoroughly. Put green, red and yellow food color in three individual bowls. Stir approximately 4 tablespoons batter in every bowl.
- Pour original batter in muffin cups filling them 3/4-full. Drizzle green, red and yellow batters over. Put muffin cups carefully in steamer. Put a clean kitchen towel under the lid for steam to not drip on cakes. Cook for 20 minutes, with cover, till surfaces bounces back once pressed.

Nutrition Information

- Calories: 118 calories;
- Sodium: 45
- Total Carbohydrate: 23.8
- Cholesterol: 51
- Protein: 2.9
- Total Fat: 1.2

488. Strawberry Champagne Cupcakes

Serving: 18 | Prep: 25mins | Cook: 21mins | Ready in:

Ingredients

- 1 1/2 cups all-purpose flour, sifted
- 1/4 cup instant vanilla pudding mix
- 1 teaspoon baking powder
- 1/2 teaspoon baking soda
- 1/4 teaspoon kosher salt
- 1/2 cup frozen unsweetened strawberries, thawed
- 1/4 cup whole milk, at room temperature
- 1 teaspoon vanilla extract
- 1 cup white sugar
- 1/2 cup unsalted butter, at room temperature
- 2 egg whites, at room temperature
- 1 egg, at room temperature
- 1/4 cup Champagne
- 1/2 teaspoon red food coloring

Direction

- Heat oven to 350°F (175°C). Line 18 muffin cups with paper liners.
- In a bowl, stir salt, baking soda, baking powder, vanilla pudding mix, and flour together.
- In a blender or food processor, blend strawberries. Scale 1 quarter cup puree into a bowl. Stir in vanilla extract and milk.
- In the bowl of a stand mixer fitted with the paddle attachment, mix sugar and butter. Whip on medium-high speed until light and fluffy. Turn speed down to medium; whip in whole egg and egg whites until just combined.
- Into the batter, stir 1/2 of the flour mixture on low speed. Pour food coloring, Champagne, and milk mixture; whip until just combined. Whip in flour mixture remaining until just blended. To make sure batter is smooth, scrape the sides of the bowl with a spatula.
- Split batter between prepared muffin cups.
- Bake in the heated oven for about 21 minutes until a toothpick inserted in the middle comes out clean. Rest for 5 minutes to cool; turn to a wire rack for about 20 minutes to rest and cool completely.

Nutrition Information

- Calories: 151 calories;
- Total Fat: 5.6
- Sodium: 146
- Total Carbohydrate: 22.9
- Cholesterol: 24
- Protein: 2

489. Strawberry Cupcakes With Strawberry Icing

Serving: 24 | Prep: | Cook: | Ready in:

Ingredients

- Cake:
- 1 (18.25 ounce) package white cake mix
- 3 large eggs
- 4 ounces Mott's® Strawberry Applesauce
- 1 1/4 cups Mott's® Strawberry Boom
- Icing:
- 4 ounces cream cheese, room temperature
- 1/4 cup Mott's® Strawberry Boom
- 2 cups confectioners' sugar
- 1/2 teaspoon vanilla extract

Direction

- Set the oven to 350°F for preheating.
- Combine the cake mix, Mott's Strawberry Boom, applesauce, and eggs in a mixer and whisk them for 3 minutes until well-combined.
- Distribute the batter among the lined or greased cupcake tin holder.
- Bake them for 23-25 minutes until the inserted toothpick into the cupcake will come out clean. Allow them to cool completely before adding the icing.

- While you're baking the cupcakes, mix all the ingredients for the icing in a mixing bowl using the electric mixer. Ice the cupcakes, and then serve.

Nutrition Information

- Calories: 163 calories;
- Cholesterol: 28
- Protein: 2.1
- Total Fat: 4.6
- Sodium: 166
- Total Carbohydrate: 28.7

490. Strawberry Shortcake Cupcakes

Serving: 24 | Prep: 30mins | Cook: 15mins | Ready in:

Ingredients

- Cupcakes:
- 1 (18.25 ounce) box yellow cake mix (such as Betty Crocker®)
- 1 cup water
- 3 eggs
- 1/2 cup vegetable oil
- 7 tablespoons strawberry jam
- Strawberry Topping:
- 1 pound fresh strawberries, hulled and quartered
- 3 tablespoons white sugar
- 2 teaspoons lemon juice
- Whipped Cream:
- 2 cups heavy whipping cream
- 3 tablespoons confectioners' sugar
- 1 tablespoon vanilla extract

Direction

- Preheat an oven to 175°C/350°F. Grease/line paper liners on 12 muffin cups.
- Use an electric mixer to beat oil, eggs, water and cake mix for 30 seconds on low speed; put speed on medium. Beat for 2 more minutes till batter is smooth. Put batter into the prepared muffin cups.
- In the preheated oven, bake for 12-17 minutes till toothpick inserted in middle exits clean. Cool cupcakes for 5 minutes in the tin.
- In bowl, mix strawberry jam till you get a spreadable and smooth texture. Spread a thin jam layer on each cupcake; refrigerate the cupcakes for 3 hours to overnight till jam sets into cake.
- Mix lemon juice, white sugar and strawberries till combined evenly in a bowl. Refrigerate for 3 hours minimum till strawberries break down slightly.
- Use an electric mixer to beat vanilla extract, confectioners' sugar and cream till whipped cream is fluffy and light and soft peaks form in a bowl.
- Put 2 tablespoons of whipped cream and 3-4 strawberry slices on each cupcake.

Nutrition Information

- Calories: 243 calories;
- Protein: 2.3
- Total Fat: 15.1
- Sodium: 158
- Total Carbohydrate: 25.3
- Cholesterol: 51

491. Surprise Pumpkin Cupcakes

Serving: 2 dozen. | Prep: 25mins | Cook: 20mins | Ready in:

Ingredients

- 1 can (15 ounces) solid-pack pumpkin
- 2 cups sugar
- 1 cup canola oil
- 4 large eggs
- 2 cups all-purpose flour

- 2 teaspoons baking powder
- 2 teaspoons ground cinnamon
- 1 teaspoon baking soda
- 1/2 teaspoon salt
- FILLING:
- 1 package (8 ounces) cream cheese, softened
- 1/3 cup sugar
- 1 large egg
- Confectioners' sugar, optional

Direction

- Beat eggs, oil, pumpkin and sugar until well blended in a large bowl. Combine salt, baking soda, cinnamon, baking powder and flour in a small bowl; beat into pumpkin mixture gradually until blended.
- To prepare filling, beat sugar and cream cheese until smooth in another small bowl. Add egg; whisk until just combined on low.
- Fill the batter 1/3 full in paper-lined muffin cups. Drop filling into center of each cupcake by tablespoonfuls. Place the rest of the batter on top.
- Bake at 350° until the inserted toothpick in the pumpkin portion is clean when coming out or for 20-25 minutes. Cool for 10 minutes; transfer from pans to wire racks to completely cool. Sprinkle with confectioners' sugar if preferred. Keep the leftovers in the fridge.

Nutrition Information

- Calories: 250 calories
- Protein: 3g protein.
- Total Fat: 14g fat (3g saturated fat)
- Sodium: 179mg sodium
- Fiber: 1g fiber)
- Total Carbohydrate: 29g carbohydrate (20g sugars
- Cholesterol: 54mg cholesterol

492. Surprise Inside Cupcakes

Serving: 2 dozen. | Prep: 25mins | Cook: 20mins | Ready in:

Ingredients

- CAKE:
- 2 cups sugar
- 2 cups water
- 2/3 cup canola oil
- 2 tablespoons white vinegar
- 2 teaspoons vanilla extract
- 3 cups all-purpose flour
- 1/2 cup baking cocoa
- 2 teaspoons baking soda
- FILLING:
- 1 package (8 ounces) cream cheese, softened
- 1/3 cup sugar
- 1 egg
- Dash salt
- Chocolate frosting, optional

Direction

- Beat the oil, vanilla, water, sugar, and vinegar in a large bowl until well-combined. In a separate bowl, mix the baking soda, flour, and cocoa, and then beat the mixture gradually into the sugar mixture until well-blended. Pour the mixture into the paper-lined muffin cups, filling them 2/3 full.
- In a small bowl, whisk the salt, cream cheese, egg, and sugar for the filling until smooth. Fill the cupcake with a drop of a teaspoonful of the filling.
- Let them bake at 350° for 20 to 24 minutes until the inserted toothpick into the center will come out clean. Allow them to cool for 10 minutes. Remove them from the pans and place them on wire racks. Let them cool completely. If desired, pipe the frosting onto the cupcakes.

Nutrition Information

- Calories: 227 calories

- Sodium: 142mg sodium
- Fiber: 1g fiber)
- Total Carbohydrate: 33g carbohydrate (19g sugars
- Cholesterol: 19mg cholesterol
- Protein: 3g protein.
- Total Fat: 10g fat (3g saturated fat)

493. Tres Leches Cupcakes

Serving: 12 | Prep: 15mins | Cook: 12mins | Ready in:

Ingredients

- Cake:
- 2 eggs, separated
- 1/2 cup white sugar, divided
- 1/4 cup milk
- 1 dash vanilla extract
- 1/2 cup cake flour
- 1/2 teaspoon baking powder
- 1 pinch salt
- 1/4 teaspoon cream of tartar
- Tres Leches:
- 1 (6 ounce) can evaporated milk
- 1/2 cup heavy whipping cream
- 1/2 cup sweetened condensed milk
- 1 dash vanilla extract, or to taste
- Frosting:
- 2 ounces cream cheese, softened
- 2 tablespoons white sugar
- 1/2 teaspoon vanilla extract
- 1/4 cup cold heavy whipping cream

Direction

- Set the oven to 325°F or 165°C for preheating. Use the paper liners to line 12 muffin cups.
- Use an electric mixer to whisk 1/3 cup of white sugar and eggs in a bowl until fluffy and pale. Stir in 1 dash of vanilla extract and milk. In a separate bowl, mix the salt, cake flour, and baking powder and whisk the mixture into the egg mixture.
- In a separate bowl, whisk the cream of tartar and egg whites using the electric mixer until it forms soft peaks. Add the remaining sugar gradually and whisk the mixture until firm and glossy. Mix the egg whites mixture into the flour mixture until the batter is just blended. Pour the batter into the prepared muffin cups.
- Let them bake in the preheated oven for 12-15 minutes until the inserted toothpick into the center will come out clean. Let them cool slightly.
- In a bowl, mix the sweetened condensed milk, a dash of vanilla extract, evaporated milk, and a half cup of the cream. Prick some holes into the cupcake. Spread 4-5 spoonfuls of milk mixture all over each cupcake.
- In a bowl, beat 2 tbsp. of white sugar, 1/2 tsp. of vanilla extract, and cream cheese until smooth. Add 1/4 cup of the cold cream. Whisk the mixture until it forms stiff peaks. Spread this frosting all over the cupcake.

Nutrition Information

- Calories: 205 calories;
- Protein: 4.3
- Total Fat: 10.3
- Sodium: 98
- Total Carbohydrate: 24.4
- Cholesterol: 65

494. Truffle Chocolate Cupcakes

Serving: 2 dozen. | Prep: 40mins | Cook: 20mins | Ready in:

Ingredients

- 1-1/2 cups semisweet chocolate chips
- 1/2 cup plus 2 tablespoons sweetened condensed milk
- 1 teaspoon butter

- 2 teaspoons vanilla extract
- CUPCAKES:
- 1 package devil's food cake mix (regular size)
- 4 large eggs
- 1 cup (8 ounces) sour cream
- 3/4 cup canola oil
- 1/2 cup water
- 2 teaspoons vanilla extract
- 1 cup heavy whipping cream, whipped, optional

Direction

- To make the truffles, melt butter, milk and chocolate in a small saucepan over low heat; stir until blended. Take the saucepan away from the heat. Stir in vanilla. Pour into a small bowl; put in the fridge with a cover until firm; approximately 1 hour. Round into twenty-four 1-inch balls; let it chill for 1 more hour.
- For cupcakes, mix vanilla, water, oil, sour cream, eggs and cake mix in a big bowl; beat for 30 seconds on low speed. Switch to medium speed and beat for 2 more minutes.
- Pour into muffin cups lined with papers, filling one-third full. Put a truffle in the middle of each cupcake. Pour remaining batter on top. Bake at 350° for 17 to 22 minutes or until a toothpick comes out clean when inserted in the center.
- Allow to cool for 10 minutes before transferring from the pan to the wire racks to let them cool completely. Put whipped cream on top if you like.

Nutrition Information

- Calories: 275 calories
- Total Fat: 17g fat (6g saturated fat)
- Sodium: 195mg sodium
- Fiber: 2g fiber)
- Total Carbohydrate: 29g carbohydrate (21g sugars
- Cholesterol: 52mg cholesterol
- Protein: 4g protein.

495. Vanilla Cupcakes With Rhubarb Compote

Serving: 1-1/2 dozen. | Prep: 50mins | Cook: 20mins | Ready in:

Ingredients

- 1/2 cup unsalted butter, softened
- 1-1/2 cups sugar
- 3 large eggs
- 3 teaspoons vanilla extract
- 1-1/2 cups all-purpose flour
- 1/2 teaspoon baking soda
- 1/4 teaspoon salt
- 1/3 cup sour cream
- TOPPING:
- 1 carton (8 ounces) mascarpone cheese
- 3/4 cup fat-free vanilla Greek yogurt
- 1 tablespoon honey
- STRAWBERRY RHUBARB COMPOTE:
- 2 cups chopped fresh rhubarb
- 2 tablespoons sugar
- 1 tablespoon water
- 1/4 teaspoon ground ginger
- 1/2 cup quartered fresh strawberries

Direction

- Set oven to 350 degrees and start preheating. Prepare 18 muffin cups lined with paper liners.
- Beat sugar and butter until fluffy and light in a big bowl. Put in eggs, one by one, whisk thoroughly before adding another one. Beat vanilla into the mixture. Mix together salt, baking soda and flour in a different bowl, then put into the creamed mixture alternately with sour cream; cream well between each addition.
- Pour batter into prepped cups until it reaches 2/3 full. Bake until a toothpick pricked into the middle comes out clean, or for 18 to 20 minutes. Allow to cool in pans for 10 minutes, then transfer to wire racks to cool thoroughly.

- Stir together honey, yogurt and mascarpone cheese in a small bowl to make topping. Leave in the fridge until using.
- Boil ginger, water, sugar and rhubarb in a small saucepan to make compote. Lower the heat; simmer without a cover for about 6-8 minutes until rhubarb starts to tenderize.
- Mix in strawberries; bring to a gentle simmer for about 5 minutes until slightly thick and strawberries are just tender. Let it cool thoroughly.
- Serve cupcakes with topping and compote.

Nutrition Information

- Calories:
- Sodium:
- Fiber:
- Total Carbohydrate:
- Cholesterol:
- Protein:
- Total Fat:

496. Vanilla Cupcakes With Vanilla Whipped Cream Frosting

Serving: 12 | Prep: 10mins | Cook: 20mins | Ready in:

Ingredients

- 1/2 cup unsalted butter, softened
- 1/2 cup Pyure Organic All Purpose Stevia Blend
- 1/2 teaspoon Pyure Organic Liquid Stevia Extract, vanilla flavor
- 2 eggs
- 1 teaspoon vanilla extract
- 1 3/4 cups all-purpose flour
- 1 1/2 teaspoons baking powder
- 1/4 teaspoon salt
- 3/4 cup milk
- Billowy Vanilla Whipped Cream:
- 1 cup 35% cream
- 1/4 teaspoon Pyure Organic Liquid Stevia Extract, vanilla flavor

Direction

- Before starting, preheat the oven to 350 degrees F. Arrange parchment paper liners into 12 cupcake cups and spray some oil on it, set aside.
- Whisk the butter and Pyure Organic All Purpose Stevia Blend and Pyure Organic Liquid Stevia Blend, Vanilla Flavor until soft in texture.
- Pour and blend the eggs one by one into the mixture. Add vanilla and pour in salt, baking powder and flour and stir well.
- Combine the butter mixture and the milk. Make sure to pour the flour mixture three times and the milk two times alternately, combining evenly.
- Scoop out and put the batter into cupcake cups. Oven-bake for 20 to 22 minutes or tested using a toothpick thrusted in the center. It should come out clearly if it's cooked. Place on a wire baking shelf for 10 minutes to cool thoroughly.
- In a separate bowl, mix Pyure Organic Liquid Stevia Blend, Vanilla flavor and the cream using a hand blender to form a stiff peak. Spread instantly on the cupcakes.

Nutrition Information

- Calories: 223 calories;
- Cholesterol: 80
- Protein: 3.9
- Total Fat: 16.3
- Sodium: 136
- Total Carbohydrate: 15.5

497. Vegan Cupcakes

Serving: 18 | Prep: 10mins | Cook: 15mins | Ready in:

Ingredients

- 1 tablespoon apple cider vinegar
- 1 1/2 cups almond milk
- 2 cups all-purpose flour
- 1 cup white sugar
- 2 teaspoons baking powder
- 1/2 teaspoon baking soda
- 1/2 teaspoon salt
- 1/2 cup coconut oil, warmed until liquid
- 1 1/4 teaspoons vanilla extract

Direction

- Preheat an oven to 175°C/350°F. Grease/line 18 paper baking cups on 2 12-cup muffin pans.
- Measure apple cider vinegar into 2-cup measuring cup; to get 1 1/2 cups, add almond milk. Stand for 5 minutes till curdled. Whisk salt, baking soda, baking powder, sugar and flour in a big bowl. Whisk vanilla, coconut oil and almond milk mixture in another bowl. Put wet ingredients into dry ingredients; mix till just blended. Put batter into prepped cups, evenly dividing.
- In preheated oven, bake for 15-20 minutes till tops spring back when pressed lightly; cool in pan set above wire rack. Put cupcakes onto serving platter when cool; frost with preferred frosting.

Nutrition Information

- Calories: 152 calories;
- Total Fat: 6.4
- Sodium: 167
- Total Carbohydrate: 22.6
- Cholesterol: 0
- Protein: 1.5

498. Vegan Red Velvet Cupcakes

Serving: 24 | Prep: 15mins | Cook: 20mins | Ready in:

Ingredients

- 2 cups soy milk
- 2 teaspoons apple cider vinegar
- 1/3 cup applesauce
- 1/4 cup vegetable oil
- 1/4 cup beet juice
- 2 teaspoons vanilla extract
- 2 1/2 cups all-purpose flour
- 1 2/3 cups white sugar
- 1/4 cup cocoa powder
- 1 teaspoon baking powder
- 1 teaspoon baking soda
- 1 teaspoon salt

Direction

- Preheat an oven to 175°C/350°F then line cupcake liners on 2 muffin tins.
- Mix apple cider vinegar and soymilk in big bowl; stand for about 5 minutes till curdled. Mix vanilla extract, beet juice, oil and applesauce in.
- Mix salt, baking soda, baking powder, cocoa powder, sugar and flour in big bowl; whisk to get rid of lumps. Put soy milk mixture in; mix till batter just combines.
- Fill every cupcake liner with batter to 3/4 full.
- In preheated oven, bake for about 20 minutes till an inserted toothpick in middle exits clean and top springs back when touched; cool for 5 minutes. Transfer from tins to wire racks; completely cool.

Nutrition Information

- Calories: 138 calories;
- Total Carbohydrate: 26.3
- Cholesterol: 0
- Protein: 2.2
- Total Fat: 2.9
- Sodium: 185

499. Winter Fantasy Cupcakes

Serving: varies. | Prep: 60mins | Cook: 0mins | Ready in:

Ingredients

- 1 to 2 cans vanilla frosting (16 ounces each)
- Cupcakes of your choice
- SNOWMEN:
- Coarse sugar
- Chocolate wafers
- Semisweet chocolate chips and miniature semisweet chocolate chips
- Orange candy slices
- Additional vanilla frosting
- Blue food coloring, pearl dragees, blue jumbo diamond sprinkles and edible glitter, optional

Direction

- Start frosting the cupcakes, saving some frosting for later use for decorating as preferred.
- For making snowmen cupcakes: Dip the surface of each cupcake in a coarse sugar; lightly shake off to remove excess sugar. For making a stovepipe hats, put the chocolate wafers in the microwave and heat for a few seconds to make it slightly soft as necessary. Slice two thin strips from the opposite sides of every wafer using a serrated knife. (The big center piece will form the crown of hat and the other strip will form the brim.) Put the chips and mini chips to the cupcake to make the eyes and the mouth. Slice a small piece of orange to make the nose.
- Stick the edge of the hat, with its' rounded side facing up, in the surface of the cupcake; insert the hat crown in the top edge. Seal with extra frosting. Color the frosting if preferred; put them in a resealable plastic bag. Trim a tiny hole in the corner of the bag. Pipe a pretty hat band; add some sprinkles and dragees if preferred. Sprinkle the cupcakes with glitter if preferred.

Nutrition Information

- Calories:
- Protein:
- Total Fat:
- Sodium:
- Fiber:
- Total Carbohydrate:
- Cholesterol:

500. Winter Fantasy Poinsettia Cupcakes

Serving: varies. | Prep: 60mins | Cook: 0mins | Ready in:

Ingredients

- 1 to 2 cans vanilla frosting (16 ounces each)
- Cupcakes of your choice
- POINSETTIA:
- Clear decorating sugar
- Winterfresh or cinnamon chewing gum
- Additional vanilla frosting
- Yellow candy-coated sunflower kernels

Direction

- Frost the cupcakes, and reserve some frosting for your desired decoration.
- For making poinsettia cupcakes: Put the decorating sugar in a small shallow bowl; turn around the top edge of every cupcake in the sugar to create a decorative rim. Put aside.
- With a clean kitchen scissors or you can use a small sharp knife, slice the gum into shapes of leaves in different sizes. Pinch the base end of every leaf, making a curved leaf shape. Transfer the frosting on a small resealable plastic bag; trim a small hole in the corner.
- Position the leaves in a circular pattern on top of every cupcake, starting from the outer leaves in. Press the outer leaves on top of the cupcake; sealing with extra frosting as necessary. Continue to add some leaves and sealing using the frosting to make a poinsettia. Lightly press the sunflower kernels in the middle.

Nutrition Information

- Calories:
- Cholesterol:
- Protein:
- Total Fat:
- Sodium:
- Fiber:
- Total Carbohydrate:

501. Winter Fantasy Snowflake Cupcakes

Serving: varies. | Prep: 60mins | Cook: 0mins | Ready in:

Ingredients

- 1 to 2 cans vanilla frosting (16 ounces each)
- Cupcakes of your choice
- SNOWFLAKE:
- Clear decorating sugar
- Pencil, paper, scissors and waxed paper
- White candy coating
- Blue decorating sugar and edible glitter

Direction

- Frost the cupcakes and save some frosting for garnishing as you like.
- For the snowflake cupcakes: into a small shallow bowl, put clear decorating sugar and then roll the top edge of every cupcake in the sugar to make a nice rim. Reserve.
- Draw assorted snowflake designs using a pencil and paper. Slice into individual patterns. In a microwave-safe bowl, melt the candy coating and then mix until smooth. Pour into a sealable plastic bag and then prick a small hole in the corner of the bag. Put waxed paper atop the drawings and the pipe the candy coating onto the designs. Drizzle with edible glitter and blue decorating sugar. Chill until set.
- Carefully lift the candy flakes from the waxed paper and place the snowflakes into cupcakes. Drizzle with more edible glitter.

Nutrition Information

- Calories:
- Fiber:
- Total Carbohydrate:
- Cholesterol:
- Protein:
- Total Fat:
- Sodium:

502. Winter Fantasy Star Cupcakes

Serving: varies. | Prep: 55mins | Cook: 5mins | Ready in:

Ingredients

- 1 to 2 cans vanilla frosting (16 ounces each)
- Cupcakes of your choice
- STAR:
- Clear decorating sugar
- Miniature silver dragees, optional
- Nonstick foil or parchment paper
- Blue, clear and/ or white hard candies
- Additional vanilla frosting
- Blue decorating sugar

Direction

- Frost the cupcakes, and set aside some frosting for garnishing as you like.
- For the star cupcakes: Into a small shallow bowl, put clear decorating sugar and then mix in miniature dragees if you like. (The dragees aren't edible and they are just for decoration). Roll the top edge of every cupcake in the sugar to make a nice rim. Reserve.
- Line nonstick foil onto a 15x10x1-inch baking pan. Smash the candies in the color desired to make about one cup. Put in the prepared pan

and spread the candy to approximately 1/4-inch thickness. Bake for 3 to 5 minutes at 350° or until melted. In the meantime, use cooking spray to coat 6 to 8 metal star-shaped cookie cutters.
- Take out the pan from oven and then press the prepared cutters into the melted candy. Allow to stand until before candy sets. Take out the cutters. (If desired, reheat the scraps in oven). Place the frosting into a small sealable plastic bag and make a small hole in the corner of the bag. Then pipe the frosting around the edges of the stars. Add decorating sugars on top and the miniature dragees as you like. Press on top of cupcake with the stars and hold in place with more frosting if desired.

Nutrition Information

- Calories:
- Total Carbohydrate:
- Cholesterol:
- Protein:
- Total Fat:
- Sodium:
- Fiber:

503. Yazdi Cakes

Serving: 24 | Prep: 20mins | Cook: 25mins | Ready in:

Ingredients

- 2 cups all-purpose flour
- 1 teaspoon baking powder
- 4 eggs
- 1 1/4 cups white sugar
- 1 1/2 cups butter, melted
- 1 cup plain yogurt
- 1 1/2 teaspoons ground cardamom
- 1 tablespoon rose water
- 1/2 cup blanched slivered almonds
- 1 1/2 tablespoons chopped pistachio nuts

Direction

- Preheat an oven to 175 degrees C (350 degrees F). Into a bowl, sift the baking powder and flour and set aside. Coat the cups of a cupcake/muffin pan with grease. You will require 24 cups.
- In a large heatproof bowl, mix the sugar and eggs and assemble on top of a pan of simmering water. Use a whisk or electric mixer to beat continuously for about 8 minutes until pale and thick. Take out from heat and continue beating for about 10 minutes until cooled. Stir in rose water, butter, cardamom, and yogurt. Use your hand to mix in the flour mixture and then roll in slivered almonds. Scoop into the prepared cupcake molds and fill to 3/4 full. Drizzle some chopped pistachios on top.
- Bake for 25 to 30 minutes in the preheated oven until golden brown and firm to touch.

Nutrition Information

- Calories: 215 calories;
- Total Fat: 14
- Sodium: 121
- Total Carbohydrate: 19.9
- Cholesterol: 62
- Protein: 3.4

504. Zucchini Chip Cupcakes

Serving: about 2 dozen. | Prep: 15mins | Cook: 20mins | Ready in:

Ingredients

- 1/2 cup butter, softened
- 1/2 cup canola oil
- 1-3/4 cups sugar
- 2 eggs
- 1/2 cup milk
- 1 teaspoon vanilla extract

- 2-1/2 cups all-purpose flour
- 1/4 cup baking cocoa
- 1 teaspoon baking soda
- 1/2 teaspoon salt
- 1/2 teaspoon ground cinnamon
- 2 cups shredded zucchini
- 1/4 cup miniature semisweet chocolate chips
- 1/4 cup chopped pecans

Direction

- Cream sugar, oil, and butter in a large bowl until they are fluffy and light. Whisk in vanilla, milk, and eggs. Mix cinnamon, salt, baking soda, cocoa, and flour; add into the creamed mixture gradually Fold in chocolate chips and zucchini.
- Add into paper-lined or greased muffin cups to 2/3 full. Place pecans on top. Bake at 375 degrees until a toothpick comes out clean, for 20-25 minutes. Let cool for 10 minutes, then transfer from the pans onto wire racks to cool entirely

Nutrition Information

- Calories: 208 calories
- Total Fat: 11g fat (4g saturated fat)
- Sodium: 149mg sodium
- Fiber: 1g fiber)
- Total Carbohydrate: 27g carbohydrate (16g sugars
- Cholesterol: 29mg cholesterol
- Protein: 3g protein.

505. Zucchini Cupcakes With Cream Cheese Frosting

Serving: 24 | Prep: 20mins | Cook: 20mins | Ready in:

Ingredients

- 1 1/3 cups all-purpose flour
- 2/3 cup whole-wheat pastry flour
- 2 tablespoons baking powder
- 1 tablespoon ground cinnamon
- 2 cups white sugar
- 1 cup coconut oil
- 3 eggs
- 1 tablespoon vanilla extract
- 2 cups shredded zucchini
- 1 cup chopped walnuts
- 1 (8 ounce) package cream cheese, softened
- 1/2 cup butter, softened
- 4 cups confectioners' sugar

Direction

- Preheat oven to 350 °F (175 °C). Use paper muffin liners to line or grease 24 muffin cups.
- In a bowl, sift whole-wheat flour, all-purpose flour, cinnamon and baking powder together.
- In a large bowl, beat coconut oil, sugar, vanilla extract and eggs together using an electric mixer on medium speed for nearly 4 minutes till smooth; fold in walnuts and zucchini. Stir flour mixture into egg mixture till batter is mixed well. Fill about half full into the prepared muffin cups with batter.
- In the preheated oven, bake for 20 to 25 minutes till a toothpick pricked into the center comes out clean. Allow 15 minutes to cool in the pans before taking away to complete cooling on a wire rack.
- In a bowl, beat butter and cream cheese together using an electric mixer until smooth. Beat confectioners' sugar gradually into cheese mixture till frosting is fluffy and light. Spread frosting over completely cooled cupcakes.

Nutrition Information

- Calories: 372 calories;
- Total Fat: 20.4
- Sodium: 187
- Total Carbohydrate: 46.6
- Cholesterol: 44
- Protein: 3.5

Index

A

Almond 4,5,90,106

Apple 5,6,7,8,95,96,166,211,242,260,267,268,310,312

B

Bacon 3,31,37

Baking 23,72,135,136,139

Banana 3,6,7,8,11,162,173,184,190,197,211,212,220,231,266,267,268,269,270,279,292,298,299

Basil 100

Beer 3,7,18,202

Berry 6,7,163,196,213

Blackberry 4,79

Blueberry 8,271,277

Bran 59

Bread 5,117

Butter 3,4,5,6,7,8,9,25,32,34,36,39,40,45,48,51,52,53,74,79,92,93,94,106,117,125,133,147,165,170,178,186,188,190,193,198,199,209,223,246,247,248,270,273,274,275,276,304,310

C

Cake 3,4,5,6,7,8,9,16,23,25,42,43,44,50,56,64,66,95,97,104,107,114,115,122,138,139,141,142,155,163,189,190,216,273,275,278,280,296,301,302,305,308,312,315,321

Caramel 3,4,5,6,7,9,21,35,87,88,95,103,106,166,168,200,284,306,309

Carrot 3,5,6,7,8,16,107,114,115,116,139,163,215,216,241,242,260,277,278

Champ 5,9,117,312

Cheese 3,4,5,6,7,8,9,11,16,27,36,39,47,51,57,60,61,62,63,64,65,66,67,68,69,70,71,72,73,74,75,76,80,81,92,97,102,114,115,118,139,140,143,149,151,155,157,159,216,221,252,262,270,278,285,286,310,322

Cherry 4,5,7,8,63,69,88,89,98,117,118,218,219,279

Chickpea 3,37

Chocolate 3,4,5,6,7,8,9,10,11,15,16,18,19,20,21,22,23,24,25,27,28,30,31,32,33,34,35,36,37,39,43,44,45,47,48,50,51,52,53,55,56,57,58,59,60,64,65,69,72,89,90,107,119,120,133,143,144,157,160,165,167,168,169,170,171,175,185,187,188,200,214,218,220,221,222,223,224,225,228,229,233,238,246,247,255,256,257,259,265,270,276,279,280,281,282,283,285,288,292,314,315,319

Cinnamon 7,8,9,115,122,135,136,226,252,282,310

Coconut 3,4,6,7,8,28,38,90,100,130,174,218,220,227,228,229,238,255,268,282,296,298,299

Coffee 276

Crackers 74

Cranberry 4,59

Cream 3,4,5,6,7,8,9,11,16,18,27,28,29,30,35,36,39,47,49,51,56,57,60,62,67,68,72,78,80,81,85,86,97,100,102,108,111,114,115,122,132,137,139,140,143,149,151,155,157,159,166,169,171,172,175,176,177,178,179,182,183,184,186,188,191,194,196,197,202,204,207,209,210,212,213,216,219,220,221,222,226,228,231,232,238,239,240,242,243,244,245,247,248,250,251,252,255,257,260,261,262,264,265,266,267,269,270,272,276,278,279,281,285,286,287,296,300,306,309,310,311,313,317,322

Curd 7,100,240

Curry 100

D

Dab 164

Date 7,9,244,309

Dijon mustard 66

E

Egg 3,5,46,127,128,129

F

Fat
4,10,11,12,13,14,15,16,17,18,19,20,21,22,23,24,25,26,27,28,29,30,31,32,33,34,35,36,37,38,39,40,42,43,44,45,46,48,49,50,51,52,53,54,55,56,57,58,59,60,61,62,63,64,65,66,67,68,69,70,71,72,73,74,75,76,77,78,79,80,81,82,83,84,85,86,87,88,89,90,91,92,93,94,95,96,97,98,99,100,101,102,103,104,105,106,107,108,109,110,111,112,113,114,115,116,117,118,119,120,121,122,123,124,125,126,127,128,129,130,131,132,133,134,135,136,137,138,139,140,141,142,143,144,145,146,147,148,149,150,151,152,153,154,155,156,157,158,159,160,161,162,163,164,165,166,167,168,169,170,171,172,173,174,175,176,177,178,179,180,181,182,183,184,185,186,187,188,189,190,191,192,193,194,195,196,197,198,199,200,201,202,203,204,205,206,207,208,209,210,211,212,213,214,215,216,217,218,219,220,221,222,223,224,225,226,227,228,229,230,231,232,233,234,235,236,237,238,239,240,241,242,243,244,245,246,247,248,249,250,251,252,253,254,255,256,257,258,259,260,261,262,263,264,265,266,267,268,269,270,271,272,273,274,275,276,277,278,279,280,281,282,283,284,285,286,287,288,289,290,291,292,293,294,295,296,297,298,299,300,301,302,303,304,305,306,307,308,309,310,311,312,313,314,315,316,317,318,319,320,321,322

Flour 3,4,34,55,69,77,292

Fruit 5,6,8,105,131,163,184,208,209,299

Fudge 3,4,22,44,90

G

Gin 3,5,6,7,36,119,131,135,150,187,219,234

H

Hazelnut 3,4,8,22,69,90,294

Honey 8,66,295

I

Icing 3,5,6,8,9,16,18,25,76,77,113,114,128,157,239,299,312

Irish stout 18

J

Jam 3,42

Jelly 5,7,9,138,198,232,302

Jujube 105

Jus 71,102

L

Lamb 3,32

Lemon 3,4,5,6,7,8,43,77,78,79,80,81,82,83,84,100,115,132,139,140,141,147,157,188,189,206,207,238,239,240,262,297

Lime 4,5,7,8,81,138,234,237,296

M

Marmalade 9,301

Marshmallow 3,4,6,43,53,58,130,158,169,190

Marzipan 9,303

Mascarpone 5,114,142,234

Meringue 3,4,51,84

Milk 8,28,233,268

Mint 3,4,5,6,7,48,49,92,118,144,145,192,225

Mustard 66

N

Nut 8,10,11,12,13,14,15,16,17,18,19,20,21,22,23,24,25,26,27,28,29,30,31,32,33,34,35,36,37,38,39,40,41,42,43,44,45,46,47,48,49,50,51,52,53,54,55,56,57,58,59,60,61,62,63,64,65,6

6,67,68,69,70,71,72,73,74,75,76,77,78,79,80,81,82,83,84,85,86,87,88,89,90,91,92,93,94,95,96,97,98,99,100,101,102,103,104,105,106,107,108,109,110,111,112,113,114,115,116,117,118,119,120,121,122,123,124,125,126,127,128,129,130,131,132,133,134,135,136,137,138,139,140,141,142,143,144,145,146,147,148,149,150,151,152,154,155,156,157,158,159,160,161,162,163,164,165,166,167,168,169,170,171,172,173,174,175,176,177,178,179,180,181,182,183,184,185,186,187,188,189,190,191,192,193,194,195,196,197,198,199,200,201,202,203,204,205,206,207,208,209,210,211,212,213,214,215,216,217,218,219,220,221,222,223,224,225,226,227,228,229,230,231,232,233,234,235,236,237,238,239,240,241,242,243,244,245,246,247,248,249,250,251,252,253,254,255,256,257,258,259,260,261,262,263,264,265,266,267,268,269,270,271,272,273,274,275,276,277,278,279,280,281,282,283,284,285,286,287,288,289,290,291,292,293,294,295,296,297,298,299,300,301,302,303,304,305,306,307,308,309,310,311,312,313,314,315,316,317,318,319,320,321,322

O

Oil 51,79,81,97,105,136,150

Orange 3,6,7,8,9,25,116,135,167,174,180,186,201,206,242,243,244,261,280,284,301,319

P

Pastry 190

Peach 8,253

Pecan 6,7,8,35,146,227,251

Pepper 3,4,6,7,53,65,94,148,250

Pie 6,7,8,136,146,150,237,267

Pineapple 4,5,6,9,80,102,115,146,303

Pistachio 3,7,9,25,205,305

Plum 8,263

Potato 5,6,8,113,158,265

Pulse 54

Pumpkin 4,5,6,7,8,9,64,70,73,107,109,130,136,149,150,151,159,160,200,201,251,252,286,304,313

R

Raspberry 3,4,6,8,9,23,24,53,60,83,153,253,254,280,305

Rhubarb 9,306,316

Rice 4,55

S

Salad 4,55

Salt 5,9,103,106,306

Strawberry 3,4,5,6,7,8,9,24,57,76,82,130,141,142,152,154,156,157,189,196,205,206,262,289,291,298,300,312,313

Sugar 3,5,8,39,50,113,130,166,196,199,201,207,213,216,217,262,263,271,277,288

T

Tea 5,6,8,141,153,189,280,293

Toffee 7,224

Tonic 7,234

Truffle 7,8,9,208,248,294,315

V

Vegan 3,8,9,45,292,317,318

W

Walnut 4,8,91,241,266,270

White chocolate 114,250

Wine 5,8,120,255

Y

Yam 5,111

Z

Zest 6,157

Conclusion

Thank you again for downloading this book!

I hope you enjoyed reading about my book!

If you enjoyed this book, please take the time to share your thoughts and post a review on Amazon. It'd be greatly appreciated!

Write me an honest review about the book – I truly value your opinion and thoughts and I will incorporate them into my next book, which is already underway.

Thank you!

If you have any questions, **feel free to contact at:** *author@ashkenazirecipes.com*

Angela Lopez

ashkenazirecipes.com

CPSIA information can be obtained
at www.ICGtesting.com
Printed in the USA
LVHW050934190622
721610LV00016B/200

9 798697 131572